BEYOND THE LINE

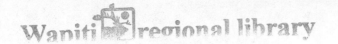

Beyond the Line

MILITARY AND VETERAN HEALTH RESEARCH

Edited by
ALICE B. AIKEN and
STÉPHANIE A. H. BÉLANGER

Published for the Canadian Institute for
Military and Veteran Health Research
by
McGill-Queen's University Press
Montreal & Kingston | London | Ithaca

© McGill-Queen's University Press 2013

ISBN 978-0-7735-4279-2 (cloth)
ISBN 978-0-7735-4280-8 (paper)
ISBN 978-0-7735-9021-2 (ePDF)
ISBN 978-0-7735-9022-9 (ePUB)

Legal deposit fourth quarter 2013
Bibliothèque nationale du Québec

Printed in Canada on acid-free paper that is 100% ancient forest free (100% post-consumer recycled), processed chlorine free

McGill-Queen's University Press acknowledges the support of the Canada Council for the Arts for our publishing program. We also acknowledge the financial support of the Government of Canada through the Canada Book Fund for our publishing activities.

LIBRARY AND ARCHIVES CANADA CATALOGUING IN PUBLICATION

Beyond the line : military and veteran health research / edited by Alice B. Aiken and Stéphanie A.H. Bélanger.

Includes bibliographical references and index.
Issued in print and electronic formats.
ISBN 978-0-7735-4279-2 (bound).
ISBN 978-0-7735-4280-8 (pbk.).
ISBN 978-0-7735-9021-2 (ePDF).
ISBN 978-0-7735-9022-9 (ePUB).

1. Veterans – Services for – Canada.   2. Veterans – Health and hygiene – Canada.
3. Veterans – Medical care – Canada.   4. Soldiers – Services for – Canada.
5. Soldiers – Health and hygiene – Canada.   6. Soldiers – Medical care – Canada.
7. Military dependents – Services for – Canada.   8. Military dependents – Health and hygiene – Canada.   9. Military dependents – Medical care – Canada.   10. Medicine, Military – Research – Canada.   I. Aiken, Alice, 1965–, author, writer of introduction, editor of compilation   II. Bélanger, Stéphanie A. H., author, writer of introduction, editor of compilation

UB369.5.C3B49 2013   362.86'80971   C2013-904818-9
                                                C2013-904819-7

Set in 10/12.5 Minion Pro with Humanist 777
Book design & typesetting by Garet Markvoort, zijn digital

Contents

PART TWO | VETERAN AND TRANSITION HEALTH

Acknowledgments

This collective brings together some of the different research challenges that have been undertaken by researchers from across Canada on the topic of military and veteran health. The researchers who contributed to this volume were part of the third Military and Veteran Health Research (MVHR) Forum that took place in November 2012, hosted by Queen's University and the Royal Military College of Canada in Kingston, Ontario, under the auspices of the Canadian Institute for Military and Veteran Health Research (CIMVHR).

This volume is one of the many ways CIMVHR is connecting researchers, government stakeholders, and, most importantly, the beneficiaries – still-serving military members, veterans, and their families – through knowledge exchange, while also working towards our mission: *To optimize the health and well-being of Canadian military personnel, veterans, and their families by harnessing and mobilizing the national capacity for high-impact research, knowledge creation, and knowledge exchange.*

A special thank you is extended to our Board of Directors; without their support, CIMVHR could not undertake such high-impact projects as the annual forum and the publication of some of the best research it showcased. Our sincere gratitude to the chair of the Board, Dr Richard Reznick, dean of the Faculty of Health Sciences at Queen's University, and the Board members; Dr Jean Fugère, vice-principal research at the Royal Military College of Canada; General (Retired) Walter Natynczyk, former chief of the Defence Staff; Commodore (Retired) Dr Hans Jung, former Canadian Forces surgeon general; Mr Michael Burns, co-founder and vice-chair of the True Patriot Love Foundation; Mr Tim Patriquin, president of the Treble Victor Group; Honorary Captain (Navy) The Honourable Myra Freeman, former lieutenant governor of Nova Scotia; Mr Michael Brennan, CEO of the Canadian Physiotherapy Association; Dr Dennis Fitzpatrick, vice-president research at University of Regina; and Dr Bill Montelpare, professor and chair in Human Development and Health, University of Prince Edward Island.

A special thank you is also extended to our colleagues in the Canadian Forces (CF), especially the surgeon general, Brigadier General Jean-Robert Bernier, and his advisor Lieutenant Colonel Robert Poisson; Veterans Affairs Canada (VAC) director of the Research Directorate, Dr David Pedlar, and his policy advisor Mr Stewart MacIntosh; the scientists of Defence Research Development Canada, especially Dr Jacques Lavigne, Dr Kurtis Simpson, Dr Kelly Farley, and Mr Keith Hendy; the Royal Canadian Legion, especially Lieutenant Colonel (Retired) Shelley Carey; and the Canadian Institutes for Health Research (CIHR), especially Mr Erik Blache. Without your support this volume would not have been possible to create.

Many aspects of this project would not have been possible without the combined support of Queen's University, Principal Daniel Woolf and Dr Steven Liss, vice-principal research, and of the Royal Military College of Canada, Brigadier General Éric Tremblay, the commandant, Principal Joel Sokolsky, as well as Dr Jean Fugère, vice-principal research.

Kingston is the hub of the institute; however, we would not exist were it not for the collaborative efforts of all our university partners. Twenty-six universities from all provinces have joined us in collaborating on military and veteran health research. This has allowed us unprecedented accomplishment toward our goal of affecting the health of military members, veterans, and their families, as well as first responders who have many of the same concerns as this population, and indeed all Canadians who stand to benefit from the excellent research being done by CIMVHR researchers.

We would also like to acknowledge the support and patience of the members of the CIMVHR College of Peer Reviewers who were instrumental in ensuring this volume is of the highest quality: Lieutenant Colonel Dr Markus Besemann, Canadian Forces Health Services Group; Dr Richard Birtwhistle, director of the Centre for Studies in Primary Care, Faculty of Health Sciences, Queen's University; Dr Ibolja Cernak, Faculty of Rehabilitation Medicine, University of Alberta; Dr Marc Corbière, School of Rehabilitation, University of Sherbrooke; Dr Eva Dickson, Science Department, Royal Military College of Canada; Dr Allan English, Department of History, Queen's University; Dr Kelly Farley, director general military personnel research and analysis; Dr Steve Fischer, School of Kinesiology and Health Studies, Queen's University; Dr James Gomes, Interdisciplinary School of Health Sciences, University of Ottawa; Dr Michael Greenwood, Department of Chemistry, Royal Military College of Canada; Dr Dianne Groll, Department of Psychiatry, Queen's University; Dr Kate Harkness, Department of Psychology, Queen's University; Dr Luc Hebért, Faculty of Medicine, Université Laval; Dr Geoffrey Hodgetts, School of Medicine, Queen's University; Colonel Dr Rakesh Jetly, Canadian Forces Health Services Group; Dr Cheryl King Van-Vlack, School of Rehabilitation Therapy, Queen's University; Dr Ruth Lanius, Department of Psychiatry, Western University; Dr Mélanie Lavoie-Tremblay, School of Nursing, McGill University; Dr Ed Lemaire, Faculty of Health Sciences, University of Ottawa; Dr Christian Leuprecht, Department of Politics and Economics, Royal

Military College of Canada; Dr Victor Marshall, School of Sociology, University of North Carolina; Dr Bob Martyn, fellow, Queen's Centre for International and Defence Policy; Dr Mary Ann McColl, Centre for Health Services and Policy Research, Queen's University; Dr Bradford McFadyen, Centre Interdisciplinaire de Recherche en Réadaptation et Intégration Sociale (CIRRIS), Laval University; Dr Roumen Milev, Department of Psychiatry, Queen's University; Dr Patrick Neary, Faculty of Kinesiology and Health Studies, University of Regina; Dr Luc Noreau, CIRRIS; Dr Deborah Norris, Faculty of Professional Studies, Mount Saint Vincent University; Dr Lucie Pelland, School of Rehabilitation Therapy, Queen's University; Dr Richard Preuss, School of Physical and Occupational Therapy, McGill University; Dr Don Richardson, Department of Psychiatry, McMaster University; Dr Elizabeth Taylor, Faculty of Rehabilitation Medicine, University of Alberta; Colonel Dr James Taylor, Canadian Forces Dental Corps; Dr Jim Thompson, Research Directorate, Veterans Affairs Canada; Dr Elizabeth van den Kerkoff, School of Nursing, Queen's University; and Dr Oshin Vartanian, Defence Research and Development Canada.

As editors, we are very proud of the final product. The layout and formatting were handled in expert fashion by Michelle U. Daigle, Angela Whitehead, and Selina Wang: their professionalism and attention to detail have made this final product the work that it is. The edit, layout, and design have resulted in a volume in which we can all take great pride.

We are grateful to the team at McGill-Queen's University Press, especially Philip Cercone, Ryan Van Huijstee, and Ian MacKenzie whose gracious acceptance of our request and expert advice has helped us produce such an outstanding volume of work.

But none of this would have been possible without the great support that we have from our military colleagues, from the community of veterans who have approached us in the past few years, and from their families who also provided us with great inspiration. This collective hopes to be a humble tribute to the ones who have gone beyond the line to serve us. Thank you.

Dr Alice B. Aiken and Dr Stéphanie A. H. Bélanger, editors

Foreword

PETER MACKAY

It is an honour for me to introduce the report of the third Military and Veterans Health Research Forum organized by the Canadian Institute for Military and Veteran Health Research (CIMVHR). *Beyond the Line: Military and Veteran Health Research* is of great importance, not just in its content but in its demonstration of the academic research community's support for the health of serving and retired Canadian Forces (CF) members and their families.

Given the special and evolving conditions, hardships, and health hazards of service in the CF, research that is specific to military exposures and populations has long been recognized as essential to enhancing and protecting military and veterans' health. In fact, the first research scientist in what is now Canada was a military medical officer, Surgeon-Major Michel Sarrazin of the colonial regular troops of New France. His modern-day successors with the Surgeon General and at Defence Research and Development Canada continue to conduct internationally recognized health research, often in collaboration with Veterans Affairs Canada and military allies. Much high-impact research to improve military and veterans' health is conducted, such as the Canadian Forces Cancer and Mortality Study, to elucidate the causes of death and cancer among serving and retired military personnel. With the government's support and a $440 million military health budget, CAF research chairs in military trauma and critical care have also been established over the past year in academic medical centres, while mental health surveillance and research capabilities will be significantly enhanced by my re-allocation of $11.4 million annually, bringing the total military mental health budget to $50 million annually.

The Canadian academic community's capabilities, capacity, and collaboration have long been important to conducting and supplementing military and veterans' health research. The organization whose successor is now the Canadian Institutes of Health Research was, in fact, established by Lieutenant-General Andrew McNaughton in 1938 to address the medical problems of warfare. I therefore strongly endorsed the initiative of Queen's University and the Royal Military College in establishing the CIMVHR as a means of guiding relevant research while enhancing education, collaboration, and synergy. I am particularly pleased to see its extraordinary growth into an exemplary network of 26 universities dedicated to the health of those Canadians who uniquely commit to risking and, if necessary, losing their own lives to protect those of others.

Health-related sciences and capabilities have greatly advanced since Surgeon-Major Sarrazin's time, but military personnel continue to face unusual, dangerous, and evolving hazards, while military life presents their families with extraordinary stresses. Given the risks and sacrifices that they accept for our sake, the important research published in these pages represents a gratifying commitment to protecting their health and is a testament to the authors' scientific excellence. I congratulate and thank them all.

The Honourable Peter MacKay
Former Minister of National Defence

Preface

MARC FORTIN

It is with delight that I introduce the third edition of the Canadian Institute of Military and Veteran Health Research (CIMVHR) collective, *Beyond the Line: Military and Veteran Health Research*. This book is a compilation of research done by some of the brightest minds in the field of military and veteran health science. It brings together publications from researchers across Canada who investigate the health care of active and retired members of the Canadian Forces (CF).

This volume exemplifies the high quality of military and veteran health research being undertaken in Canada. The 2012 MVHR Forum gave researchers an opportunity to showcase their work while building professional relationships and future collaborations with fellow colleagues. The existence of the forum speaks to the success and importance of creating science and technology (S&T) partnerships and how valuable knowledge sharing is. Through these enhanced collaborative opportunities, the synergies created between government scientists, academia, and members of industry can further improve and support the health of CF members, veterans, and their families and deliver impact for them.

The health challenges faced by our military and our veterans are in many cases unique. They collectively form a large population at the national level that is faced with health issues that need more research. The scientific community has much to contribute to better understand, better diagnose, and better treat these health issues. At Defence Research and Development Canada (DRDC) we are committed to the development of research partnerships between academia, the federal government, and other providers to mobilize knowledge and achieve progress and to continue to work with all partners in achieving those goals.

There is a wealth of expertise in Canada, and through collaboration with our allies, that must be mobilized to address those health challenges. CIMVHR has developed a network of 26 Canadian universities with expertise that will allow all of us to make progress on military and veteran health. CIMVHR has been an important player in helping to build trusted relationships with and within the research community.

We need to continue to strive to generate but also mobilize science and knowledge to best serve the needs of those who serve Canada.

Marc Fortin, PhD
ADM (Science & Technology), Department of National Defence
CEO Defence Research and Development Canada

Introduction

ALICE B. AIKEN, STÉPHANIE A. H. BÉLANGER,
AND MICHELLE U. DAIGLE

The Canadian Institute for Military and Veteran Health Research (CIMVHR) is a network of Canadian researchers from across the country who are strongly committed to working together to improve the health and well-being of military personnel, veterans, and their families. We are proud to say that our network includes over 300 researchers and clinicians from 26 universities and defence scientists across the country, and we are growing.

The words of two of our eminent keynote speakers at the Third Annual Military and Veteran Health Research (MVHR) Forum (26–28 November 2012, Kingston, ON), highlight the importance of the work being done, and the continuing need for new research on the unique health-care challenges of the military, veterans, and their families. In the words of the Honourable Peter Mackay, Minister of National Defence, "The health of our men and women in uniform is my central priority for this government, and research efforts such as this contribute to the critical evidence informing the quality of care they receive ... The level of participation in this event is a testament to the support from Canadians for the health of Canadian Forces members and their families."[1]

And in the words of Lieutenant-General Peter Devlin, commander of the Canadian Army, "Military personnel, veterans, and their families are the foundation of the Canadian Forces' success, which is why we are committed to providing the best possible support to current and former military members and their loved ones ... The Military and Veteran Health Research Forum helps us to not only understand the health concerns of military personnel and veterans, but also address challenges in a collaborative way."[2]

Mental and physical health challenges prevent many Canadians from participating fully in society. Military personnel, veterans, and their families are particularly vulnerable. The goal of CIMVHR, and the MVHR Forum, is to optimize the potential of every one of the over 700,000 veterans and 100,000 serving personnel living in Canada, and the evidence shows that this issue needs our focused attention. If we consider the number of people serving, those who have served, and their families, we are talking about two to three million Canadians who can be positively affected by the work we are doing, not to mention all the others in similar professions such as police, firefighters, paramedics, and their families.

In its third year, the MVHR Forum continues to be the premiere conference of its kind in Canada. The 2012 MVHR Forum brought together a network of over 500 academics, military and veteran health experts, clinicians, defence scientists, and beneficiaries from Canada and around the world. This volume brings together research covering the fields of mental health, physical health, social health, rehabilitation, transitioning from military life, family health, combat care, and occupational health, all of which formed a portion of the material presented at the 2012 MVHR Forum. The foreword from the Honourable Peter MacKay, minister of national defence, and the preface from Dr Mark Fortin, the ADM Science and Technology for the Department of National Defence, lay the groundwork for the research presented in this volume, and offer an excellent glimpse into the importance of the research being done on military and veteran health.

The remainder of this volume is arranged into two sections: "Military and Family Health" and "Veterans and Transition Health," providing the reader with a clear guide to the areas of research that have been and are being explored within these areas. The topics are diverse, ranging from technology to programs for children, but all relevant to the readership of this volume, as well as to those to whom it pertains.

This volume is just one way that CIMVHR engages the research community and helps to build the Canadian momentum in military and veteran health research. We continue to provide new opportunities for research growth and the translation of that research into new policies, programs, and practices that benefit the population we serve. We invite you to visit our website www.cimvhr.ca to see published books, as well as the myriad other ways we are engaging those who need this information.

We hope you enjoy this volume and that it inspires all of you to continue the great work in the pursuit of rigorous research in military, veteran, and family health.

Alice B. Aiken and Stéphanie A. H. Bélanger, editors, and Michelle U. Daigle, editorial assistant

Notes

1 MacKay, P., Minister of National Defence, Speech presented at the MVHR Forum (November) 2012, Kingston, ON.
2 Devlin, P., Lieutenant-General, Speech presented at the MVHR Forum (November) 2012, Kingston, ON.

PART ONE

Military and Family Health

1

Differentiation of Physiological Measures of Neck Myalgia by Principal Component Analysis

MICHAEL F. HARRISON, J. PATRICK NEARY, WAYNE J. ALBERT, VICTORIA L. CHESTER, AND JAMES C. CROLL

CORRESPONDING AUTHOR: J. PATRICK NEARY

Abstract

Principal component analysis (PCA) is a powerful statistical tool capable of multivariate data reduction, used here to analyze electromyography (EMG) root mean square (RMS) reconstructed waveform results from military aircrew with and without reported neck pain. We hypothesized PCA would identify significant modes of variability between groups.

Methods: Twenty-nine aircrew (25 males, 4 females) participated in an isometric testing protocol, including maximal voluntary contraction (MVC) and a submaximal ramping protocol of cervical extension. Bilateral EMG monitoring of the upper trapezius, sternocleidomastoid, and splenius capitis occurred, and the resultant EMG waveforms were analyzed with PCA. Principal component (PC) scores were analyzed with one-way analysis of variance.

Results: PC scores were significantly different between groups for the left ($p = 0.021$) and right ($p = 0.016$) splenius capitis only. Reconstructed curves of RMS results corresponding to force production indicated symptomatic subjects displayed lower RMS values as compared to subjects without neck pain, suggesting a possible mechanism of injury.

Conclusion: The application of PCA to the results of a submaximal isometric ramping protocol made it possible to differentiate between neck pain symptomatic and asymptomatic individuals using a physiological parameter. Further physiological investigations of neck pain should be aware of this technique where more conventional statistical methods do not detect differences.

Introduction

Neck strain among military helicopter aircrew has been a focus topic, and a number of published papers have proposed different mechanisms of injury.[1] Some authors suggest that pain is a result of forces acting on the skeletal structures – in particular the vertebral bodies and the intervertebral discs.[2] We propose that the issue stems from a muscle physiology component, and our investigations have proceeded under that assumption. This hypothesis is based on other published works that indicate EMG is useful in measuring in-flight stress related to neck pain in fast jet aircrew[3] as well as fatigue in the musculature of the lumbar region of helicopter pilots.[4] Our initial work with military helicopter aircrew focused on using near infrared spectroscopy (NIRS) response of the trapezius muscles of aircrew employing night vision goggles (NVG) during training missions in a full-motion flight simulator.[5] Our follow-up work has involved the collection of electromyography (EMG) and isometric force with the same population.[6] From this research we demonstrated that the additional mass of the NVG does increase the metabolic activity of the trapezius muscles during simulated flight in helicopter pilots, regardless of left or right seat position.[7] Other research has demonstrated that the additional mass of NVG can elicit a quantifiable neuromuscular response for the cervical region of helicopter aircrew that corresponds with values that are well below what would be considered a maximal value in voluntary force production for this region.[8] Coupled with our maximal voluntary contraction (MVC) results,[9] and the summary of forces and loads experienced by helicopter aircrew in the Canadian Forces (CF),[10] it appears that NVG-induced neck strain in Canadian aircrew is the result of chronic exposure to low-level forces and the associated submaximal activity related to flight duties.[11]

However, while we have a logistic regression equation to identify and predict those aircrew who suffer neck pain as a result of NVG use,[12] this equation did not incorporate any of the physiological variables in the larger data set.[13] Our previous publications have included a great number of physiological results, but these are made available only through the analysis of submaximal endurance testing that is somewhat lengthy and has been reported to be uncomfortable for the subject in the day(s) that followed testing. Regardless, our current methods of statistical evaluation of results provided evidence only of increased metabolism as a result of exposure to the mass of NVG without providing a physiological variable by which to differentiate between aircrew with self-reported pain symptoms and aircrew without pain symptoms. At least two studies have failed to identify differences between muscle function in aircrew with and without symptoms as assessed with EMG.[14] For this link, we propose the use of principal components analysis (PCA).

PCA is a data-reduction technique that allows "a large number of independent variables [to be] systematically reduced to a smaller, conceptually more coherent set of variables."[15] This aim is met through the identification of the fewest orthogonal factors or vertices that best describe the correlations and minimize variance among those original variables.[16] PCA, for n variables, returns n components that explain a successively smaller proportion of the variation within the data set. Obviously n components are not retained, but the successive ordering by magnitude of variance within the data set allows the researcher to retain fewer variables (k) that are indicative of the vast majority of the vital information within the data. From these k components that are deemed retainable, principal component (PC) scores that combine results from multiple variables into one number that is relative to the principal component scores of all other individual subjects within the sample population can be calculated. These values can then be used for subsequent analysis to test for statistically significant differences or relationships.

PCA, in kinesiological studies, has been used with success in investigations ranging from climbing performance to hockey player skating-stride fatigue, to gait analysis and biomechanical lifting fatigue.[17] Wrigley et al.[18] have twice been successful in applying PCA to biomechanical waveforms related to lifting techniques. Through their analyses, PCA was shown to be sensitive enough to detect important differences within the variables of lifting mechanics, where traditional methods failed, while remaining insensitive to confounding factors. Further, Wrigley et al.[19] were the first to discriminate lifting technique patterns between workers who later developed lower back pain from those who did not. Deluzio and Astephen[20] used PCA to identify the discriminating factors in knee kinematics related to osteoarthritis of that joint, while Chester and Wrigley[21] have further applied PCA to identify differences in gait mechanics across four age groups to describe the maturational process of bipedal walking. Given how effectively PCA has identified subtle but important differences in various waveform results related to human performance, we are proposing an expansion of PCA's application with the present study. Other researchers have successfully used PCA to identify differences in recruitment patterns during trunk stability testing for low-back pain subjects as compared to healthy controls.[22]

We now propose that a single maximal voluntary contraction and a single submaximal isometric ramping protocol in which EMG signals are collected at relative workloads and analyzed with PCA would allow both a quicker testing session and less post-testing subject discomfort. Perhaps most importantly, this could be used to differentiate healthy from injured aircrew on the basis of their EMG signals. Therefore, we hypothesized that the responses as measured with EMG reconstructed waveforms related to submaximal isometric force production in the sagittal plane (extension) would differ significantly between aircrew reporting to suffer or experiencing NVG-induced neck strain and aircrew reporting to be asymptomatic.

Methods

Subjects

Ethical approval was obtained from the University of Regina's Review of Ethics Board, and subjects were provided verbal and written summaries of the goal of the project by both CF personnel and the members of the research team. Twenty-nine CF helicopter aircrew (25 M, 4 F), representing all Canadian tactical helicopter squadrons and levels of experience, agreed to participate in the study and signed informed consent. Fifteen pilots (12 M, 3 F; age = 32.9 ± 5.6 yrs; ht = 1.77 ± 6.68 cm; wt = 78.0 ± 10.4 kg; flight experience = 1531.9 ± 1485.5 hrs) and fourteen flight engineers (FE: 13 M, 1 F; age = 37.5 ± 5.6 yrs; ht = 1.77 ± 7.86 cm; wt = 85.1 ± 11.8 kg; flight experience = 1128.3 ± 707.3 hrs) volunteered to participate in this study. This created the following groups: asymptomatic pilots ($n = 8$), asymptomatic flight engineers ($n = 5$), symptomatic pilots ($n = 7$), and symptomatic flight engineers ($n = 9$).

Electromyography Monitoring

Six EMG channels, with surface electrodes in a bipolar arrangement, were collected with a commercially available eight-channel system (Bortec Biomedical Ltd, Calgary, Alberta) over the right and left splenius capitis, right and left sternocleidomastoid, and right and left upper trapezius muscles. Placement sites were cleaned with 70% alcohol swab and lightly abraded with fine sandpaper. A reference electrode was affixed over the bony protuberance of C7, and signal quality was visually assessed with custom oscilloscope software (US Army Aeromedical Research Laboratory, Ft Rucker, AL) through the subject's performance of a series of test movements such as neck flexion/extension and shoulder shrugs.

Isometric Testing

Isometric testing was performed with subjects seated in a standard CH-146 helicopter cockpit seat with the appropriate four-point safety harness tightened and secured to minimize trunk movements during testing. As per figure 1.1, a two-inch webbing strap was secured around the subject's head and attached to a SSM-AJ-100 force transducer (Interface, Scottsdale, AZ) that was attached at head level to a one-inch square steel pole. The pole was positioned sixteen inches directly in front of the subject and secured in place (figure 1.1).

Maximal Voluntary Contractions

Subjects were instructed to cross their arms on their chest to prevent them from generating additional leverage by grabbing the arm rests of the cockpit chair during the isometric contractions. During the maximal voluntary contractions (MVC) testing sequence, subjects were provided verbal instructions to "gradually ramp" their force up to maximal force production (approximately 2 s) to avoid an injury of the neck muscles through a "jerking" movement and the large rate of force development and application related to those types of movements. Each subject performed three five-second isometric extension contractions, with a

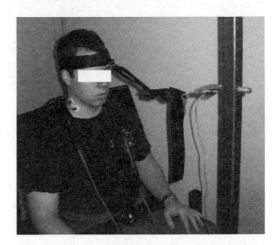

Figure 1.1 | Apparatus for testing
of isometric cervical extension

two-minute rest between contractions. The MVC trial with the largest peak force
during the five-second contraction was saved as the true MVC score, and this value
was used to calculate the subsequent 70% MVC submaximal target forces for the
submaximal ramping protocol.

Submaximal Ramping Protocol

Subjects performed one submaximal ramping protocol trial in which they were
instructed to increase force production by 7% of their MVC value every two seconds
for ten equal intervals until they reached a value equivalent to 70% of their MVC
value (i.e., rest, 7%, 14%, 21% … 70%). At this time, subjects were instructed to decrease force production by the same magnitude at the same rate until they were no
longer producing isometric force (i.e., 70%, 63%, 56% … rest). Visual feedback was
provided with numeric indicators and colour-coded graphs that corresponded to
actual force production and target force production in real time. Verbal feedback
related to force production and relaxation was also provided in real time by the
tester. The same tester was present for all subjects for all data collection sessions.

Data Analysis

Statistical analysis was performed with SPSSV 14.0 (SPSS, Chicago, IL). The EMG
variable results included the RMS values that corresponded to each target force
value (i.e., 7%, 14%, 21% … 70% of MVC) of the submaximal ramping protocol for
the splenius capitis, sternocleidomastoid, and upper trapezius muscles, bilaterally.
This resulted in six variables being used in the PCA. In the current methodology, which represents a subset analysis of data from a larger project,[23] the EMG
RMS was normalized to a value of 1.0, as compared to the average RMS of the

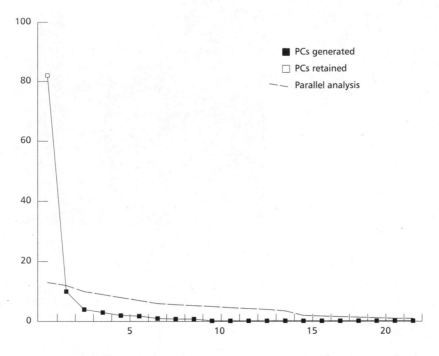

Figure 1.2 | Parallel analysis applied to the scaled eigenvalues of the 21 principal components (PCS) for root mean square (RMS) results of the left splenius capitis during submaximal ramping protocol with isometric extension. Only PCS for which the associated eigenvalue fell above the line generated by parallel analysis were retained for further analysis.

first fifteen seconds of the EMG signal from each subject's volitional fatigue trial at a force equal to 70% of his or her MVC. This technique was selected specifically to reflect the submaximal workload represented by the task of helicopter flight while wearing NVG. Even though the EMG data collected were continuous, each waveform was divided into twenty-one data points. This was necessary because the duration of the test was the same for all subjects, but the exact timing at which subjects achieved the appropriate percentage of their MVC differed very slightly (i.e., < 0.5s). To match the RMS value with the appropriate force value and to make certain that another source of variability was not introduced to the dataset, the curves were then reconstructed using the normalized twenty-one points. Each waveform was stored in a matrix with dimensions 29 × 21 (no. of subjects x no. of time points). The reconstructed waveform data were transformed into principal components through an eigenvector analysis of the covariance matrix using custom written MATLAB program software.[24] A scree plot was generated, and component retention for statistical comparison was determined using paral-

Table 1.1 | Summary of PCA results for EMG RMS variables

Variable	PC number	Captured variance (%)	PC scores	
			Asymptomatic	Symptomatic
Splenius capitis (left)	1	81.62	56.28 ± 108.26*	-22.34 ± 63.41*
Splenius capitis (right)	1	84.95	66.66 ± 122.68*	-26.20 ± 69.92*
Sternocleidomastoid (left)	1	94.41	11.28 ± 35.54	9.00 ± 57.15
Sternocleidomastoid (right)	1	96.09	9.91 ± 32.81	7.36 ± 54.19
Upper trapezius (left)	1	95.32	8.74 ± 34.52	6.47 ± 56.19
Upper trapezius (right)	1	75.20	-4.24 ± 39.49	1.55 ± 50.02
Upper trapezius (right)	2	18.21	-4.71 ± 14.42	4.51 ± 21.34

Only the scores for the significant PCs are presented as means and standard deviations.
* Denotes a significant difference between the asymptomatic and symptomatic populations ($p < 0.05$).

lel analysis[25] (figure 1.2). This method retains only the principal components that captured an amount of variability that was greater than what would be expected by chance. The retained PC scores were then stratified based on aircrew position, pilots ($n = 15$) or flight engineers ($n = 14$) or pain reporting, symptomatic ($n = 16$) or asymptomatic ($n = 13$). The data were also stratified by position and status of neck pain, and two-way analysis of variance (ANOVA) was performed to identify significant differences between the component scores across the stratified populations. Significance was set at $p < 0.05$.

Results

No significant differences were noted as a function of aircrew position or as a function of aircrew position and pain. Therefore, only significant PC scores performed as a function of reported neck pain are presented.

The overall mean MVC result for the twenty-nine subjects was 23.5 ± 5.4kg. No differences were found between groups as a function of position, pain, or position and pain. No significant differences were found for the results of any of the EMG RMS variables (symptomatic vs asymptomatic). A summary of the PC scores is provided in table 1.1, with means and standard deviations for the symptomatic and asymptomatic groups presented. Significant differences are noted for $p < 0.05$. Only the ANOVA of the PC scores for the RMS results of the right upper trapezius returned more than one statistically significant PC. However, of the EMG variables used in the PCA, only the PC scores for the left splenius capitis ($p = 0.021$) and the right splenius capitis ($p = 0.016$) RMS results were found to be statistically significant as a function of pain. The reconstructed curves for the RMS of the submaximal ramp protocol and the variance explained by the PC (81.62%) with the data for left splenius capitis are included in figure 1.3. Figure 1.4 provides the same information for the right splenius capitis PC, which captured 84.95% of the variance within the data set. In both cases, the symptomatic aircrew demonstrated suppressed RMS values as compared to their healthy counterparts.

When the curves are analyzed as one entity, the top portions of figures 1.3 and 1.4 demonstrate that the variability between the symptomatic and asymptomatic aircrew is most prominent at isometric forces between 14% and 28% of MVC. This variability remains stable as force continues to increase to 70% and subsequently decreases back to 2% to 14%.

Discussion

We were successful in using PCA and the resultant PC scores to identify differences between helicopter aircrew with and without reported neck pain. To the best of our knowledge, this is the first time that PCA has been applied to data curves reconstructed from both EMG RMS data as they relate to standardized force production of the cervical spine. Previous publications using PCA with waveforms have had success in analyzing gait to identify differences as a result of maturation that had been too subtle for detection with more conventional statistics,[26] and to identify lifting mechanics related to back pain.[27] Hubley-Kozey and Vezina[28] noted a lack of uniformity as assessed with EMG within their low-back pain population with respect to recruitment co-activation across seven muscle groups.

Perhaps more importantly, we were able to use the PC scores to differentiate aircrew reporting neck pain symptoms from aircrew who reported to be asymptomatic for neck pain using a physiological variable. We had previously been unable to differentiate aircrew who reported neck pain from their reportedly healthy colleagues using parameter-based analyses with various physiological measures including MVC, EMG (RMS and median frequency), and NIRS results.[29] In this publication, we have found success with the application of PCA to curves generated by only one isometric submaximal ramping protocol in differentiating neck-pain reporters from non-reporters. With respect to the continuation of a muscular

Figure 1.3 (*right*) | The PC coefficient and proportion of variance explained by first PC of the left splenius capitis are presented above (top). The difference ($p = 0.021$) between the reconstructed curves for symptomatic and asymptomatic subjects is also presented (bottom). The submaximal ramping protocol was standardized to 21 points and presented with time as a percentage of the trial: ramping protocol time < 50% corresponds to gradual increases in force (i.e., 7%, 14%, 21% … 63% MVC); ramping protocol time = 50% corresponds to 70% MVC; ramping protocol time > 50% corresponds to the gradual decreases in force (i.e., 63%, 56%, 49% … 7% MVC).

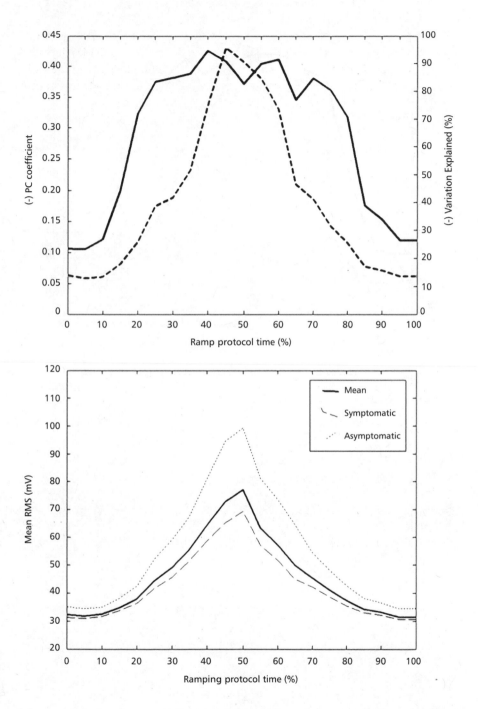

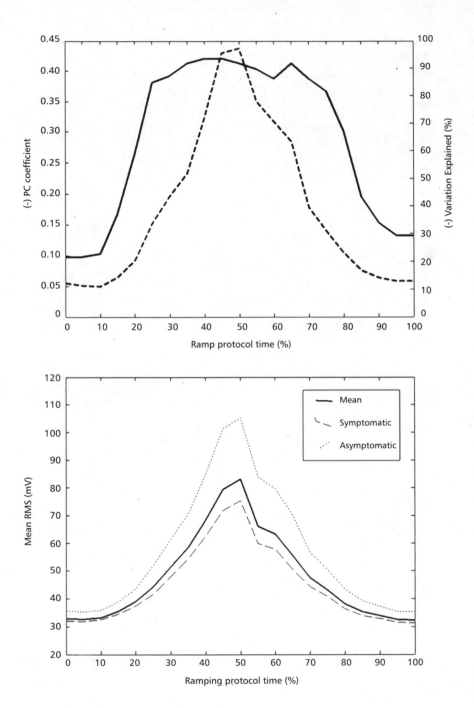

physiology component of neck pain investigations, this finding is of great importance for a number of reasons.

The decrease in cost and time in this current methodology in assessing neck pain is significant. Lopez-Lopez et al.[30] measured a change in EMG signal from the lumbar musculature of helicopter pilots, flying an aircraft that was similar in cockpit ergonomics, over the course of actual flights that demonstrated side differences in the insidious onset of fatigue. Flight time – especially for research purposes – is a costly endeavour and would potentially decrease the availability of aircrew for military training exercises. Our previous publications using laboratory testing protocols have been lengthy and have involved both maximal force production and maximal endurance of a submaximal force in four isometric directions.[31] Our logistic regression paper indicated that these test protocols were more involved than was needed to accurately predict neck pain.[32] However, the resulting logistic regression equation did not provide sufficient physiological insight. Data were collected from subjects performing a series of isometric tests of varying intensities in four different directions, with the corresponding EMG and NIRS channels monitored. The resulting logistic regression equation, much to our surprise, did not provide any physiological insight. That is to say, of all the information collected, only the most basic of information was required to accurately identify aircrew as symptomatic or asymptomatic on the basis of their self-reported neck pain status. Once again, this demonstrates that perhaps our original methodology was beyond what was needed to identify and monitor neck pain status among this aircrew population. While EMG and NIRS channels were monitored during submaximal trials that saw force increased and decreased in a successive manner that was proportional to each subject's maximal capacity for force production in each of the four directions (for the scope of this chapter and lack of significance offered by the NIRS results, these have been omitted but are available in the full dissertation by Harrison[33] at the University of Regina), only the splenius capitis EMG RMS results for extension trial was required to differentiate the asymptomatic aircrew from their symptomatic colleagues. The result is a testing methodology that is simple, quick, and detailed in the physiological sense.

While the entire protocol involved in the collection of this segment of data consisted of nearly 90 minutes of testing per subject as described elsewhere,[34] the

Figure 1.4 (*left*) | The PC coefficient and proportion of variance explained by first PC of the right splenius capitis are presented above (top). The difference ($p = 0.016$) between the reconstructed curves for symptomatic and asymptomatic subjects is also presented (bottom). The submaximal ramping protocol was standardized to 21 points and presented with time as a percentage of the trial: ramping protocol time < 50% corresponds to gradual increases in force (i.e., 7%, 14%, 21% … 63% MVC); ramping protocol time = 50% corresponds to 70% MVC; ramping protocol time > 50% corresponds to the gradual decreases in force (i.e., 63%, 56%, 49% … 7% MVC).

physiological variables that were most telling in the final PCA required less than fifteen minutes of collection time per subject. For a military unit that must continue to engage in the performance of regular duties, this is of benefit. Using results for our laboratories parallel training study projects,[35] testing efficacy of training studies may become more focused and efficient.

We selected to use only the extension isometric contraction to keep with the intent of PCA to achieve data reduction and parsimony. While we collected and could have analyzed results from the same four isometric contractions as we have previously reported,[36] our intent was to present the most meaningful data with the fewest tests. The extension protocol seemed the most logical test to include for a variety of reasons. First, research has indicated that the mass of the NVG is often forward and above the centre of gravity of the head, and the extensors are the muscles that are primarily responsible for maintaining a heads-up posture.[37] Second, there is evidence that the postures of aircrew using NVG often involve a head-down posture.[38] Third, we wanted to make certain we collected data from the musculature on the left and right side of the cervical spine. Our results have consistently noted a left and right difference that is independent of cockpit seat side[39] and complement the work of others in the assessment of lumbar spinal muscular activity in the same population.[40] Our use of the extension trial allowed us to monitor the key neck muscles bilaterally with one test and to do so in the appropriate plane.

Our PCA of the RMS of the primary antagonist during isometric extension has provided a novel finding that may provide insight into some mechanisms of neck pain. The symptomatic aircrew demonstrated a decreased RMS response, bilaterally, in the splenius capitis, as compared to the asymptomatic aircrew. Several hypotheses could explain this phenomenon. The relative workloads (7%, 14%, 21% ... 70% of MVC) were not statistically different between the two groups (i.e., asymptomatic vs symptomatic). Therefore, the level of muscular recruitment is decreased in the prime agonist for the symptomatic aircrew as compared to their healthy peers. This did not correspond with any increases in neuromuscular function in other muscles monitored by our protocol (incidentally, this also occurred independent of any change in metabolism as assessed by NIRS and presented previously[41]). Our first hypothesis is that the symptomatic aircrew members might be relying on fewer muscle fibres to do the same amount of work. This postulation bears similarities to the "Cinderella Hypothesis"[42] that we have discussed as being a possibility in this population in their occupational settings.[43] Alternatively, our decrease in RMS could be indicative of an impairment of muscular recruitment coordination. The symptomatic aircrew population could be utilizing a comparable number of muscle fibres and associated motor units as the asymptomatic subjects but the firing sequences may be dysfunctional.

Another hypothesis may further explain the apparent link between decrease in muscular activity in the splenius capitis during submaximal extension and neck pain. Panjabi[44] suggests that ligament sub-failure injuries may lead to pain in the cervical and lumbar spine. These injuries are purported to be the result of micro-trauma from a source that is either acute or cumulative. The ligaments, the facet capsules, or the discs themselves are damaged and muscle control dysfunction results. The author suggests that "muscle coordination and individual muscle force characteristics, i.e., onset, magnitude, and shut-off, are disrupted." He further suggests that this increases the stress and strain on a number of structures, including the slow-healing spinal ligaments and the imbedded mechanoreceptors. This line of thought complements the abnormal muscle recruitment patterns recorded with EMG in low-back pain subjects by Hubley-Kozey and Vezina[45] as compared to healthy controls.

The injury model involving cumulative micro-trauma and resulting impact on muscular response to load in the cervical spine described by Panjabi[46] seems to have been arrived at as a result of research in military flight involving NVG. Other studies have noted that the mass of the NVG-equipped helmet is submaximal as compared to the strength capacity of the neck in all directions.[47] But the cumulative effects have been attributed to neck strain, in literature using helicopter aircrew.[48] Thresholds of total flight hours logged with NVG have been identified,[49] and thresholds for maximum duration of single mission exposure have been determined.[50] In this chapter, we now provide evidence of decreased muscle activity in conjunction with reported neck pain among that aircrew population, despite previous studies failing to identify muscular function and strength between symptomatic and asymptomatic helicopter aircrew.[51]

It is possible that structures other than those monitored with EMG and hypothesized by Panjabi[52] may be assisting in force production in the extension movement in ways that we were not able to measure in this study. It is possible, in the sense that our results do not allow us to refute the suggestion that non-superficial muscles such as the longissimus capitis or semispinalis capitis are more active in the symptomatic subjects as compared to their asymptomatic counterparts during extension. We can, though, suggest that this is unlikely to be true. Research has suggested that training programs should aim to recruit the deep flexors and extensors to address neck myalgia,[53] and our research group has recently completed a project that complements those findings.[54] It is therefore unlikely that our subjects who were reporting neck pain were recruiting their non-superficial muscles to a greater degree than their healthy colleagues and still reporting neck pain.

Follow-up research should endeavour to evaluate the causes of our results. We cannot state definitively whether we are observing a decreased RMS in splenius capitis muscles as determined with PC scores in the symptomatic group as a *cause* of injury or as a *result* of injury. We also cannot say with certainty that this decrease in activity results in increased stress on the structures postulated by Panjabi[55] or whether the deficit in muscular activity is being addressed by other deeper muscles that are not easily measured with EMG.

Conclusion

We have successfully used PCA to differentiate between the neuromuscular activity curves created by the RMS of a progressive submaximal isometric cervical extension task by aircrew who did and who did not report suffering from neck pain. This finding provides dual benefit: it provides evidence to support the further use of physiological data analyses as well as provides the pre-existing and compelling hypothesized mechanism of cervical pain.

Notes

1 D. M. Salmon, M. F. Harrison, and J. P. Neary, "Neck Pain in Military Helicopter Aircrew and the Role of Exercise Therapy," *Aviation, Space and Environmental Medicine* 82, no. 10 (2011): 978–87; M. van den Oord, V. De Loose, T. Meeuwsen, J. K. Sluiter, and M. H. W. Frings-Dresen, "Neck Pain in Military Helicopter Pilots: Prevalence and Associated Factors," *Military Medicine* 175, no. 1 (2010): 55–60.

2 W. Fraser, K. Behdinan, F. Jahanshah, H. Ghaemi, L. Ziren, A. Ma, and A. Kapps, "Integration of Multiple Approaches to Modeling the Stresses in the Neck Due to Head Mounted Mass," *Aviation, Space and Environmental Medicine* 77, no. 3 (2006): 290.

3 K. J. Netto and A. F. Burnett, "Neck Muscle Activation and Head Postures in Common High Performance Aerial Air Combat Maneuvers," *Aviation, Space and Environmental Medicine* 77, no. 10 (2006): 1049–55.

4 C. G. de Oliviera and J. Nadal, "Back Muscle EMG of Helicopter Pilots in Flight: Effects of Fatigue, Vibration, and Posture," *Aviation, Space and Environmental Medicine* 75, no. 4 (2004): 317–22.

5 M. F. Harrison, J. P. Neary, W. J. Albert, D. W. Veillette, N. P. McKenzie, and J. C. Croll, "Trapezius Muscle Metabolism Measured with NIRS in Helicopter Pilots Flying a Simulator," *Aviation, Space and Environmental Medicine* 78, no. 2 (2007): 110–16; M. F. Harrison, J. P. Neary, W. J. Albert, D. W. Veillette, N. P. McKenzie, and J. C. Croll, "Physiological Effects of Night Vision Goggle Counterweights on Neck Musculature of Military Helicopter Pilots," *Military Medicine* 172, no. 8 (2007): 864–70; M. F. Harrison, J. P. Neary, W. J. Albert, D. W. Veillette, N. P. McKenzie, and J. C. Croll, "Helicopter Cockpit Seat Side and Trapezius Muscle Metabolism with Night Vision Goggles," *Aviation, Space and Environmental Medicine* 78, no. 10 (2007): 995–8.

6 M. F. Harrison, J. P. Neary, W. J. Albert, and J. C. Croll. "Neck Pain and Muscle Function in a Population of CH-146 Helicopter Aircrew," *Aviation, Space and Environmental Medicine* 82, no. 12 (2011): 1125–30, M. F. Harrison, J. P. Neary, W. J. Albert, U. Kuruganti, J. C. Croll, V. C. Chancey, and B. A. Bumgardner, "Measuring Neuromuscular Fatigue in Cervical Spinal Musculature of Military Helicopter Aircrew," *Military Medicine* 174, no. 11 (2009): 1183–9.

7 Harrison et al., "Trapezius Muscle Metabolism"; Harrison et al., "Helicopter Cockpit Seat Side and Trapezius Muscle Metabolism."

8 B. Ang and K. Harms-Ringdahl, "Neck Pain and Related Disability in Helicopter Pilots: A Survey of Prevalence and Risk Factors," *Aviation, Space and Environmental Medicine* 77, no. 7 (2006): 713–19; M. Thuresson, B. Ang, J. Linder, and K. Harms-Ringdahl, "Neck Muscle Activity in Helicopter Pilots: Effect of Position and Helmet-Mounted Equipment," *Aviation, Space and Environmental Medicine* 74, no. 5 (2003): 527–34.

9 Harrison et al., "Neck Pain and Muscle Function"; Harrison et al., "Measuring Neuromuscular Fatigue."

10 B. Visser and J. H. van Dieën, "Pathophysiology of Upper Extremity Muscle Disorders," *Journal of Electromyography and Kinesiology* 16, no. 1 (2006): 1–16.

11 K. A. Forde, W. J. Albert, M. F. Harrison, J. P. Neary, J. C. Croll, and J. P. Callaghan, "Neck Loads and Postures Experienced by Canadian Forces Helicopter Pilots during Simulated Day and Night Flights," *International Journal of Industrial Engineering* 41, no. 2 (2011): 128–35.

12 M. F. Harrison, J. P. Neary, W. J. Albert, and J. C. Croll, "A Predictive Logistic Regression Equation for Neck Pain in Helicopter Aircrew," *Aviation, Space and Environmental Medicine* 83, no. 6 (2012): 604–8.

13 Harrison et al., "Neck Pain and Muscle Function."

14 Ibid.; M. van den Oord, V. De Loose, T. Meeuwsen, J. K. Sluiter, and M. H. W. Frings-Dresen, "Neck Pain in Military Helicopter Pilots: Prevalence and Associated Factors," *Military Medicine* 175, no. 1 (2010): 55–60.

15 G. H. Dunteman, *Principal Components Analysis* (Newbury Park, CA: Sage Publications, 1989), 1–92.

16 Ibid.; I. T. Jolliffe, *Principal Component Analysis*, 2nd ed. (Secaucus, NJ: Springer-Verlag New York, 2002), 1–405.

17 V. L. Chester and A. T. Wrigley, "The Identification of Age-Related Differences in Kinetic Gait Parameters Using Principal Component Analysis," *Clinical Biomechanics* 23, no. 2 (2008): 212–20; M. F. Harrison, *Using Principal Component Analysis to Investigate the Influence of Hip Flexors on Ice-Hockey Skating Acceleration* (Fredericton, NB: University of New Brunswick, 2005), 1–62; A. T. Wrigley, W. J. Albert, K. J. Deluzio, and J. M. Stevenson, "Differentiating Lifting Technique between Those Who Develop Low Back Pain and Those Who Do Not," *Clinical Biomechanics* 20, no. 3 (2005): 254–63; A. T. Wrigley, W. J. Albert, K. J. Deluzio, and J. M. Stevenson, "Principal Component Analysis of Lifting Waveforms," *Clinical Biomechanics* 21, no. 6 (2006): 567–78.

18 Wrigley et al., "Differentiating Lifting Technique"; Wrigley et al., "Principal Component Analysis."

19 Wrigley et al., "Differentiating Lifting Technique."

20 K.J. Deluzio and J.L. Astephen, "Biomechanical Features of Gait Waveform Data Associated with Knee Osteoarthritis: An Application of Principal Component Analysis," *Gait and Posture* 25, no. 1 (2007): 86–93.

21 V.L. Chester and A.T. Wrigley, "The Identification of Age-Related Differences in Kinetic Gait Parameters Using Principal Component Analysis," *Clinical Biomechanics* 23, no. 2 (2008): 212–20.

22 C.L. Hubley-Kozey and M.J. Vezina, "Differentiating Temporal Electromyographic Waveforms between Those with Chronic Low Back Pain and Healthy Controls," *Clinical Biomechanics* 17, nos 9–10 (2002): 621–9.

23 Harrison et al., "Neck Pain and Muscle Function"; Harrison et al., "Measuring Neuromuscular Fatigue."

24 Wrigley et al., "Differentiating Lifting Technique."

25 J. E. Jackson, *A User's Guide to Principal Components* (New York: John Wiley & Sons, 1991), 1–436; Wrigley et al., "Differentiating Lifting Technique."

26 V. L. Chester and A. T. Wrigley. "The Identification of Age-Related Differences in Kinetic Gait Parameters Using Principal Component Analysis," *Clinical Biomechanics* 23, no. 2 (2008): 212–20.

27 Wrigley et al., "Differentiating Lifting Technique."

28 Hubley-Kozey and Vezina, "Differentiating Temporal Electromyographic Waveforms."

29 Harrison et al., "Neck Pain and Muscle Function"; Harrison et al., "Predictive Logistic Regression Equation"; Harrison et al., "Measuring Neuromuscular Fatigue."

30 J. A. Lopez-Lopez, P. Vallejo, F. Rios-Tejada, R. Jimenez, I. Sierra, and L. Garcia-Mora, "Determination of Lumbar Muscular Activity in Helicopter Pilots: A New Approach," *Aviation, Space and Environmental Medicine* 72, no. 1 (2001): 38–43.

31 Harrison et al., "Neck Pain and Muscle Function."

32 M.F. Harrison, J.P. Neary, W.J. Albert, and J.C. Croll, "Predictive Logistic Regression Equation."

33 M.F. Harrison, *The Investigation of Muscular Factors in Night Vision Goggle Induced Neck Strain in the Canadian Forces Helicopter Aircrew* (Regina, SK: University of Regina; 2009), 1–117.

34 Harrison et al., "Neck Pain and Muscle Function"; Harrison et al., "Predictive Logistic Regression Equation."

35 D. M. Salmon, *The Efficacy of Exercise Therapy in Reducing Neck Pain and Fatigue in CH-146 CF Aircrew* (Regina, SK: University of Regina, 2009), 1–96.

36 Harrison et al., "Neck Pain and Muscle Function"; Harrison et al. "Predictive Logistic Regression Equation"; Harrison et al., "Measuring Neuromuscular Fatigue."

37 Netto and Burnett, "Neck Muscle Activation and Head Postures"; Thuresson et al., "Neck Muscle Activity in Helicopter Pilots."

38 Forde et al., "Neck Loads and Postures."

39 Harrison et al., "Trapezius Muscle Metabolism"; Harrison et al., "Helicopter Cockpit Seat Side and Trapezius Muscle Metabolism"; Harrison et al., "Neck Pain and Muscle Function"; Harrison et al., "Measuring Neuromuscular Fatigue."

40 Lopez-Lopez et al., "Determination of Lumbar Muscular Activity"; de Oliviera and Nadal, "Back Muscle EMG of Helicopter Pilots."

41 Harrison, *Investigation of Muscular Factors*, 1–117.

42 W. Eriksen, "Linking Work Factors to Neck Myalgia: The Nitric Oxide / Oxygen Ratio Hypothesis," *Medical Hypotheses* 62, no. 5 (2004): 721–6; G. Sjogaard, U. Lundberg, and R. Kadefors, "The Role of Muscle Activity and Mental Load in the Development of Pain and Degenerative Processes at the Muscle Cell Level during Computer Work," *European Journal of Applied Physiology* 83, nos 2–3 (2000): 99–105;

S. Thorn, *Muscular Activity in Light Manual Work: With Reference to the Development of Muscle Pain among Computer Users* (Göteborg, Sweden: Chalmers University of Technology, 2005), 1–132; B. Visser and J. H. van Dieën, "Pathophysiology of Upper Extremity Muscle Disorders," *Journal of Electromyography and Kinesiology* 16, no. 1 (2006): 1–16.

43 M. F. Harrison et al., "Measuring Neuromuscular Fatigue."

44 M. M. Panjabi, "A Hypothesis of Chronic Back Pain: Ligament Subfailure Injuries Lead to Muscle Control Dysfunction," *European Spine Journal* 15, no. 5 (2006): 668–76.

45 Hubley-Kozey and Vezina, "Differentiating Temporal Electromyographic Waveforms."

46 Panjabi, "Hypothesis of Chronic Back Pain."

47 Ang and Harms-Ringdahl, "Neck Pain and Related Disability in Helicopter Pilots"; B. Ang, J. Linder, and K. Harms-Ringdahl, "Neck Muscle Strength and Myoelectric Fatigue in Fighter and Helicopter Pilots with a History of Neck Pain," *Aviation, Space and Environmental Medicine* 76, no. 4 (2005): 375–80; Harrison et al., "Neck Pain and Muscle Function."

48 J. Adam, *Results of NVG-Induced Neck Strain Questionnaire Study in CH-146 Griffon Aircrew* (Toronto: DRDC Toronto), 1–75; Fraser et al., "Integration of Multiple Approaches to Modeling"; Harrison et al., "Predictive Logistic Regression Equation"; S. Wickes and J. Greeves, "Epidemiology of Flight-Related Neck Pain in Royal Air Force (RAF) Aircrew," *Aviation, Space and Environmental Medicine* 76, no. 3 (2005): 298.

49 Adam, *Results of NVG-induced Neck Strain Questionnaire*; Fraser et al., "Integration of Multiple Approaches to Modeling."

50 Harrison et al., "Predictive Logistic Regression Equation."

51 M. H. van den Oord, V. De Loose, J. K. Sluiter, and M. H. W. Frings-Dresen, "Neck Strength, Position Sense, and Motion in Military Helicopter Crew with and without Neck Pain," *Aviation, Space and Environmental Medicine* 81, no. 1 (2010): 46–51.

52 Panjabi, "Hypothesis of Chronic Back Pain."

53 G. Jull, C. Barrett, R. Magee, and P. Ho, "Further Clinical Clarification of the Muscle Dysfunction in Cervical Headache," *Cephalalgia* 19, no. 3 (1999): 179–85.

54 Salmon, *Efficacy of Exercise Therapy*.

55 Panjabi, "Hypothesis of Chronic Back Pain."

2

Novel Functional Magnetic Resonance Imaging to Quantify Neuronal Hemodynamic and Metabolic Underpinnings of Cognitive Impairment in Mild Traumatic Brain Injury and Amyotrophic Lateral Sclerosis

CLARISSE ILDIKO MARK AND GILBERT BRUCE PIKE

Abstract

Mild traumatic brain injury (mTBI) is a cerebral disorder still poorly understood and initially believed to be solely a temporary and reversible loss of consciousness. Yet recent clinical evidence shows that even concussion, TBI's mildest form, can result in long-term disability because of the development of cerebral hemodynamic and metabolic dysfunctions as well as associated cognitive impairments.[1] Individuals at high risk of concussions have been found to suffer increased cases of amyotrophic lateral sclerosis (ALS): a two-fold increase has been reported in veterans, irrespective of the war or military branch of service,[2] and an eight-fold increase in Italian soccer players and American footballers.[3] While the origins of ALS remain unknown, this fatal progressive disease causing the degeneration of cerebral and spinal motor neurons is believed to be triggered primarily by environmental factors rather than family history. Consistent with this unusually high ALS incidence and mortality among military personnel and professional contact-sport athletes, the strongest risk has been suspected to be trauma to the brain.[4] At the moment, mTBI and ALS are most often diagnosed on the basis of symptoms, which are subjective, under-reported, and appearing once brain damage is already well underway. Novel and safe techniques to image the brain are hence desperately needed for the early detection, investigation, and understanding of the pathological condition of concussion, including its potential association with ALS. We hypothesize that our latest advances in quantitative functional magnetic resonance imaging (fMRI) will offer the sensitivity required to detect the precise physiological mechanisms underlying brain dysfunctions associated with specific cognitive defects in mTBI and ALS. In this chapter we present our proof-of-concept in healthy humans, demonstrating precise measurement of metabolic and hemodynamic changes in specifically activated brain regions. We propose to extend our methodology to concussed individuals, with and without a history of ALS, to shine light into the specific and shared physiological dysfunctions underlying cognitive impairments, representing early bio-markers of invaluable diagnostic value.

Diagnosis of Mild Traumatic Brain Injury and Amyotrophic Lateral Sclerosis

Current Assessment Tools

Mild TBI are diagnosed on the basis of symptoms. Although sometimes the signs are clear (acute headache, dizziness, confusion, and nausea), in many instances they are more covert, manifesting as mild cognitive deficits difficult to detect. Organizations generally use two types of assessment: Sport Concussion Assessment Tool version 2 (SCAT2) and/or a neurocognitive assessment such as Immediate Post-Concussion Assessment and Cognitive Testing (ImPACT). The SCAT2 is a symptom inventory and screening assessment for orientation, alertness, cognitive function, and balance. ImPACT is a very brief test designed to measure a variety of cognitive functions including processing speed, attention, and working memory. While these tests provide post-injury cognitive and symptom data to help clinicians determine safe return-to-duty or return-to-play time,[5] there is insufficient medical evidence on their reliability to make them the sole diagnostic factor,[6] and their usefulness in predicting long-term impairments associated with multiple concussions is still under debate.[7]

More robust and complementary diagnostic tools are hence clearly needed, as an exclusive reliance on symptoms for diagnosis and management is prone to bias and inconsistent reporting. In the case of athletes, concussion is seldom reported because they can fail to recognize an injury or be reluctant to report it for fear of exclusion from play.[8] Furthermore, it is thought that purely symptomatic assessment fails to reveal residual brain injury and can lead to premature return-to-duty or return-to-play decisions,[9] which are associated with an increased risk of repeated injury.[10] Studies have suggested that multiple concussions might later lead to catastrophic disability – not only ALS, but also chronic traumatic encephalopathy (CTE),[11] manifested as alterations in behaviour and personality such as increased irritability or aggressiveness, short-term memory loss, frontal-lobe dysfunction, and increasing cognitive impairment progressing to dementia with symptoms similar to Alzheimer's and Parkinson's diseases.[12] If present, these potential additional long-term sequelae from repeated concussions greatly affect the lives of brain-injured individuals. Whether ALS onset could be triggered by head injury remains unclear, and ALS is also currently diagnosed only once symptoms appear, at which point it might already be too late to stop the rapid degeneration of motor neurons, which leads to death within three to five years.

The Premise of Neuroimaging Tools

Recently developed neuroimaging methods may be more sensitive to the patho-physiology of concussion than current assessment tools, allowing the identification of bio-markers to improve the evaluation and management of concussed individuals and make informed return-to-duty and return-to-play decisions. This will lead to the best possible health and safety outcomes for both military personnel and athletes. Yet the utility of neuroimaging for diagnosis and establishment of prognosis in concussion has been limited. Conventional computed tomography (CT) and structural magnetic resonance imaging (MRI), often performed for the clinical identification of head trauma, detect only severe anatomical damage, usually absent in concussion,[13] making concussion an "invisible" injury. MRI techniques for measuring subtle structural integrity of white-matter connections (i.e., diffusion tensor imaging, or DTI) appear more sensitive to concussion, although the results are variable, and the link to severity of injury and prognosis remains to be clearly established.[14] For imaging of brain function, rather than brain structure, the most spatially specific and readily available tool is functional MRI (fMRI), a non-invasive technique to map cerebral function that has found widespread use in cognitive neuroscience since its inception in the nineties. fMRI is an appealing imaging technique for probing the pathophysiology of concussion, for several reasons. First, it is sensitive to *functional* changes. This accords well with the fact that concussion is recognized as being a functional disorder.[15] Also, fMRI can be used to assess function simultaneously in a widely distributed network of brain regions. Given that the brain damage in concussion and ALS is most often distributed and diffuse, casting a "wide functional net" yields the best chance of observing abnormalities. fMRI neuronal tasks provide a sensitive way to probe specific aspects of sensory, motor, and cognitive function and hence offer promising neurophysiological assessment of concussion and ALS by recruiting a distributed network of brain regions.

Need for Calibration in Functional Magnetic Resonance Imaging

Traditional fMRI does not measure neuronal activity directly but rather relies on a complex interplay of underlying physiological changes that are reflected in a measure of blood oxygenation: the blood oxygen level dependent (BOLD) effect.[16] BOLD indirectly reflects cerebral blood flow (CBF) and the metabolic rate of oxygen consumption by brain tissue ($CMRO_2$). These hemodynamic and metabolic changes are all prone to poorly understood variations under pathological conditions. Accordingly, although exciting and novel, it is not sufficient to use BOLD to investigate the origin of cognitive impairments in neurological pathologies such as mTBI and ALS; it is essential to also quantify its determinants, CBF and $CMRO_2$.

Fortunately, recent advances in quantitative fMRI allow CBF to be acquired simultaneously with BOLD and used to estimate $CMRO_2$ on the basis of a simple mathematical formulation.[17] The biophysical model involves a calibration step to evaluate the maximal BOLD signal under full venous oxygenation, traditionally obtained from a vasodilation induced by subjects breathing an increased level of carbon dioxide (CO_2) through a clinical facemask. However, manual gas manipulation of this high CO_2 condition, termed hypercapnia (HC), suffers from large intra- and inter-subject as well as inter-session variations, questioning the validity of $CMRO_2$-estimates.[18] An improved automated gas delivery system (RespirAct™, Thornhill Research, Toronto) can be employed to rigorously control the flow and composition of CO_2 to achieve precise, predictable, and repeatable HC stimuli.[19] Yet, already poorly tolerated in healthy subjects, the HC calibration step limits the methodology's applicability to, amongst others, patients with impaired cerebrovascular reactivity. In such cases, the computerized system could offer a better-tolerated non-vasoactive calibration alternative involving increases in oxygen (O_2), termed a hyperoxic condition (HO).[20] We thereby sought to compare computer-controlled HC calibration to traditional manual HC calibration and computer-controlled HO calibration. As a proof-of-concept, the calibrations were performed in the same set of healthy subjects in the same scanning session and followed by robust and simple visual and sensorimotor tasks. Our hypothesis was of an improved calibration under computer-controlled HC, and better yet under HO, with significantly reduced variability in regional $CMRO_2$ estimates.

Methods

Nine healthy adults (4 males; mean age 26 years) were studied on a 3T MRI scanner (Siemens, Erlangen, Germany) using a thirty-two-channel head coil. After consent and safety screening, participants first underwent a structural scan to position and analyze nine oblique axial slices through the visual and sensorimotor cortices during pulsed arterial spin labelling (PASL). The imaging PASL sequence termed quantitative imaging of perfusion using single subtraction echo planar imaging (QUIPSS II–EPI) was used to simultaneously acquire BOLD and CBF images during calibration and neuronal tasks.

Calibration Tasks

Prior to entering the scanner room, participants were given the opportunity to become familiar with the breathing tasks and practice keeping a constant relaxed breathing rate. For the first scanning session, participants were fitted with a non-re-breathable mask (figure 2.1 – left) into which CO_2 and O_2 gases were infused through manual manipulation of randomized graded levels of high CO_2 challenges (hypercapnia – HC). For the second scanning session, the mask was replaced by

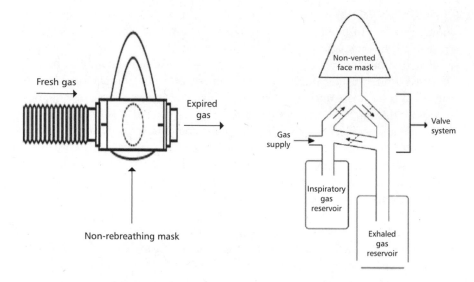

Figure 2.1 | Manual (left, courtesy of Nicholas Blockley) and RespirAct™ computerized (right, courtesy of TRI) gas delivery methods used to induce graded calibration levels of high CO_2 and high O_2 challenges

a sealed re-breathable breathing circuit (figure 2.1 – right) controlled by a feed-forward computerized algorithm (RespirAct™, TRI). Participants then completed graded hypercapnic (high CO_2) as well as hyperoxic (high O_2) respiratory stimulation in a randomized fashion.

Neuronal Tasks

Following the gas calibration sessions, a yellow/blue checkerboard alternating at 8 Hz, in four OFF/ON/OFF blocks was presented to the participants to activate their visual cortex (figure 2.2 – left). During the ON periods, subjects were asked to perform voluntary bilateral finger-to-thumb apposition to activate their sensorimotor cortex (figure 2.2 – right).

Data Analysis

Two subjects were excluded as a result of head motion. BOLD and CBF responses under all tasks were analyzed as described previously.[21] $CMRO_2$ responses in both activated visual and sensorimotor brain regions were estimated based on individual- and group-calibrated hypercapnic as well as hyperoxic data.

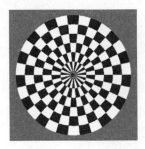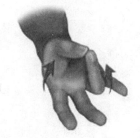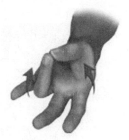

Figure 2.2 | Visual (left) and sensorimotor (right) tasks used to induce activity-localized responses.

Results

Manual versus Computerized Calibration

The cerebral blood flow (CBF) vasodilation induced by hypercapnic-stimulation, and the resulting BOLD response, were more uniformly distributed across the brain and more linear in gradation through the computerized system than the conventional manual manipulation (figure 2.3). Such robust control of respiratory stimuli is vital not only to calibrated-fMRI studies but also to investigate cerebro-vascular reactivity under healthy and pathological conditions.[22]

Hypercapnic versus Hyperoxic Calibration

While both challenges induced similar BOLD activation in all subjects, the hyper-oxic protocol (HOP) consistently lacked a CBF response (figure 2.4). Hence by eliminating this intrinsically noisy measurement, hyperoxia consistently produced markedly lower calibration variance with reduced dispersion across individuals compared to standard hypercapnic calibration studies.[23]

Visual and Sensorimotor Activation

While most fMRI-calibrated studies have been limited to group calibration because of excessively large errors, our reduced calibration variability allowed a per-subject calibration for proper quantification of individual metabolic responses on a per-brain-region basis (e.g., visual and sensorimotor cortices [figure 2.5]). Moreover, by eliminating the variability in individual vascular reactivity, hyperoxic calibration avoided the uncertainty in a flow–volume relationship often overestimated in the bio-physical model and shone light on a more accurate parametrization under the hypercapnic calibration.[24]

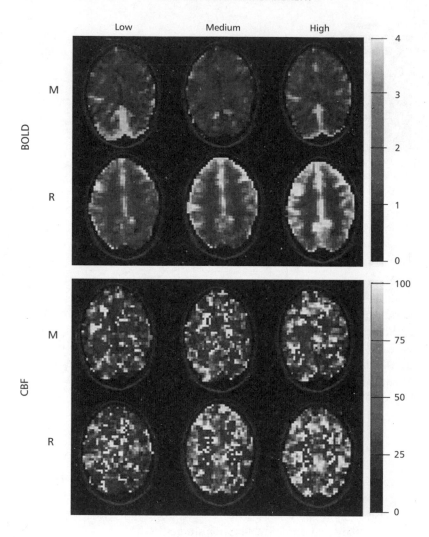

Figure 2.3 | Whole brain BOLD (top) and CBF (bottom) responses to graded levels (left to right: low, medium, and high) of manual (M) and RespirAct™ computerized (R) hyper-capnic (HC) calibration. Greyscales indicate the % signal change from baseline.

Discussion

As clinically useful physiological concomitants of concussion have not yet been reliably identified, current clinical assessment tools focus solely on reported symptoms and structural neuroimaging. There is growing evidence that the resulting return-to-duty and return-to-play decisions may be premature,[25] especially since conventional structural neuroimaging is often normal, making mild TBI an "in-

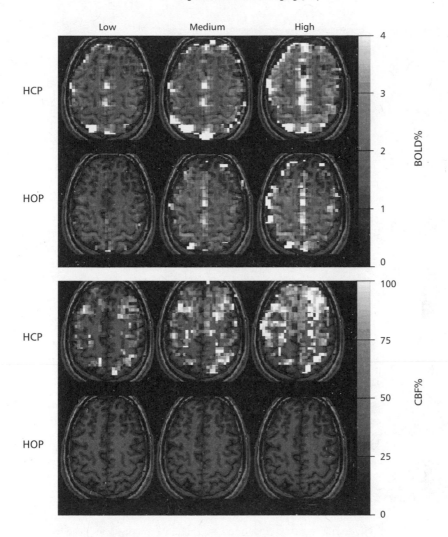

Figure 2.4 | Whole brain BOLD (top) and CBF (bottom) responses to graded levels (left to right: low, medium, and high) of RespirAct™ computerized hypercapnic (HCP) and hyperoxic protocols (HOP). Greyscales indicate the % signal change from baseline.

visible" injury. Our results in healthy subjects indicate the appropriateness of our methodology in enabling fMRI's full clinical potential in the pursuit of detecting cerebral dysfunctions associated with specific mTBI cognitive impairments and their potential association to ALS. fMRI offers fast, non-invasive, high spatial and temporal resolution images, highly appropriate to the patient population, including those with compromised cerebral blood flow, as demonstrated by numerous fMRI studies of stroke cases. Our gas calibration methodology has a small

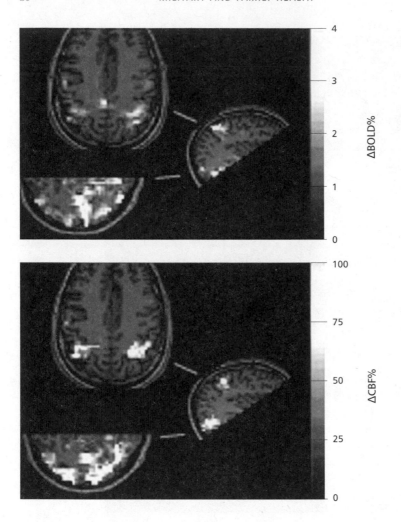

Figure 2.5 | Activity-localized BOLD (top) and CBF (bottom) responses induced by visual and sensorimotor tasks. Greyscales indicate the % signal change from baseline.

footprint and low gas requirement, and provides an inherent passive compensation to hyperventilation, making its use highly tolerable by patients, compared to the common manual gas delivery method, which limits respiratory ventilation. From a safety point of view, the computerized gas system does not use any hypoxic source gases; they all contain a minimum of 10% O_2, so that malfunction of any single or combination of gas controller cannot result in complete hypoxia. This is in contrast to most systems that employ pure O_2, CO_2, and N_2, two of which are anoxic. The RespirAct™ has been used in over 500 patients in a number of centres to study cerebrovascular reactivity. The hypercapnic challenges required for our calibration are safe and well within the range of changes encountered in everyday life. Yet hypercapnia might be poorly tolerated by some patients with impaired cerebrovascular reactivity. In such cases, the computerized system could offer the better-tolerated and non-vasoactive hyperoxic calibration alternative.

Quantitative Functional Magnetic Resonance Imaging "Proof-of-Concept" in Healthy Subjects

Through precisely controlled calibration in healthy individuals, our work demonstrates unique fMRI acquisition, calibration, and modelling methods to extend the conventional BOLD signal by the added robust quantification of underlying hemodynamic and metabolic responses to brain activation. As mentioned earlier, fMRI does not measure neuronal activity directly: BOLD indexes the ratio of oxyhemoglobin (diamagnetic) to deoxyhemoglobin (paramagnetic), typically in deoxygenated venous brain vessels. This ratio depends primarily on cerebral blood flow (CBF) and the metabolic rate of oxygen consumption by brain tissue ($CMRO_2$) required for the oxidative breakdown of glucose into energy. CBF determines the supply of oxygen to tissue (*perfusion*), whereas $CMRO_2$ reflects tissue consumption of oxygen (*metabolism*). In healthy tissue, the balance between O_2 perfusion and metabolism, called the oxygen flow–metabolic coupling, provides sufficient nutrients to brain cells, regardless of their state of activity. Perfusion and metabolism are hence confounded in the BOLD signal, as it probes the overall oxygenation state of brain tissues. Worse, independent of actual changes in perfusion and metabolism, if their balance was maintained, BOLD would be minimally altered.[26] Our recent advances in quantitative fMRI (qfMRI) described here allow the accurate, non-invasive measurement of these key aspects of cerebral hemodynamic and metabolic physiology, which can be registered to structural MRI acquired during the same session for precise localization. Our group has been a pioneer in developing these quantitative methods,[27] by acquiring CBF simultaneously with BOLD (avoiding a potential physiological change of state between measurements) to estimate $CMRO_2$ on the basis of a simple biophysical model and a gas calibration procedure.[28] Our improved calibration methodology extends the information provided by conventional BOLD imaging with the added robust quantification of underlying cerebrovascular reactivity (CVR), and hemodynamic (CBF) and metabolic ($CMRO_2$) responses to brain activation.

Quantitative Functional Magnetic Resonance Imaging in Mild Traumatic Brain Injury and Amyotrophic Lateral Sclerosis

On the basis of extensive prior animal and human research, our measured responses to brain activation (i.e., CVR, CBF, and $CMRO_2$) appear to be key bio-markers in mTBI and ALS. Although the pathophysiology of concussion is complex and its association with ALS is unclear, both appear to have consistent metabolic "signatures." Studies in animal models indicate that concussion results in mitochondrial dysfunction,[29] which decreases oxygen metabolism.[30] Concussion also appears to upregulate the expression and receptor distribution of endothelin, a powerful vasoconstrictor,[31] altering CVR and reducing CBF.[32] Indeed, studies in both rodents and humans report reduced CBF after concussion.[33] Positron emission tomography (PET) and single-photon emission computerized tomography (SPECT), two other imaging techniques, have revealed decreased blood flow and oxygen metabolism in concussed patients.[34] Because the neuropathological processes underlying changes in perfusion and metabolism are somewhat independent, it is unlikely that the balance between them remains unchanged after injury, and indeed studies indicate that the flow-metabolic coupling is altered in concussion.[35] Nevertheless, since pathological changes in perfusion and metabolism are in the same direction (hypo-perfusion and hypo-metabolism), they will, to some extent, "balance each other out," yielding potentially misleadingly small or negligible alteration in BOLD compared to the unconcussed healthy state. Clearly, the direct measurement of these BOLD determinants, perfusion and metabolism, is essential for maximal specificity and sensitivity to the metabolic and physiological abnormalities underlying mTBI-induced dysfunctions and their association with the onset of ALS. While the exact mechanism of motor neuron death in ALS remains unknown, recent in vivo capillary imaging also showed early and progressive uncoupling of flow-metabolism preceding sequential pathological changes in spinal cords of mice.[36] A study on post-mortem brains of athletes with a history of multiple concussions, diagnosed for CTE and with signs of motor neuron disease, revealed metabolic alterations in specific proteins associated with degenerated fronto-temporal cerebral regions contributing to memory loss, and behavioural and cognitive changes.[37] Non-invasive measurements of cerebral blood flow and oxygen metabolism to assess cerebral dysfunction under mTBI and ALS could hence offer early bio-markers of tremendous diagnostic value. A recent investigational attempt to reveal hemodynamic and metabolic defects induced by brain damage in children through fTBI employed standard measurements of blood flow and whole brain oxygen extraction.[38] Such global quantification cannot detect the spatial distribution of abnormalities, expected to be heterogeneous, whereas our qfMRI methodology can be used for precise regional measurements of blood flow and metabolism. Our quantitative fMRI results support this extremely powerful non-invasive tool, invaluable for basic neuroscience and for the clinical assessment, prevention, therapy, and management of brain pathologies.

The sensitivity of qfMRI indices of localized brain damage can be potentiated by measuring them under neuronal activation that induces relevant metabolic responses and accurately calibrating the measured signal responses in the non-activated state. In physiologically healthy brain tissue, increased neuronal activity results in a rapid increase in CBF followed by a smaller and more localized increase in CMRO$_2$, which reduces the concentration of paramagnetic deoxyhemoglobin and hence yields a positive BOLD signal change. By introducing cognitive activation tasks during concurrent measurement of CBF and CMRO$_2$ in hypoperfused and hypo-metabolic tissue, such as appears to occur following injury to the brain, we will increase our sensitivity to physiological abnormality. Quantitative fMRI can be easily integrated into current clinical MR practice: it is efficient and complements BOLD-fMRI with physiological measurements of greater functional and spatial specificity.

We hence propose to apply our fMRI methods through the use of neuro-functionally specific, clinically validated, cognitive tasks in mTBI. By recruiting concussed and un-concussed ALS patients, our imaging methodology will have the sensitivity required to explore the specificity and possible causality of the physiological dysfunctions underpinning these conditions. Non-invasive and sensitive methods such as described herein are desperately needed to quantify bio-markers for early diagnosis, improved treatment, and patient management in cases of mTBI and to investigate the potential association with ALS.

Notes

1 E. Matser, A. Kessel, M. Lezak, B. Jordan, and J. Troost, "Neurological Impairment in Amateur Soccer Players," *Journal of the American Medical Association* 282, no. 10 (1999): 971–3.

2 ALS Association, "ALS in the Military: Unexpected Consequences of Military Service," ALS in the Military White Paper, http:/www.alsa.org/als-care/veterans.

3 E. Abel, "Football Increases the Risk for Lou Gehrig's Disease, Amyotrophic Lateral Sclerosis," *Perceptual and Motor Skills* 104 (2007): 1251–4.

4 A. McKee, B. Gavett, R. Stern, C. Nowinski, R. Cantu, N. Kowall, D. Perl, E. Hedley-Whyte, B. Price, C. Sullivan, P. Morin, H. Lee, C. Kubilus, D. Daneshvar, M. Wulff, and A. Budson, "TDP-43 Proteinopathy and Motor Neuron Disease in Chronic Traumatic Encephalopathy," *Journal of Neuropathology and Experimental Medicine* 69, no. 9 (2010): 918–29.

5 A. B. Ashare, "Returning to Play after Concussion," *Acta Paediatrica* 98, no. 5 (2009): 774–6; P. Schatz, J. E. Pardini, M. R. Lovell, M. W. Collins, and K. Podell, "Sensitivity and Specificity of the Impact Test Battery for Concussion in Athletes," *Archives of Clinical Neuropsychology* 21, no. 1 (2006): 91–9.

6 L. Mayers and T. Redick, "Clinical Utility of Impact Assessment for Postconcussion Return-to-Play Counseling: Psychometric Issues," *Journal of Clinical and Experimental Neuropsychology* 34, no. 3 (2012): 235–42.

7 E. Breedlove, M. Robinson, T. Talavage, K. Morigaki, U. Yoruk, K. OKeefe, J. King, L. Leveren, J. Gilger, and E. Nauman, "Biomechanical Correlates of Symptomatic and Asymptomtic Neurophysiological Impairment in High School Football," *Journal of Biomechanics* 45 (2012): 1265–72.

8   J. Delaney, V. Lacroix, S. Leclerc, and K. Johnston, "Concussions among University Football and Soccer Players," *Clinical Journal of Sport Medicine* 12 (2002): 331–8.

9   Mayers and Redick, "Clinical Utility of Impact Assessment for Postconcussion Return-to-Play Counseling."

10 K. Guskiewicz and S. Broglio, "Sport-Related Concussion: On Field and Sideline Assessment," *Physical Medicine and Rehabilitation Clinics of North America* 22, no. 4 (2011): 603–17; K. M. Guskiewicz, M. McCrea, S. W. Marshall, R. C. Cantu, C. Randolph, W. Barr, J. A. Onate, and J. P. Kelly, "Cumulative Effects Associated with Recurrent Concussion in Collegiate Football Players: The Ncaa Concussion Study," *Journal of the American Medical Association* 290, no. 19 (2003): 2549–55; D. Stuss, P. Ely, H. Hugenholtz, M. Richard, S. LaRochelle, C. Poirier, and I. Bell, "Subtle Neuropsychological Deficits in Patients with Good Recovery after Closed Head Injury," *Neurosurgery* 17 (1985): 41–7.

11 S. Shively, A. I. Scher, D. P. Perl, and R. Diaz-Arrastia, "Dementia Resulting from Traumatic Brain Injury," *Archives of Neurology*, doi:10.1001/archneurol.2011.3747.

12 A. McKee, R. Cantu, C. Nowinski, E. Hedley-Whyte, B. Gavett, A. Budson, V. Santini, H. Lee, C. Kubilus, and R. Stern, "Chronic Traumatic Encephalopathy in Athletes: Progressive Tauopathy after Repetitive Head Injury," *Journal of Neuropathology and Experimental Neurology* 68 (2009): 709–35.

13 D. Hughes, A. Jackson, D. Mason, E. Berry, S. Hollis, and D. Yates, "Abnormalitites on Magnetic Resonance Imaging Seen Acutely Following Mild Traumatic Brain Injury: Correlation with Neuropsychological Tests and Delayed Recovery," *Neuroradiology* 46 (2004): 550–8.

14 A. Gardner, K. Kay-Lambkin, P. Stanwell, J. Donnelly, W. Huw Williams, A. Hiles, P. Schofield, C. Levi, and D. K. Jones, "A Systematic Review of Diffusion Tensor Imaging Findings in Sports-Related Concussion," *Journal of Neurotrauma* 29, no. 16 (2012): 2521–38.

15 D. Pulsipher, R. Campbell, R. Thoma, and J. King, "A Critical Review of Neuroimaging Applications in Sports Concussion," *Current Sports Medicine Reports* 10, no. 1 (2011): 14–20.

16 S. Ogawa, T. Lee, A. Kay, and D. Tank, "Brain Magnetic Resonance Imaging with Contrast Dependent on Blood Oxygenation," *Proceedings of the National Academy of Sciences of the United States of America* 87 (1990): 9868–72.

17 T. L. Davis, K. K. Kwong, R. M. Weisskoff, and B. R. Rosen, "Calibrated Functional MRI: Mapping the Dynamics of Oxidative Metabolism," *Proceedings of the National Academy of Sciences of the United States of America* 95, no. 4 (1998): 1834–9; R. Hoge, J. Atkinson, B. Gill, G. Crelier, S. Marrett, and G. Pike, "Investigation of BOLD Signal Dependence on Cerebral Blood Flow and Oxygen Consumption: The Deoxyhemoglobin Dilution Model," *Magnetic Resonance in Medicine* 42, no. 5 (1999): 849–63.

18 P. A. Chiarelli, D. P. Bulte, S. Piechnik, and P. Jezzard, "Sources of Systematic Bias in Hypercapnia-Calibrated Functional MRI Estimation of Oxygen Metabolism," *NeuroImage* 34, no. 1 (2007): 35–43.

19 M. Slessarev, J. Han, A. Mardimae, E. Prisman, D. Preiss, G. Volgyesi, C. Ansel, J. Duffin, and J. A. Fisher, "Prospective Targeting and Control of End-Tidal CO_2 and O_2 Concentrations," *Journal of Physiology* 581, no. 3 (2007): 1207–19.

20 P. A. Chiarelli, D. P. Bulte, R. Wise, D. Gallichan, and P. Jezzard, "A Calibration Method for Quantitative BOLD fMRI Based on Hyperoxia," *NeuroImage* 37, no. 3 (2007): 808–20.

21 C. Mark, M. Slessarev, I. Shoji, J. Han, J. Fisher, and B. Pike, "Precise Control of End-Tidal Carbon Dioxide and Oxygen Improves BOLD and ASL Cerebrovascular Reactivity Measures," *Magnetic Resonance in Medicine* 64, no. 3 (2010): 749–56; C. Mark and B. Pike, "Indication of BOLD-Specific Venous Flow-Volume Changes from Precisely Controlled Hyperoxic versus Hypercapnic Calibration," *Journal of Cerebral Blood Flow and Metabolism* 23, no. 4 (2012): 709–19; C. Mark, J. Fisher, and G. Pike, "Improved fMRI Calibration: Precisely Controlled Hyperoxic versus Hypercapnic Stimuli," *Neuroimage* 54, no. 2 (2011): 1102–11.

22 Mark, Slessarev et al, "Precise Control of End-Tidal Carbon Dioxide and Oxygen."

23 Mark, Fisher, and Pike, "Improved fMRI Calibration."

24 Mark and Pike, "Indication of BOLD-Specific Venous Flow-Volume Changes."

25 Mayers and Redick, "Clinical Utility of Impact Assessment for Postconcussion Return-to-Play Counseling."

26 R. Buxton, "Interpreting Oxygenation-Based Neuroimaging Signals: The Importance and the Challenge of Understanding Brain Oxygen Metabolism," *Frontiers in NeuroEnergetics* 2 (2010): 1–16.

27 B. Stefanovic, J. M. Warnking, K. M. Rylander, and G. B. Pike, "The Effect of Global Cerebral Vasodilation on Focal Activation Hemodynamics," *NeuroImage* 30, no. 3 (2006): 726–34; Mark, Fisher, and Pike, "Improved fMRI Calibration"; Mark and Pike, "Indication of BOLD-Specific Venous Flow-Volume Changes"; Mark, Slessarev et al., "Precise Control of End-Tidal Carbon Dioxide and Oxygen"; J. J. Chen and G. Pike, "Global Cerebral Oxidative Metabolism during Hypercapnia and Hypocapnia in Humans: Implications for BOLD fMRI," *Journal of Cerebral Blood Flow and Metabolism* 30 (2010): 1094–9; Hoge et al., "Investigation of BOLD Signal Dependence."

28 Davis et al., "Calibrated Functional MRI"; R. D. Hoge, J. Atkinson, B. Gill, G. Crelier, S. Marrett, and G. B. Pike, "Stimulus-Dependent BOLD and Perfusion Dynamics in Human V1," *NeuroImage* 9 (1999): 573–85.

29 T. Clausen, A. Zauner, J. E. Levasseur, A. C. Rice, and R. Bullock, "Induced Mitochondrial Failure in the Feline Brain: Implications for Understanding Acute Post-Traumatic Metabolic Events," *Brain Research* 908, no. 1 (2001): 35–48; J. Lifshitz, H. Friberg, R. W. Neumar, R. Raghupathi, F. A. Welsh, P. Janmey, K. E. Saatman, T. Wieloch, M. S. Grady, and T. K. McIntosh, "Structural and Functional Damage Sustained by Mitochondria after Traumatic Brain Injury in the Rat: Evidence for Differentially Sensitive Populations in the Cortex and Hippocampus," *Journal of Cerebral Blood Flow and Metabolism* 23, no. 2 (2003): 219–31; B. H. Verweij, J. P. Muizelaar, F. C. Vinas, P. L. Peterson, Y. Xiong, and C. P. Lee, "Impaired Cerebral Mitochondrial Function after Traumatic Brain Injury in Humans," *Journal of Neurosurgery* 93, no. 5 (2000): 815–20.

30 P. Vespa, M. Bergsneider, N. Httori, C. Wu, S.-C. Huang, N. Martin, T. Glenn, D. McArthur, and D. Hovda, "Metabollic Crisis without Brain Ischemia Is Common after Traumatic Brain Injury: A Combined Microdialysis and Positron Emission Tomography Study," *Journal of Cerebral Blood Flow and Metabolism* 25, no. 6 (2005):

763–74; M. N. Diringer, K. Yundt, T. O. Videen, R. E. Adams, A. R. Zazulia, E. Deibert, V. Aiyagari, R. G. Dacey, R. L. Grubb, and W. J. Powers, "No Reduction in Cerebral Metabolism as a Result of Early Moderate Hyperventilation Following Severe Traumatic Brain Injury," *Journal of Neurosurgery* 92, no. 1 (2000): 7–13.

31 S. Kallakuri, C. Kreipke, P. Schafer, S. Schafer, and J. Rafols, "Brain Cellular Localization of Endothelin Receptors a and B in a Rodent Model of Diffuse Traumatic Brain Injury," *Neuroscience* 168 (2010): 820–30.

32 J. A. Rafols, C. W. Kreipke, and T. Petrov, "Alterations in Cerebral Cortex Microvessels and the Microcirculation in a Rat Model of Traumatic Brain Injury: A Correlative Em and Laser Doppler Flowmetry Study," *Neurological Research* 29, no. 4 (2007): 339–47; C. W. Kreipke, P. C. Schafer, N. F. Rossi, and J. A. Rafols, "Differential Effects of Endothelin Receptor a and B Antagonism on Cerebral Hypoperfusion Following Traumatic Brain Injury," *Neurological Research* 32, no. 2 (2010): 209–14.

33 I. Yamakami and T. McIntosh, "Alterations in Regional Cerebral Blood Flow Following Brain Injury in the Rat," *Blood Flow and Metabolism* 11, no. 4 (1991): 655–60; I. Yamakami and T. K. McIntosh, "Effects of Traumatic Brain Injury on Regional Cerebral Blood Flow in Rats as Measured with Radiolabeled Microspheres," *Blood Flow and Metabolism* 9, no. 1 (1989): 117–24; H. Tenjin, S. Ueda, N. Mizukawa, Y. Imahori, A. Hino, T. Yamaki, T. Kuboyama, T. Ebisu, H. Hirakawa, and M. Yamashita, "Positron Emission Tomographic Studies on Cerebral Hemodynamics in Patients with Cerebral Contusion," *Neurosurgery* 26, no. 6 (1990): 971–9; Kallakuri et al., "Brain Cellular Localization of Endothelin Receptors a and B."

34 T. Glenn, D. Kelly, W. Boscardin, D. McArthur, P. Vespa, M. Oertel, D. Hovda, M. Bergsneider, L. Hillered, and N. Martin, "Energy Dysfunction as a Predictor of Outcome after Moderate or Severe Head Injury: Indices of Oxygen, Glucose, and Lactate Metabolism," *Journal of Cerebral Blood Flow and Metabolism* 23, no. 10 (2003): 1239–50; N. Hattori, S. Huang, H. Wu, W. Liao, T. Glenn, P. Vespa, M. Phelps, D. Hovda, and M. Bergsneider, "Acute Changes in Regional Cerebral ^{18}F-Fdg Kinetics in Patients with Traumatic Brain Injury," *Journal of Nuclear Medicine* 45 (2004): 775–83; Vespa et al., "Metabollic Crisis without Brain Ischemia."

35 W. Obrist, T. Langfitt, J. Jaggi, J. Cruz, and T. Gennarelli, "Cerebral Blood Flow and Metabolism in Comatose Patients with Acute Head Injury," *Journal of Neurosurgery* 1 (1984): 241–53.

36 K. Miyazaki, K. Masamoto, N. Morimoto, T. Kurata, T. Mimoto, T. Obata, I. Kanno, and K. Abe, "Early and Progressive Impairment of Spinal Blood Flow-Glocuse Metabolism Coupling in Motor Neuron Degeneration of ALS Model Mice," *Journal of Cerebral Blood Flow and Metabolism* 32 (2012): 456–67.

37 McKee et al., "TDP-43 Proteinopathy and Motor Neuron Disease."

38 D. Ragan, R. McKinstry, T. Benzinger, J. Leonard, and J. Pineda, "Alterations in Cerebral Oxygen Metabolism after Traumatic Brain Injury in Children," *Journal of Cerebral Blood Flow and Metabolism* 33, no. 1 (2013): 48–52.

3

Incidence and Risk Factors for Venous Gas Emboli Formation in Canadian Forces Experimental Divers

....

KAIGHLEY BRETT AND PETER ZEINDLER

Abstract

This study aims to investigate the relationship of self-reported pre-dive behaviours of Canadian Forces (CF) divers and detected venous gas emboli (VGE) post-experimental dive. A retrospective chart review of pre-dive questionnaires and matching post-dive venous Doppler bubble scores of 1,092 CF experimental dives was completed. Non-parametric categorical statistics were used to measure the effect of independent variables of age, exercise, alcohol, medication, smoking, food, fluid, fatigue, and infectious symptoms on maximum bubble grades (BG) measured precordially and at any site. Dives were analyzed as a single group and stratified into high-, moderate-, and low-stress dives, as well as exercise / no exercise during the dive subsets.

Results: 12.6% of precordial BG and 26.1% of maximum any-site BG recorded as ≥ 3. Within 48 hours of diving, 45% exercised, 16.7% used oral medications, 38.25% consumed alcohol, 15.4% smoked, and 9.7% experienced infectious symptoms. Prior to the dive, 88.1% consumed food, 91.8% consumed liquids, and 26.3% felt fatigued. There was a statistically significant difference in BG among divers based on age ($p = 0.043$, binary logistic regression All Dives, MaxBG) and smoking ($p = 0.045$, Fisher's exact test, All Dives MaxBG). These differences did not continue in the other diving subsets, and no statistically significant effects attributed to the other variables were noted in any dive subset. CF experimental divers do report exposure to potential pre-dive risk factors for VGE. Significant association is detected between age, smoking status, and BG in one subset (all dives, MaxBG any site). No significant effect attributed to the remaining risk factors and BG is found. This study suggests that these factors may not affect VGE formation and its attendant risk of decompression sickness (DCS) in this military experimental diver population. However, as the result of study limitations, future studies are required to evaluate each risk factor prospectively to determine its impact on VGE formation during diving.

Introduction

Compressed gas divers are at risk for developing decompression sickness (DCS) – a syndrome caused by injury from circulating and tissue-borne inert gas bubbles that evolve in body tissues and the intravascular system as the result of inadequate decompression. The increased partial pressures of inert gases inhaled at depth results in increased tissue uptake of those gases (nitrogen for most diving, helium in mixed-gas diving). With ascent (decompression) the inhaled partial pressures decrease and inert gas flow is reversed from tissue to vasculature and then exhaled. If decompression is inadequate, inert gas bubbles may form either de novo or from pre-existing micronuclei precursors. Aside from the rate of ascent, this process is dependent upon gas solubility, tissue perfusion, and tolerance for supersaturation and individual physiologic differences. The physiologic consequence of bubble formation is still unresolved, but mechanical (obstructive and direct injury effects) and immunological/inflammatory cascades are thought to play important roles. It has been noted that the incidence of DCS is low when few or no bubbles are present in circulation, and increased with higher levels of circulating bubbles.[1]

The incidence of DCS among recreational scuba divers has ranged from zero to ten cases per 10,000 dives since 1995;[2] however, many mild cases of DCS are thought to go unreported or misdiagnosed. Symptoms of DCS range from mild cases of pruritus, lymphedema, and joint pain, to severe cases involving the neurological, cardiac, pulmonary, and vestibular systems.[3]

Research into the risk factors for DCS is an evolving field. Inadequate decompression is a known cause of DCS; however, the impact of individual physiologic factors on venous gas emboli (VGE) remains unclear. It is perceived that age, fatigue, exercise prior and after a dive, dehydration, smoking, hypothermia, substance use, and flying after diving are risk factors for DCS, while light exercise during decompression could be protective.[4] There is little research into many of these risk factors, and recommendations against them remain controversial.

While DCS is a relatively rare condition amongst the general population, it is an important health consideration among Canadian Forces (CF) divers because of its potentially significant impact on diver health, as well as the subsequent negative operational consequences. The aim of this study is to investigate the relationship of self-reported pre-dive behaviours of CF divers and detected VGE post–experimental dive, in order to determine what individual factors might increase a diver's susceptibility to DCS on a given dive table.

Methods

This study was a retrospective chart review of 1,194 CF experimental Canadian Underwater Mine Countermeasures Apparatus (CUMA) Helium-Oxygen (Heliox) pre-dive questionnaires and matching post-dive venous Doppler bubble scores completed between 1998 and 2005 within the Canadian Forces Environmental Medicine Establishment (CFEME), Defence Research & Development Canada (DRDC), Toronto. This included CUMA AGS Series 1-5, CUMA 84MSW Series 1-2, and the CUMA Repet Series 4-12 experimental dives carried out in the wet dive chamber at DRDC Toronto. Study divers ranged in age from 19 to 48 years old, with a mean of 33.06 years (SD 5.5). There were 1,086 dives completed by male divers, 6 dives completed by female divers. Canadian Underwater Mine Countermeasures Apparatus (CUMA) is a self-contained, semi-closed-circuit breathing device employed by the CF, which uses helium and oxygen (Heliox) as the air supply.[5]

Excluded from our study were 102 repetitive dives with a surface interval (SI) of less than six hours, as residual gas effects from the first dive may be experienced in the second dive, potentially increasing VGE formed. Repeat dives during the same day but with an SI of greater than six hours are considered new dives without residual gas effects, and were included in the data analysis.[6]

The Queen's University Health Sciences Research Ethics Board, and the Human Research Ethics Committee, DRDC Toronto, granted ethics approval for this study. All information collected was stored in the study database without identifying information, to protect diver confidentiality.

Pre-Dive Questionnaire

Prior to diving, each study diver completed a pre-dive questionnaire (Appendix 3.1) in which each was asked to indicate whether he or she had exercised, taken any medications, consumed any alcohol, used any tobacco products within the last forty-eight hours; fatigue level; whether he or she had consumed food or fluids; and the presence of any cold/other infectious symptoms or physical complaints prior to the dive.

Dive Protocols

Within the CUMA Heliox series indicated above, No Decompression (NOD), In Water Oxygen with Surface Decompression (IWO_2 + SD), and In Water Oxygen (IWO_2) dives were included. Dive profiles included IWO_2 + SD dive depths of sixty to eighty metres sea water (MSW) for a bottom time (BT) of ten to twenty minutes, IWO_2 dive depths of fifty-one to seventy-five MSW for BT of five to twenty minutes, and NOD dive depths of eighteen to sixty-nine MSW for BT of 5–20 minutes.

Prior work for the development of the CUMA Heliox dive tables has provided an algorithm for stratifying dives into high, medium, and low stress, based on the percentage of dives with BW > 2. Based on this prior work, this study stratified dives as high-decompression-stress dives, including IWO$_2$ BT > 90 minutes, IWO$_2$ + SD BT > 60 minutes; moderate-stress dives, including IWO$_2$ BT 60–90 minutes, IWO$_2$ + SD BT 40–60 minutes; low-stress dives, including IWO$_2$ BT < 60 minutes, IWO$_2$ + SD BT < 40 minutes, all NOD dives.[7]

For divers assigned to work during the dive, the exercise protocol consisted of repeat cycles of five minutes of cycling followed by five minutes of rest on electromagnetically braked bicycle ergometers modified for underwater use.[8] The standby diver sat immersed in water up to the waist in full dive gear, and the team leader remained dry during the dive.

Bubble Formation Assessment

As the incidence of DCS is low, and the risk of DCS increases with increased bubble formation, Doppler bubble grade assessment is often used as a surrogate for risk of DCS.[9] In each of the dives included, Doppler ultrasound was used to monitor post-dive bubble formation or venous gas emboli, using the Kisman-Masurel (K-M) scoring system. Doppler monitoring was conducted at the precordial and subclavian sites at rest and with movement at approximately thirty-minute intervals for a minimum of three measurements. Continued Doppler monitoring was conducted if bubble grade was ranked at 3 or higher during the third session, and continued every thirty minutes until the BG dropped below 3 or a downward trend was apparent. The K-M scoring system synthesizes the number of bubbles seen in each cardiac cycle, the percentage of cardiac cycles containing bubbles at rest, and the amplitude of bubble signals into a bubble grade of 0, 1-, 1, 1+, 2-, 2, 2+, 3-, 3, 3+, 4-, 4. The precordial site estimates rate of bubble formation for the entire venous system, whereas the subclavian site provides the rate of bubble formation for a limited section of the venous system. Of all possible Doppler monitoring sites, increased maximum BG at the precordial site as well as maximum BG at any site have been shown to have the highest association with increased risk of DCS;[10] these were the two bubble grades recorded for this study.

Data Points Extracted

For each subject, the following information was extracted from the chart:

- Diver characteristics at time of dive: age
- Dive characteristics: depth, time, dive number, exercise during the dive
- Pre-dive self-report variables (recorded as yes or no): exercise, medication use, alcohol consumption, tobacco product use, sleep, food intake, fluid intake, infection status, physical complaints

- Precordial and subclavian bubble formation scores at rest and
  with movement at approximately thirty-minute intervals for three
  measurements

Statistical Analysis

Doppler data scores are categorical data; as such, non-parametric categorical statistics were used to measure the effect of the independent variables on bubble grade. Risk factors of exercise, medication use, alcohol consumption, tobacco product use within forty-eight hours of the dive, fatigue level, food intake, fluid intake, infectious status prior to the dive were recorded in a binary fashion of yes or no and recorded as dummy code of yes = 1, no = 0. Age was recorded in years. It has been demonstrated that the risk of DCS is low with BG $\leq$ 2 and increases with BG $\geq$ 3;[11] in this study BG were classified and analyzed as being $\leq$ 2 or $\geq$ 3. Contingency tables were created for each of the risk factors and precordial BG as well as maximum BG at any site.

Statistical analysis was carried out for the following subsets: all dives; high-stress, moderate-stress, and low-stress dives; and exercise or no exercise during the dive. Fisher's exact test (2-sided) was utilized to analyze the effect of the independent variables of exercise, medication use, alcohol, tobacco, fatigue level, food, fluid, and infectious symptoms individually on bubble grade. T test for equality of means was used to assess differences in age means between BG $\leq$2, and $\geq$ 3. As the dependent variable of BG was dichotomous, binary logistic regression was used to analyze the effect of the independent variables together on bubble grade, as well as each independent variable when controlling for the remaining risk factors. A confidence level of 0.05 was chosen as significant.

Results

Of the 1,092 dives included, 12.6% of precordial BG and 26.1% of maximum any site BG recorded as $\geq$ 3. There was one recorded mild DCS event. Table 3.1 shows the pre-dive behaviours as reported on the pre-dive questionnaire by study divers.

The individual effects of the independent variables upon BG are listed in table 3.2. When analyzing maximum BG at any site for all dives, smoking was statistically significant ($p = 0.045$); however, smoking was not statistically significant for all dives at the precordial site, or when analyzing dives by stress or exercise ($p > 0.05$). As all Fisher's exact test p-values for all other variables were greater than 0.05 in all dive subsets, no statistical significance may be applied to these risk factors. Similarly the p-value of the t test for equality of means for BG based on age for each dive subset was greater than 0.05 and was not statistically significant.

Binary logistic regression was performed on the nine potential predictor variables to determine whether they could statistically significantly predict bubble formation (table 3.3). As all p-values were greater than 0.05 for each dive subset, this

Table 3.1 | Pre-dive behaviours in experimental divers: Incidence of potential risk factors

Risk factor	Yes		No	
	n	%	n	%
Exercise[a]	491	45.0	601	55.0
Medications[a]	182	16.7	910	83.3
Alcohol[a]	417	38.2	675	61.8
Smoking[a]	168	15.4	924	84.6
Fatigued[b]	287	26.3	805	73.7
Food[b]	962	88.1	130	11.9
Fluids[b]	1003	91.8	89	8.2
Infection[a]	106	9.7	986	90.3

[a] within 48 hours preceding study dive
[b] experienced/consumed prior to dive

model was not significantly able to predict the outcome of BG based on the risk factors studied.

Table 3.4 shows the logistic coefficient Wald test significance (p-value) of each risk factor when controlling for the remaining risk factors. Age was statistically significant for increased bubble formation when analyzing all dives and maximum BG any site ($p = 0.043$); however, age was not statistically significant in the remainder of the dive subsets. There was no statistically significant association between the remaining individual risk factors on bubble grade when controlling for all other risk factors.

The above results were calculated on the basis of dives completed by both males and females (1,086 males, 6 females). Statistical analysis was repeated, excluding the six female dives, with no effect found on the results.

Discussion

In this study, CF experimental divers do report exposure to potential pre-dive risk factors for VGE (table 3.1). A statistically significant difference was observed in BG among divers who smoked ($p = 0.045$ Fisher's exact test) in the all Dives MaxBG any site subset. Binary logistic regression also detects a significant difference in BG based on age ($p = 0.043$) in the All Dives MaxBG any site subset when controlling for the remaining risk factors. No significant differences were observed in BG among divers based on age or smoking status in the remainder of the dive subsets, or for exercise, medications, alcohol, infectious symptoms, food, fluid, or fatigue level ($p > 0.05$) in any of the dive subsets. These findings differ from the currently held beliefs of DCS risk factors.

Table 3.2 | Fisher's exact test (2-sided) and *t* test for equality of means analysis of bubble grade based on risk factors as analyzed for all dives, dives by stress level, and exercise during the dive

		Ex^a	Med^a	$EtOh^a$	$Smoke^a$	$Fatigue^a$	$Food^a$	$Fluids^a$	Inf^a	Age^a
All dives	MaxBG	0.097	0.310	0.524	0.045	0.814	0.070	0.900	0.563	0.720
	BGPR	0.144	0.464	0.513	0.315	0.837	0.090	1.000	1.000	0.726
High stress	MaxBG	0.512	0.303	0.771	0.891	0.265	1.000	1.000	0.199	0.852
	BGPR	0.747	0.377	0.876	1.000	1.000	0.682	0.569	0.854	0.531
Moderate stress	MaxBG	1.000	1.000	0.426	1.000	1.000	1.000	1.000	1.000	0.318
	BGPR	Unable to compute, all BG $\leq$ 2								
Low stress	MaxBG	0.781	0.215	1.000	0.093	1.000	1.000	0.805	1.000	0.501
	BGPR	0.632	0.364	0.341	0.751	0.054	1.000	0.181	1.000	0.196
Exercise	MaxBG	0.183	0.153	1.000	0.508	0.280	1.000	0.348	0.135	0.552
	BGPR	0.165	0.315	1.000	0.873	0.407	0.559	0.704	0.719	0.691
No exercise	MaxBG	1.000	1.000	0.897	0.248	0.465.	0.299	0.099	0.284	0.937
	BGPR	0.686	1.000	0.681	1.000	0.479	0.782	0.435	0.497	0.187

[a] Fisher's exact test (2-sided)
[b] *t* test for equality of means

Note: BG = bubble grade; MaxBG = maximum recorded BG any site; BGPR = precordial BG; Ex = exercise; Med = medications; EtOh = alcohol consumption; Inf = infection

Table 3.3 | Binary logistic regression: Omnibus test of model coefficients

Dive subset		χ^2	df	p-value
All dives	MaxBG	15.798	9	0.516
	BGPR	8.185	9	0.071
High stress	MaxBG	4.984	9	0.836
	BGPR	3.522	9	0.940
Moderate stress	MaxBG	7.256	9	0.611
	BGPR	Unable to compute, all BG $\leq$ 2		
Low stress	MaxBG	6.572	9	0.682
	BGPR	11.181	9	0.263
Exercise	MaxBG	9.730	9	0.373
	BGPR	5.767	9	0.763
No exercise	MaxBG	7.664	9	0.568
	BGPR	4.647	9	0.864

Note: BG = bubble grade; MaxBG = maximum recorded BG any site; BGPR = precordial BG

Current research into risk factors for bubble formation is limited for many of the potential risk factors included in this study. Of those that have been previously examined, results remain controversial. A brief overview of the current research will be discussed here.

Substance Use

The use of medications, alcohol, and tobacco products are generally considered contraindicated prior to diving, largely on the basis of a theoretical impact to the central nervous system and VGE formation.[12] In this study, 16.7% of our study divers reported using oral medications prior to the study dive; in the general population, it is estimated that up to 25% of divers take medications prior to diving, most commonly decongestants, anti-emetics, and bronchodilators.[13] Antihistamines, decongestants, and hallucinogens have been shown to decrease mental flexibility, coordination, and performance, while stimulants are known to increase anxiety and impair judgment at depth.[14] Their objective effects on bubble formation are unknown; we found no statistically significant association between medication use and bubble formation.

In this study, 38.25% of divers reported consuming alcohol within forty-eight hours of the study dive. In addition to the absolute risk posed by intoxication during a dive, the consumption of alcohol within twenty-four hours of a dive

Table 3.4. Binary logistic regression: Wald test value for coefficient significance of variable (p-value)

		Ex	Med	EtOh	Smoke	Fatigue	Food	Fluids	Inf	Age
All dives	MaxBG	0.053	0.328	0.948	0.086	0.920	0.088	0.606	0.906	0.043
	BGPR	0.097	0.337	0.818	0.552	0.795	0.076	0.948	0.626	0.652
High stress	MaxBG	0.371	0.264	0.594	0.799	0.272	0.858	0.896	0.252	0.949
	BGPR	0.549	0.289	0.413	0.970	0.857	0.446	0.400	1.000	0.424
Moderate stress	MaxBG	0.198	0.999	0.203	0.998	0.998	0.998	0.999	0.999	0.198
	BGPR	Unable to compute, all BG ≤ 2								
Low stress	MaxBG	0.582	0.168	0.788	0.094	0.873	0.992	0.907	0.457	0.380
	BGPR	0.594	0.283	0.497	0.707	0.066	0.998	0.216	0.699	0.121
Exercise	MaxBG	0.117	0.140	0.752	0.403	0.379	0.722	0.420	0.191	0.536
	BGPR	0.107	0.188	0.651	0.929	0.416	0.470	0.622	0.944	0.706
No exercise	MaxBG	0.791	0.779	0.944	0.200	0.629	0.341	0.114	0.208	0.868
	BGPR	0.851	1.008	1.297	1.101	0.766	0.790	1.493	2.702	0.209

Note: BG = bubble grade; MaxBG = maximum recorded BG any site; BGPR = precordial BG; Ex = exercise; Med = medications; EtOh = alcohol consumption; Inf = infection

is also thought to increase the risk of hypothermia due to peripheral vasodilation, and increase the risk of bubble formation by the decrease surface tension of serum.[15] However, no studies support the view that alcohol intake the night preceding a dive, or habitual alcohol intake, increases the risk of DCS.[16] No significant association between alcohol consumption prior to diving and BG were detected in this study.

Of the study divers, 15.4% reported smoking within forty-eight hours of the study dive. Smoking cessation is often advised for a patient's overall health in addition to decreasing the risk of DCS. It has been shown that the lung function of divers who smoke does deteriorate more rapidly than that of their non-smoking counterparts,[17] and that if DCS occurs, smokers experience an increased severity of symptoms;[18] however, no other study relating smoking and VGE formation was discovered. Our study found a significant difference based on smoking in the MaxBG all dives subset only; however, no significant difference was noted in the remaining dive subsets.

Hydration

Hydration status remains a controversial area in risk assessment. Pre-dive dehydration was thought to increase the risk for DCS by increasing blood viscosity and altering microcirculatory perfusion when bubbles occur, while adequate hydration could increase elimination of excess inert gas.[19] However, several recent studies have demonstrated that moderate dehydration induced by pre-dive exercise or heat stress decreases circulating bubble formation, likely through the alteration of bubble-forming precursors or decreased uptake of inert gases secondary to hypovolemia.[20] Of our study divers, 88.1% consumed solid food and 91.8% consumed liquids prior to their study dive; no statistical significance was detected based on fluid or food status prior to diving.

Exercise

There are multiple studies on the timing of exercise and its effect on VGE, and this remains a controversial area of research. It has been thought that exercise prior to diving could increase the risk for DCS due to dehydration as well as increased blood flow allowing for increased gas uptake. These same factors may allow for increased gas elimination with exercise during decompression. Exercise post decompression has been linked with increased VGE formation.[21] Recent studies suggest that exercise prior to diving, as well as after diving, could decrease post-dive VGE formation potentially through decreased gas uptake prior, and increased gas elimination post-dive.[22] This is a particularly important risk factor to consider in a population that strives for physical fitness. Of our study divers, 45% reported exercising within forty-eight hours of the study dive, with no statistically significant difference in bubble formation based on exercise status.

Sleep

CF divers are at a high risk of fatigue, particularly when engaged in potentially non-elective dives while on active duty. Fatigue has been reported as a major factor in the performance of divers and as a manifestation of DCS;[23] however, no studies assessing the effect of fatigue on bubble formation were found. Of our study divers, 26.3% reported slight to significant fatigue levels prior to diving, with no differences in bubble formation based on fatigue level detected.

While recommendations to avoid the above potential risk factors are pervasive within the diving community, they are often based on theoretical risk with limited objective research into their impact on VGE formation. With the exception of age and smoking status, no significant effect of the remaining risk factors on VGE formation was detected in this study.

Strengths

One of the foremost strengths of this study is the large sample size, with 1,092 dives included. As a result of the experimental nature of the dives studied, protocols ensure that dive profiles can be reproduced, and that each diver completed the pre-dive questionnaire as well as post-dive VGE monitoring in a reliable manner. As such, no dive was excluded as the result of incomplete pre- or post-dive assessments. Lastly, the use of Doppler bubble grade monitoring, which has been shown to be an appropriate surrogate for risk of DCS, allows for an objective measurement of risk for an otherwise rare and subjectively diagnosed clinical condition.

Limitations

The results of this study must be interpreted carefully because there are limiting factors. The reliability of self-reported questionnaires is limited for several reasons. Response bias may be involved if a study diver perceives a risk to his or her employment status by honestly reporting pre-dive behaviours. In the dives studied, divers received financial remuneration for dives completed, which could lead to under-reporting of infectious symptoms, alcohol, tobacco, and medication use prior to the dive for fear of being held from diving and loss of stipend. This would bias the results toward the null hypothesis. Additionally, recall bias is included, as the questionnaire required a forty-eight-hour window for certain behaviours. This may lead to an over- or under-reporting of behaviours based on what the participant can remember, as well as the fact that one often remembers events closest to the dive.

Although Doppler bubble monitoring is considered an appropriate surrogate for risk of DCS, and increased BG has been associated with increased risk of DCS, the occurrence of bubbles does not directly lead to DCS symptoms. Doppler monitoring is also limited by inter-observer variability and difficulty in detecting small or intermittent bubbling.[24]

As a significant portion of the pre-dive questionnaires did not indicate the quantity or quality of pre-dive behaviours, risk factors were recorded in a binary fashion of yes or no. Specifically there was no differentiation between the type and duration of exercise (aerobic vs weight-training), amount and type of alcohol, medications, food, fluid, tobacco products, and the level of fatigue (slight vs extreme). Furthermore, the questionnaires asked about risk factors within forty-eight hours of the study dive; however, a risk factor experienced as early as forty-eight hours prior to a dive may no longer affect potential VGE formation in the same way it would immediately prior to diving. For example, a study diver who consumed one beer forty-eight hours prior to a dive and a diver who consumed ten beers eight hours prior to a dive would be categorized equally as "yes." This would be the same for a diver who walked for fifteen minutes forty-eight hours prior to the dive and a diver who ran ten kilometres immediately prior. Quantification and qualification of risk factors would allow a more refined and powerful analysis of their relationship to VGE formation.

The study population comprised military experimental re-breather divers. All the divers were within a restricted age range and had been carefully medically screened. Successful completion of military dive training and continued military diving represents a degree of self-selection. Existing health conditions, including any prior dive injury, were not collected or considered in this study; however, each diver was medically cleared to dive prior to each dive. These factors limit the generalizability of this study's findings, in particular to the recreational diving population.

Conclusion

CF experimental divers are exposed to potential risk factors prior to study dives per self-reporting. Many of these behaviours are considered risk factors based on a theoretical basis, with limited research to support their contraindication prior to diving. Significant association between age, smoking status and BG was found in one subset (all dives, MaxBG any site), however no significant effect attributed to the remaining risk factors and BG was found. This study suggests that these factors may not affect bubble formation and its attendant risk of DCS in this military experimental diver population. However, due to study limitations, future studies are required to evaluate each risk factor prospectively to determine their impact on VGE formation during diving.

Appendix 3.1

Pre-Dive Questionnaire

PRE-DIVE QUESTIONNAIRE

Date: _____   Profile: _____   Name: _____

Position: Red ☐   Yellow ☐   Standby ☐   Team leader ☐   Dry subject ☐

IN THE LAST 48 HOURS:

Did you exercise?   Yes ☐   Date and time: _____   No ☐

If yes, what did you do and when? _____
Are these regular activities?   Yes ☐   No ☐

Did you take any medication in the last 48 hours?   Yes ☐   No ☐
If yes, list medication, quantity, date, and time. _____

Did you consume any alcohol in the last 48 hours? Yes ☐ Date and Time: _____ No ☐

If yes, list type, quantity: _____

Did you use any tobacco products in the last 48 hours?   Yes ☐   No ☐

If yes, list type, quantity; _____

How much sleep did you get last night? _____ Hrs.   How much do you normally get? _____Hrs.

Are you tired?   Yes ☐   No ☐   Slightly ☐   Moderately ☐   Very ☐

What did you eat before the dive, including fluids consumed? _____

Do you have a cold or any other infection?   Yes ☐   No ☐   If yes, what? _____

List any other physical complaints: _____

Participant's signature: _____

Medical Section Comments:

Complaints   Yes ☐   No ☐

TM's Normal ☐   Abnormal ☐

Bilat Valsalva Movement   Yes ☐   No ☐

DMT's signature: _____   **Doctor's signature:** _____

Revised by Dimitrih Lafleur Feb 2006

Courtesy of CFEME, DRDC Toronto

Appendix 3.2

Post-dive VGE Monitoring

SID: _____

DOPPLER SCORE SHEET

ProfNo: _____

Diver: _____ Date: _____ Profile: _____

Position: RD ☐   YD ☐   STBY ☐   TL ☐   DR ☐   DVRC: _____   Work type: _____

Monitor: 4 ☐   Guest: _____   Dive no: _____   Air/water temp: _____

Remarks: _____

Eval		Precordial		Subclavian				Comments
	Time	Rest	Move	L/Rest	L/Move	R/Rest	R/Move	
1								
	Depth	Grade						
2								
3								
4								
5								

Courtesy of CFEME, DRDC Toronto

Notes

1 Alfred A. Bove and Jefferson C. Davis. *Bove and Davis' Diving Medicine*, 4th ed. (Philadelphia, PA: Saunders, 2004); J. E. Blatteau, J. B. Souraud, E. Gempp, and A. Boussuges, "Gas Nuclei, Their Origin, and Their Role in Bubble Formation," *Aviation, Space, and Environmental Medicine* 77, no. 10 (2006): 1068–76; J. H. Lynch and Alfred A. Bove. "Diving Medicine: A Review of Current Evidence," *Journal of the American Board of Family Medicine* 22, no. 4 (2009): 399–407.

2 *Divers Alert Network Annual Diving Report, 2008 Edition* (Durham, NC: Divers Alert Network, 2008), https://www.diversalertnetwork.org/medical /report/2008DAN DivingReport.pdf.

3 Bove and Davis, *Diving Medicine*; Lynch and Bove, "Diving Medicine."

4 Bove and Davis, *Diving Medicine*..

5 R. Y. Nishi and M. R. N. Warlow, *Development of CUMA HeO₂ Decompression Tables Final Report*, DCIEM report no. 97-R-68 (North York, ON: DCIEM, 1997).

6 K. D. Sawatzky, "The Relationship between Intravascular Doppler-Detected Gas Bubbles and Decompression Sickness after Bounce Diving in Humans" (MSc thesis, York University, Toronto, 1991).

7 Nishi and Warlow, *CUMA HeO₂ Tables*.

8 Ibid.

9 Sawatzky, "Relationship between Intravascular Doppler-Detected Gas Bubbles"; B. C. Eatock and R. Y. Nishi, "Analysis of Doppler Ultrasonic Data for the Evaluation of Dive Profiles," in *9th International Symposium on Underwater and Hyperbaric Physiology*, 183–95 (Bethesda, MD: UHMS, 1987).

10 Nishi and Warlow, *CUMA HeO₂ Tables*; Sawatzky, "Relationship between Intravascular Doppler-Detected Gas Bubbles"; Eatock and Nishi, "Analysis of Doppler Ultrasonic Data."

11 Sawatzky, "Relationship between Intravascular Doppler-Detected Gas Bubbles"; Eatock and Nishi, "Analysis of Doppler Ultrasonic Data."

12 A. J. Trevette, R. F. Forbes, C. K. Rae, and C. Sheehan, *Does Alcohol Intake on the Preceding Night Predispose to Decompression Sickness in Recreational Divers in Orkney Waters?*, Undersea & Hyperbaric Medicine Meeting Abstract, 2003, http://archive.rubicon-foundation.org/xmlui/handle/123456789/1335; S. Taylor, D. Taylor, K. O'Toole, and C. Ryan, "Medications Taken Daily and Prior to Diving by Experienced Scuba Divers," *South Pacific Underwater Medicine Society Journal* 32, no. 3 (2002): 129–35; J. M. Walsh, "Should Divers Use Drugs?," *South Pacific Underwater Medicine Society Journal* 9 (1979): 16–17, http://archive.rubicon-foundation.org/6254.

13 Taylor et al., "Medications Taken Daily."

14 Walsh, "Should Divers Use Drugs?"; D. Taylor, K. S. O'Toole, T. E. Auble, C. M. Ryan, and D. R. Sherman, "The Psychometric and Cardiac Effects of Dimenhydrinate in the Hyperbaric Environment," *Pharmacotherapy* 20, no. 9 (2000): 1051–4.

15 A. C. Adair, "Drugs and Diving," *South Pacific Underwater Medicine Society Journal* 9 (1979): 59–66, http://archive.rubicon-foundation.org/6249.

16 Trevette et al., *Does Alcohol Intake*; M. Hagberg and H. Orhnhagen, "Incidence and Risk Factors for Symptoms of Decompression Sickness among Male and Female Dive

Masters and Instructors: A Retrospective Cohort Study," *Undersea and Hyperbaric Medicine* 30, no. 2 (2003): 93–102.

17 K. Tetzlaff, J. Thysohn, C. Stahl, S. Schlegel, A. Koch, and C. M. Muth, "Decline of FEV1 in Scuba Divers," *Chest* 130, no. 1 (2006): 238–43.

18 D. A. Buch, H. El Moalem, J. A. Dovenbarger, D. M. Uguccioni, and R. E. Moon, "Cigarette Smoking and Decompression Illness Severity: A Retrospective Study in Recreational Divers," *Aviation, Space, and Environmental Medicine* 74 (2003): 1271–4.

19 E. Gempp, J. E. Blatteau, J. M. Pontier, C. Balestra, and P. Louge, "Preventive Effect of Pre-Dive Hydration on Bubble Formation in Divers," *British Journal of Sports Medicine* 43 (2009): 223–8.

20 J. E. Blatteau, A. Boussuges, E. Gempp, J. M. Pontier, O. Castagna, C. Robinet, and L. Bourdon, "Hemodynamic Changes Induced by Submaximal Exercise before a Dive and Its Consequences on Bubble Formation," *British Journal of Sports Medicine* 41 (2007): 375–9; J. E. Bleatteau, E. Gemp, C. Balestra, T. Mets, and P. Germonpre, "Predive Sauna and Venous Gas Bubbles upon Decompression from 400kPa," *Aviation, Space and Environmental Medicine* 79 (2008): 1100–5; J. E. Blatteau, E. Gempp, F. M. Galland, J. M. Pontier, J. M. Sainty, and C. Robinet, "Aerobic Exercise 3 Hours before a Dive to 30 MSW Decreases Bubble Formation after Decompression," *Aviation, Space and Environmental Medicine* 76 (2005): 666–9.

21 Bove and Davis, *Diving Medicine*; R. D. Vann, F. K. Butler, S. J. Mitchell, and R. E. Moon, "Decompression Illness," *Lancet* 377 (2010): 153–64.

22 Blatteau et al., "Hemodynamic Changes Induced," 375–9; Z. Dujic, D. Duplancic, I. Marinovic-Terzic, D. Bakovic, V. Ivancev, Z. Valic, D. Etorovic, N. M. Petri, U. Wisloff, and A.O. Brubakk, "Aerobic Exercise before Diving Reduces Venous Gas Bubble Formation in Humans," *Journal of Physiology* 555, no. 3 (2004): 1319–23; Z. Dujic, I. Palada, A. Obad, D. Duplancic, D. Bakovic, and Z. Valic, "Exercise during a 3-Min Decompression Stop Reduces Postdive Venous Gas Bubbles," *Medicine & Science in Sports & Exercise* 37, no. 8 (2005): 1319–23; Z. Dujic, A. Obad, I. Palada, V. Ivancev, and Z. Valic, "Venous Bubble Count Declines during Strenuous Exercise after an Open Sea Die to 30m," *Aviation, Space and Environmental Medicine* 77, no. 6 (2006): 592–6; O. Castagna, J. Brisswalter, N. Vallee, and J. E. Blatteau, "Endurance Exercise Immediately before Sea Diving Reduces Bubble Formation in Scuba Divers," *European Journal of Applied Physiology* 111 (2011): 1047–54.

23 Bove and Davis, *Diving Medicine*; R. J. D. Harris, D. J. Doolette, D. C. Wilinson, and D. J. Williams. "Measurement of Fatigue Following 18 MSW Dry Chamber Dives Breathing Air or Enriched Air Nitrox," *Undersea and Hyperbaric Medicine* 30, no. 4 (2003): 285–91.

24 Sawatzky, "Relationship between Intravascular Doppler-Detected Gas"; Eatock and Nishi, "Analysis of Doppler Ultrasonic Data."

4

The Road to Joint Task Force Nijmegen 2012: The Soldier On Team Pilot Project

PAULINE GODSELL, MARKUS BESEMANN,
ALEXANDRA HEBER, AND NICHOLAS HAZLEDINE

Abstract

Canadian Forces (CF) members are often referred to as tactical athletes; ill and injured members are not different. Joint Task Force (JTF) Nijmegen, a rigorous and prestigious four-day marching event requires military participants to cover 160 kilometres, carrying at least 10 kilograms on their backs. A team of injured and ill CF members, the Soldier On team, trained for months developing the physical and mental stamina to meet the demands and selection for JTF Nijmegen 2012. CF Physical Rehabilitation and Mental Health Programs collected clinical data to identify trends that predict success and to measure progress in both physical and mental domains during this ground-breaking initiative. Clinical findings from this pilot initiative will be discussed.

Introduction

The Nijmegen Marches date back to 1909, originally part of the Dutch military training to increase the long-distance marching and weight-carrying abilities of infantry soldiers. With over one million spectators and 45,000 marchers, this largest marching event in the world has evolved into a prestigious, international, four-day event that includes military and civilian divisions. Nijmegen activities provide important international exposure for Canada and the CF. They are reminders of our distinguished past, and our current and future security commitments in Europe. The CF contingent participates in a ceremony at Vimy Ridge and a second at Groesbeek Cemetery commemorating Canada's honourable and respected legacy earned by our predecessors overseas. JTF Nijmegen also celebrates Canada's special relationship with the Netherlands and is a reminder to Europeans of our continued commitment to the North Atlantic Treaty Organization (NATO).

Leadership, teamwork, camaraderie, and endurance are core military values fostered during Nijmegen and the rigorous five months of training leading up to the event. The CF have participated in the Nijmegen Marches since 1952. The 2012 event, held in July, marked the sixtieth anniversary of CF participation in the Marches. It was also the first year the CF had a team of ill and injured members from the Soldier On Program. Created in 2006, Soldier On empowers both visible and non-visible injured and ill military personnel to adopt an active lifestyle by providing resources and opportunities to participate in sport and recreational activities. The 2012 Nijmegen Contingent commander's intent, emphasized and demonstrated by Brigadier-General Kevin Cotten, included four objectives:

1 Field a first-class Canadian military contingent (Excellence in all we do!).
2 Have all Canadian team members successfully complete the marches (Leave no one behind!).
3 Enhance Canada's and the CF special relationship with the Netherlands, with the goal of being the Dutch military and public's "preferred" visiting contingent (Actively engage the Dutch people and military.).
4 Include our ill and injured personnel (Together we are all stronger!).

The inaugural Soldier On team was recognized for its achievements in all four objectives, winning the Nijmegen Canadian Military Contingent Sergeant-Major Vierdaage Trophy award of excellence and determination 2012.

The medical screening team's basic premise was that ill or injured CF members are recovering athletes who need to be challenged and provided with an environment that fosters discipline and focus. The Nijmegen March offers such an environment and challenge. It was hypothesized that with appropriate training, medical supervision, and guidance, injured and ill military populations can safely resume high-level physical activity without lasting physical or psychological harm. Questions the authors set out to answer were:

1 Are there short-term physical and psychological benefits from engaging in such high-level activity?
2 If so, are these benefits maintained over time?
3 If not, is there benefit in carrying out such activities?
4 What outcome measures should be considered to measure and monitor change over time in this heterogeneous group?

Clinical data were collected from the 2012 trainees to identify trends as predictors of success and to measure and monitor progress in physical and mental health domains.

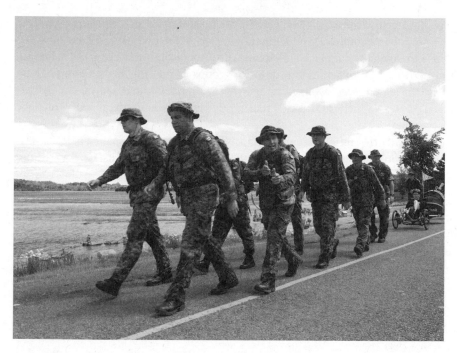

Figure 4.1 | The Soldier On Team completing their 2 x 40 km team selection camp along the Ottawa River, June 2012

Methods

All candidates for this event were volunteers; none were hand selected. This eliminated possible bias in testing and team selection. The Soldier On Program adopted a standardized clearance process to identify contraindications or safety precautions to be considered. This administrative process included approval from the candidate's local medical officer, physiotherapist, occupational therapist, or nurse practitioner; the regional adaptive fitness specialist (RAFS); and finally the CF member's approving military chain of command. Further processes for this inaugural event included objective measures administered at the 2012 February screening camp, April 2 x 20 km confirmation camp, June 2 x 40 km team selection camp, August self-administered post-event questionnaire send-out, and September post-event screening camp. One final self-administered outcome questionnaire follow-up was scheduled February 2013 for Soldier On Nijmegen participants.

At home, support staff included a team to ensure mission success and standardized collection of data: a team leader from Soldier On, one physiatrist, three physiotherapists, one physiotherapy assistant, three mental health specialists, one medical technician from Canadian Forces Health Services (CFHSvcs), and one RAFS from Personnel Support Programs (PSP). Five support staff accompanied the participants to Nijmegen to provide care and flexibility to break the team into slower/faster or longer/shorter distance groups to prevent further injury. These were the team leader, two medical marchers (a physiatry and a physiotherapy officer), and two medical bicycle orderlies (a physiotherapy officer and a medical technician).

Following the initial screening camp, all candidates were deemed able to commence training by both the physical and mental health specialists. However, those identified with specific impairments, activity limitations, or participation restrictions were afforded additional services such as conditioning, physical therapy, or mental health follow-ups at their local bases. Of the eight participants who set off for the Netherlands, three had physical health conditions, three had mental health conditions, and two had both physical and mental health conditions. As a result of the limited sample size and risk of identifying participants, authors will not disclose specific conditions or group participants by pathology in this paper.

The medical support staff chose reliable and valid outcome measures widely used within the NATO military rehabilitating population, preferably available in both English and French. The following outcome measures were chosen to track change over time:

1 Two-day, back-to-back five-, ten-, twenty-, thirty-, and forty-kilometre marches;
2 Fear Avoidance Belief Questionnaire (FABQ) (physical activity and work);
3 Tampa Scale for Kinesiophobia (TSK);
4 Lower-Extremity Functional Scale (LEFS);
5 Modified Oswestry Low Back Pain Disability Index (ODI);
6 Roland Morris Questionnaire (RMQ);
7 Comprehensive High-Activity Mobility Predictor (CHAMP);
8 Functional Movement Screen (FMS) and Selective Functional Movement Assessment (SFMA);
9 Sorensen Test;
10 Hand-Held Dynamometry (HHD) of hip abductors and extensors;
11 The Activities-Specific Balance Confidence Scale (ABC);
12 Houghton Scale;
13 Computer-Assisted Rehabilitation Environment (CAREN);
14 Outcome Questionnaire–45.2 (OQ®–45.2);
15 Post Traumatic Stress Disorder Checklist – Military Version (PCL–M);
16 The Alcohol Use Disorders Identification Test (AUDIT); and
17 Beck Depression Inventory–II (BDI–II).

Soldier On Nijmegen participants were required to meet and adhere to the Nijmegen March Training Standard, which includes both individual and team training phases. This standard was developed by the CF PSP Directorate of Fitness, Human Performance Research and Development.[1] This training standard was the single most important tool facilitating natural self-selection of the Soldier On team.

Results and Discussion

Although the cohort in this qualitative pilot study was too small and heterogeneous to allow statistically valid conclusions to be made, trends did emerge for consideration in development of the Soldier On Nijmegen program. However, no global statements on general applicability to rehabilitation in the military will be drawn. Participants were exposed to an interdisciplinary team coaching them through challenges in order to achieve personal goals. The ratio of medical support staff to participants was high for this event. However, given the fact that this was an inaugural event for Soldier On and that some of the participants had medical employment limitations (MELs) that would normally have contravened participation in Nijmegen, it seemed prudent to err on the side of caution with robust medical support.

Subjects identified the comprehensive and "holistic" nature of the medical support provided as being a pivotal factor in their success. The early identification of both physical and psychological barriers – and their remediation – by a truly interdisciplinary support team led to the implementation of corrective strategies. Participants with chronic pain and low levels of physical function showed the greatest physical improvements. This observation is compatible with the literature and recommendations on management of chronic conditions such as low back pain (LBP) and osteoarthritis. Encouraging physical activity is one of the most important aspects of long-term management of these conditions.

Severely injured participants with high levels of functioning showed the least physical improvement, as would be expected. Tests that evaluated static as opposed to dynamic strength, such as the Sorensen, appeared to be the most useful in monitoring progress. Dynamic and complex movement analyses, such as CHAMP or FMS, seemed to be less sensitive to change in this cohort. Measures of lower extremity function showed most improvements in those with pre-existing lower extremity injury. In addition, participants' fear of the unknown influenced measures of mental health and fear-avoidance behaviours.

The outcome measures and physical training schedule proved to be excellent selection tools. The Soldier On team consisted of eight participants, their team captain, and four medical support staff. All thirteen members of the Soldier On team started the four-day marching event as a team and completed it as a team.

All viewed the Nijmegen March as a very positive event on their road to recovery, rehabilitation, and reintegration to societal roles. The results of seven of the eight participants will be reviewed; one participant joined the Soldier On team less than a month before the event and will not be discussed. Three participants who completed some of the training but were unsuccessful in meeting selection for JTF Nijmegen 2012 will also be discussed in some summaries because their clinical results lend valuable insight into the training. In the accompanying figures, testing periods are shown along the x axis and average scores from each outcome measure are along the y axis. A few graphical results will include more detailed scoring data. Cut-off scores and their interpretations have been identified in each of the figures. It is to be noted that favourable or non-favourable scores are test-specific.

Physical Health

Two-Day, Back-to-Back Five-, Ten-, Twenty-, Thirty-, and Forty-Kilometre Marches in Military Boots and Fatigues, Carrying at Least Ten Kilograms on Participants' Backs

It was evident very early in the training phase that only those who could meet the gradual increases in the Nijmegen March Training Standards would reach the goal of completing Nijmegen. When a few of the members were not able to meet the forty-kilometre standard on testing day, the 2012 Nijmegen Contingent commander reviewed the data collected and decided to afford the team the flexibility to break into slower/faster or longer/shorter distance groups. It is speculated that the flexibility provided by this new directive was a key ingredient in the teams' overall success. It reduced anxiety, improved performance, and prevented the production or aggravation of injuries.

The FABQ is a sixteen-item self-report questionnaire used to assess beliefs of how physical activity and work affect LBP.[2] The TSK is a seventeen-item self-report measure for fear of movement or re-injury in chronic pain clients such as whiplash,[3] LBP, and fibromyalgia syndrome. All participants reported concerns in this domain, although no major trends or significant changes could be identified among those completing these scales. This may be due to the fact that members had volunteered for this activity and were stable in their conditions. However, of interest is one participant who progressively scored poorly on both the ODI and the RMQ for LBP while still completing the entire training and the four-day march. In contrast to the FABQ, this same participant appeared to show gradual improvement in fear of movement when using the TSK. However, the FABQ is used as a clinical prediction rule in Fritz, Cleland, and Childs's[4] approach to subgrouping patients with LBP for manipulation and stabilization interventions and should not be dismissed. Averaged results reflect participants remaining in the low score range for fear-avoidance behaviour throughout this activity.

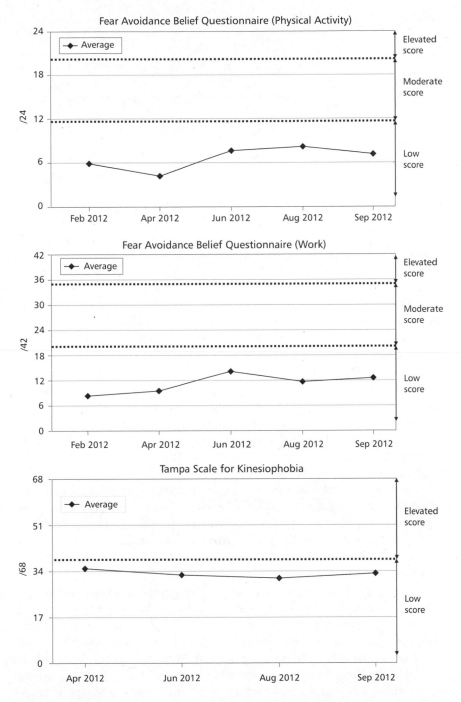

Figure 4.2 | Fear Avoidance Belief Questionnaire and Tampa Scale for Kinesiophobia data

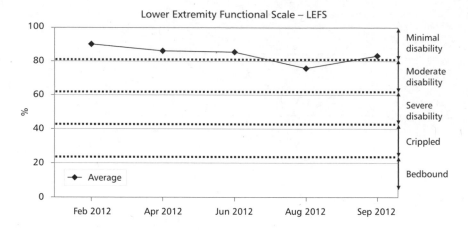

Figure 4.3 | Lower Extremity Functional Scale data

The LEFS is a twenty-item self-report condition-specific functional status measure used in lower extremity musculoskeletal (MSK) conditions.[5] Analysis of the LEFS did not reveal any general trends in participant success. Two participants demonstrated improvements on this scale. Both of these members had pre-existing, non-amputation-related MSK conditions affecting their lower extremities and gait. This supports the hypothesis that training and successful completion of Nijmegen improved the lower extremity function despite pre-existing conditions. In fact one of these candidates has since been considered for return to full duties. Lower scores in August suggest a period of post-march recovery and personal goal renewal. Overall, pre- to post-average results reflect maintenance within the minimal disability scoring range.

The LEFS is efficient to administer and score, but it is unclear what useful information this self-report measure actually provided. Three of the participants had scored better than some of their teammates on this measure, yet did not complete the training required for final selection. Given the poor prediction of cohort success, the authors recommend a trial of other outcome measures for the next Soldier On Nijmegen team.

The ODI is a ten-item self-report questionnaire of perceived level of disability for fundamental tasks of daily living as a result of LBP.[6] The RMQ is a twenty-four-item self-report questionnaire of perceived level of functional limitation for LBP.[7] Seven participants reported experiencing some form of disability in performing fundamental tasks of daily living using the ODI, in contrast to only four participants using the RMQ. Self-management was encouraged throughout the training and execution phases through constant messaging from the medical support team. Two participants had well-documented pre-existing LBP conditions. One partic-

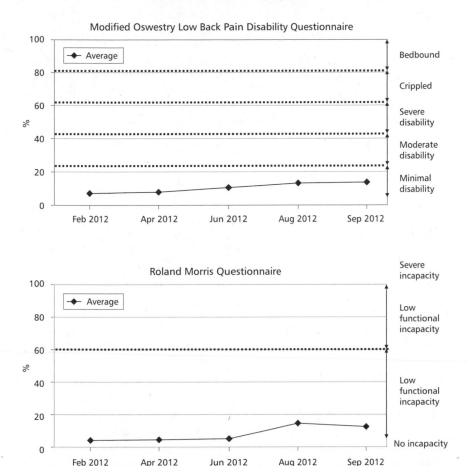

Figure 4.4 | Modified Oswestry Low Back Pain Disability Questionnaire and Roland Morris Questionnaire data

ipant did experience a gradual increase in LBP symptoms. This may have been aggravated by travel and prolonged sitting; however, it did not preclude him from completing the entire initiative. In order to compare findings of current research and to develop program benchmarking opportunities, it is suggested the ODI be more readily adopted by CF medical clinicians. It is recommended a trial comparing these two measures be completed with a larger sample size in the CF. Average results reflect participants remaining in the minimal disability scoring ranges for LBP throughout this activity.

The CHAMP was developed as a performance-based measurement tool to determine the capabilities of service members with lower limb loss who have the

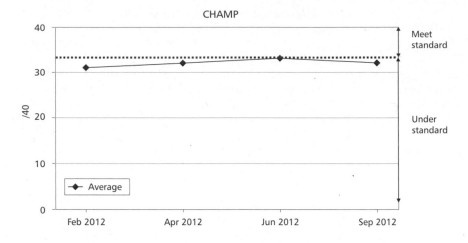

Figure 4.5 | Comprehensive High Activity Mobility Predictor (CHAMP) data

potential to participate in high-level activities.[8] Lack of ankle strategy, particularly in trans-tibial amputee participants, was a factor to be considered for this loaded 160-kilometre march. No participant achieved a perfect score, confirming that this measure is free of a ceiling effect. Of all the outcome measures utilized, the CHAMP displayed the least change across all participants. This is not surprising, in that this series of tests measures agility, strength, speed, and co-ordination and requires directional changes. None of these tasks are correlated with the unidirectional, monotonous, endurance event that is Nijmegen. The CHAMP was developed to predict outcomes in the amputee population and will likely prove its value in the context of military-specific tasks, but not for a distance event like Nijmegen. Even though CHAMP proved to be an excellent tool for team building and instilled competitive motivation among teammates, given that it requires a large gym floor to administer and no valuable information was gained from this functional measure, it is not recommended for Nijmegen testing.

The members of the Nijmegen team were screened using the FMS, a comprehensive screen that assesses quality of fundamental movement patterns to identify an individual's limitations or asymmetries.[9] This screen has not been specifically used to set a baseline for the ill and injured, but it is routinely used on both healthy and rehabilitating individuals. The screen offered the opportunity to review complete movement patterns, in contrast to the more traditional joint-focused approach. While some evidence suggests that a cut-off point of 14/21 may be an indicator of increased risk of injury, the candidates were not screened with this in mind. On initial assessment the score range was from 7 to 14, and in June just prior to the march, the score range increased to 10 to 15. Amputees retained a

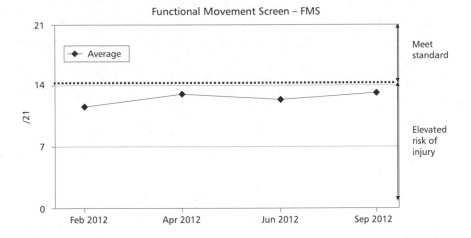

Figure 4.6 | Functional Movement Screen (FMS) data

similar score throughout the testing period. Properties of prostheses, in particular in the squatting and lunging activities, were sources of movement limitations. The remainder of the group not only maintained their scores, but average scores improved through training. They remained in the elevated risk of injury range, but very close to the cut-off standard of 14. One team member improved from 7 to 13, illustrating improvement post-march.

Utilising the FMS as a baseline enabled the medical and conditioning teams to integrate well through a common understanding of limitations. This helped develop and monitor conditioning and training programs that greatly contributed to the success of the event. Perhaps more importantly it gave the team members themselves something tangible to try to improve upon. One strong element of the test is that it not only challenges the individual being tested but allows for improvements to be recorded.

The relationship between testing the complex movements of FMS and the repetitive nature of the activity of loaded marching is unclear. While there was no improvement trend of FMS scores, members were not given specific programs to address identified deficiencies. It is recommended that future participants be prescribed individualized training programs to improve their FMS score in an effort to correlate whether injury rates, performance, and changes to movement patterns can be achieved and maintained.

The Biering-Sorensen Test is a static back endurance test that can discriminate between subjects with and without non-specific low back pain.[10] Nadeau et al. (2006)[11] final research report, "Quantification of the Levels of Effort at the Lower Limb during the Weight Load March in the Canadian Military Population," in-

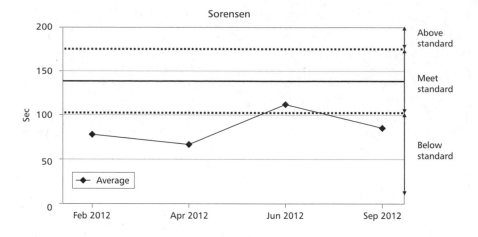

Figure 4.7 | Sorensen Test data

dicated that the endurance of trunk extensor muscles may be a relevant variable in the completion of the timed, full fighting order (24.5 kg), thirteen-kilometre rucksack march with the lowest possible risk of MSK injuries. They found the male CF members' holding time of 135 ± 38 seconds while female CF members' holding time of 207 ± 70 seconds using the Sorensen Test. According to Biering-Sorensen, holding times < 176 seconds in men are a predictor of future LBP and holding times > 198 seconds would have a protective effect in men.[12] Since back muscle endurance has been reported as a possible variable in the prevention of LBP, inclusion of this outcome measure was indicated.

All team members demonstrated an improvement in their scores, with the exception of one. This participant's uncertain diagnosis may have led to fear-avoidance behaviours, also reflected in deteriorating TSK scores. Since the Sorensen involves elements of motivation and stamina beyond simple strength, any uncertainty of diagnosis may inadvertently affect performance. Initially, only one member of the team scored within the normal range. However by June, just prior to the event, four of the seven were within normal limits. The remaining three had slightly improved or maintained their scores. Amputees improved their base scores, even when tested post-march, likely because this subgroup had already moved on to new fitness goals.

Hand-Held Dynamometry of Hip Abductors and Extensors

The use of HHD provides a quick, simple, valid, reliable, and sensitive outcome measurement of human muscle strength, and a high level of agreement can be obtained with this type of quantified muscle testing.[13] Studies of the unilateral, trans-tibial amputee population have illustrated the importance of hip abductor strength in gait.[14] As such, the medical support team chose to capture hip extensor and abductor strength as an objective measure. However, as a result of lack of sufficient experience and training in the use of HHD, common mistakes were made by the medical support team which led to flawed data collection.

Amputee-Specific Measures: The Activity-Specific Balance Confidence Scale and Houghton Scale

The ABC Scale[15] is a self-report amputee measure assessing self-confidence in performing various mobility-related tasks. The Houghton Scale[16] is a disease-specific self-report measure of functional mobility in lower extremity prosthetic users. No significant changes were noted in either of these scales. This is not surprising, given the common problem of ceiling effect on most measures of amputee function, specifically in the high-functioning amputee. Self-report measures can also be misleading in that it is the participant's perception rather than observation of task completion that is recorded. Being part of a team, along with the perceived need to perform at competitive levels that teamwork may foster, may have led to choosing the best rather than the most accurate statement in self-report measures as a whole.

Computer-Assisted Rehabilitation Environment (CAREN)

The CAREN system is an amalgamation of virtual reality and robotic systems designed to create a safe, immersive, and flexible environment to challenge patients.[17] A Nijmegen-specific standardized application was designed by the Ottawa Hospital Rehabilitation Centre virtual reality lab and CF Physical Rehabilitation Program team to provide real-time feedback to both the participants and medical support team on readiness of each participant to face both the physical and mental challenges of Nijmegen. Inclines, declines, lateral slopes, rolling hills, rough terrain, crowds, and visual and auditory surprises were part of the twenty-minute standardized self-pace application. The average speed and distance of the participants during this twenty-minute walk in various terrains and environments were 4.72 kilometres/hour and 1.58 kilometres respectively. The fastest speed was 5.65 kilometres/hour with a total distance covered of 1.9 kilometres. The slowest speed was 3.92 kilometres/hour with a total distance covered of 1.3 kilometres. This quantitative information was valuable in justifying the need for preventative flexibility to the contingent commander. Two participants reported mild, non-persistent simulator sickness symptoms that arise from the conflicting information perceived by the visual system and the vestibular system's sense of movement. Immediately following completion of CAREN session, one participant reported,

"The [simulation of] crowds cheering and the flowers being thrown, and the people walking towards me, those things triggered my vigilance, so I had to focus on my steps, use my mindfulness, and I coped okay. But it showed me how much better I am now. One year ago I would not have been able to complete [the CAREN exercise]."

The CAREN experience marked many firsts for CFHSvcs. It was the first joint application creation that attempted to simulate crowds, the first time the six degrees of freedom-marker set[18] was used to capture data in the lab, and the first time nine participants were loaded onto the CAREN in twenty-four hours, tasking the instrument to consistently perform both mechanically and optically. Finally this was the first time the CF Physical Rehabilitation and Mental Health programs worked together to provide simultaneous multidisciplinary assessment and treatment collaboration.

Mental Health

Kessler reported in the National Comorbidity Survey that post-traumatic stress disorder (PTSD) is a highly co-morbid mental health condition. Of men diagnosed with PTSD, 88.3% will have at least one other *Diagnostic and Statistical Manual of Mental Disorders* (DSM) Axis I diagnosis during their lifetime, and 59% will have at least three other Axis I diagnoses.[19] He found that approximately 47.9% of those with a diagnosis of PTSD will have a major depression, and approximately 51.9% will be diagnosed with an alcohol abuse or dependence problem at some time in their lives.[20] Knowing that a number of the candidates were likely to suffer from PTSD, it was decided to use self-report instruments that screened for conditions that are highly co-morbid with PTSD: major depression and alcohol abuse. It was also decided to include an outcome measure that could track progress of symptoms and function over time.

In addition to figures illustrating scores for each participant at each testing period, figures representing average scores have been included to represent trends over time. The authors realize interpretations are limited, since participants with and without known mental health conditions have been grouped together. The most noticeable trend are the OQ®–45.2, PCL–M, and BDI–II checklists all indicating increased post-march scores. February 2013 results are much anticipated to verify if the higher symptom scoring post-march continues or improves.

The OQ®–45.2[21] is a forty-five-item self-report instrument designed to measure clinical progress in three domains central to mental health: subjective distress, interpersonal relations, and social role performance. Four participants scored above the cut-off at which there is likely a need for mental health intervention. Not surprisingly, these were the same participants who generally scored above the clinical cut-offs for the PCL and the BDI–II. These participants were four of the five who had a known or suspected psychiatric diagnosis. The other participant

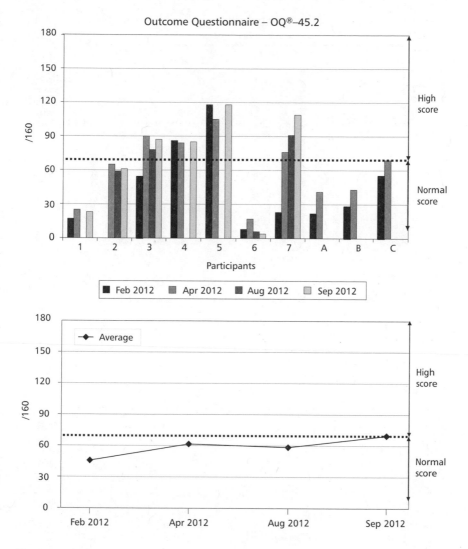

Figure 4.8 | Outcome Questionnaire–45.2 (OQ®–45.2) data

with a known diagnosis had positive but milder symptoms on the self-report instruments. He did not reach the clinical cut-off on any instrument at any screening period.

The PCL[22] is a seventeen-item self-report checklist of PTSD symptoms based on *DSM–IV* criteria for a diagnosis of PTSD. The PCL–M is a military version and questions refer to "a stressful military experience." Four participants scored above the cut-off for symptom severity consistent with a likely diagnosis of PTSD on at

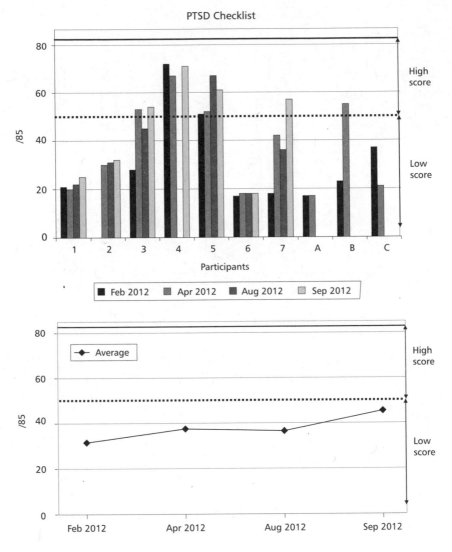

Figure 4.9 | Post Traumatic Stress Disorder Checklist – Military Version (PCL–M) data

least one of the screening periods. Interestingly, a participant with a known diagnosis of depression, but not PTSD, scored above the cut-off at all four screening periods. Another participant with a known diagnosis of PTSD, though positive for some symptoms, scored below the cut-off at all four screening periods.

The AUDIT[23] is a ten-item questionnaire developed by the World Health Organization (WHO) in 1989 as a simple way to screen for excessive and potentially

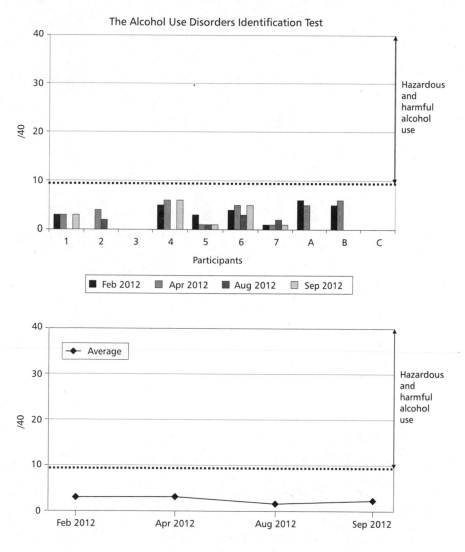

Figure 4.10 | The Alcohol Use Disorders Identification Test (AUDIT) data

harmful alcohol consumption. All members reported drinking behaviour that was below the cut-off for problematic alcohol use. This was consistent over all screening periods for all participants.

The BDI–II[24] is a twenty-one-item self-report inventory. It is one of the most widely used instruments for measuring depression severity in clinical populations. Three participants scored above the cut-off for a severe level of depressive symptoms on at least one screening. Three participants had been previously diagnosed

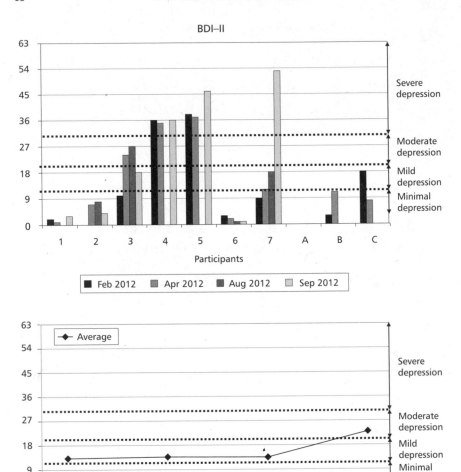

Figure 4.11 | Beck Depression Inventory–II (BDI–II) data

with PTSD and major depression, and one participant was undergoing investigation to rule out a diagnosis of PTSD and depression.

Of note, two members had an increase in symptoms post-march, which, on examination, appear to be related to issues other than the Nijmegen training and March. One related his increase in depressive symptoms to the fact that he received his military release (which had been in the process for several months) shortly after returning from Nijmegen. The other, who demonstrated a steady increase in mental health symptoms throughout the project, with another increase post-Nijmegen, continues investigations into his diagnosis.

For team members with known mental health conditions, all but one continued to be symptomatic on the mental health screens throughout the period of the Nijmegen project. It is important to note that, despite being actively symptomatic throughout most of the work-up training and the Nijmegen March itself, these four participants completed their training and finished the march with the rest of their team and with the thousands of other Nijmegen marchers, despite their mental health challenges.

Participants were interviewed after their return to Canada. One participant, talking about reactions to the crowds during the march, reported, "There were times when I really struggled with the crowds, especially when they got really close. But you know, I wasn't alone in that crowd. I was with my team. I just fought through it. It was great, the fact that I could get into crowds that big and that dense and not freak out. I guess you could say it was a confidence builder. And it's good to know that not all crowds are bad. Yeah, they were a friendly crowd. They weren't waving guns and knives in my face or anything like that."

According to another participant, "It was hard for every one of us to train because we had to train on our own. What really drove me on was that I was going to meet up with them again, and I was going to walk with them and talk with them and have some fun, and we would harass each other a little bit, like good friends do."

And finally, "I did the Nijmegen March and I did it on a team of ill and injured soldiers. We defied the odds and we silenced the critics and opened the door for future Soldier On teams. People need to realize that because we have various injuries, it doesn't make us invalids."

Recommendations and Conclusions

During this Soldier On Nijmegen pilot project, a small cohort was managed through an interdisciplinary team that collectively empowered them to change behaviours through consistent messaging and leading by example. Participants were given training goals, which naturally led to increased physical activity levels. Coming together as a team promoted both trust and teamwork, providing participants with role definition and a sense of identity within the CF they had been searching to re-establish. This qualitative study confirmed that with appropriate training, medical supervision, and guidance, injured and ill military populations can safely reintegrate high-level physical activity without lasting physical or psychological harm.

There is no indication from the data collected that ill effects resulted from participation in JTF Nijmegen in this cohort of injured and ill service members. With appropriate medical screening and supervision, such high-level activity appeared to be safe in this limited cohort. There was an overall trend for some improvement in physical measures of strength and resilience, specifically low back strength.

These gains were not maintained other than in participants with established new goals or challenges. Overall, subjective reports from participants appear to demonstrate value in such high-level participation in improved levels of self-confidence and self-efficacy. However, the following examples may point to more concrete evidence for these findings. Since participating, one member has had his MELs lifted and release proceedings halted and another has successfully passed his CF EXPRES (fitness) test. Both would otherwise have been released from the CF for medical reasons. Without new goals and challenges over a lifetime, the benefits of any activity are quickly lost. Ongoing goal-setting and -attainment is essential in the rehabilitation and reintegration of injured personnel.

Finally, outcome measures that record objective and observed tasks proved to be more useful in this population than measures that record subjective evaluation or perceptions of the individual being tested. Therefore, the following measures are recommended:

1 Activity-specific measures. For example, two-day, back-to-back five-, ten-, twenty-, thirty-, and forty-kilometre team confirmation marches in military boots and fatigues, carrying at least ten kilograms on participants' backs and activity monitoring through diaries and pedometers;

2 Mental health measures identified by mental health subject matter experts;

3 CAREN data collection and comparison at the initial screening and final selection camps;

4 The Sorensen Test;

5 A fear of movement measure;

6 Lower extremity and lower back measures should be considered and monitored. If a wheelchair participant was to join the team, the focus may need to change to upper extremity measures; and

7 Condition-specific measures as required.

Notes

1 National Defence, "NIJMEGEN March: Training Standards," http://cmp-cpm.forces.mil.ca/nij-nim/pre-pra/mts-ne-eng.asp, accessed 19 November 2012.

2 G. Waddell, M. Newton, I. Henderson, D. Somerville, and C. J. Main, "A Fear-Avoidance Beliefs Questionnaire (FABQ) and the Role of Fear-Avoidance Beliefs in Chronic Low Back Pain and Disability," *Pain* 52, no. 2 (February 1993): 157–68.

3 L. Bunketorp, J. Carlsson, J. Kowalski, and E. Stener-Victorin, "Evaluating the Reliability of Multi-Item Scales: A Non-Parametric Approach to the Ordered Categorical Structure of Data Collected with the Swedish Version of the Tampa Scale

for Kinesiophobia and the Self-Efficacy Scale," *Journal of Rehabilitation Medicine* 37 (September 2005): 330–4.

4   Julie M. Fritz, Joshua A. Cleland, and John D. Childs, "Subgrouping Patients with Low Back Pain: Evolution of a Classification Approach to Physical Therapy," *Journal of Orthopaedic & Sports Physical Therapy* 37, no. 6 (June 2007): 290–302.

5   J. M. Binkley, P. W. Stratford, S. A. Lott, and D. L. Riddle, "The Lower Extremity Functional Scale (LEFS): Scale Development, Measurement Properties, and Clinical Application, North American Orthopaedic Rehabilitation Research Network," *Physical Therapy* 79, no. 4 (April 1999): 371–83.

6   Julie M. Fritz and James J. Irrgang, "A Comparison of a Modified Oswestry Low Back Pain Disability Questionnaire and the Quebec Back Pain Disability Scale," *Physical Therapy* 81, no. 2 (February 2001): 776–88.

7   Megan Davidson and Jennifer L. Keating, "A Comparison of Five Low Back Disability Questionnaires: Reliability and Responsiveness," *Physical Therapy* 82, no. 1 (January 2002): 8–24.

8   R. S. Gailey, C. Scoville, M. Raya, I. Gaunaurd, A. Linberg, S. M. Campbell, J. Daniel, and K. Roach, "The Comprehensive High-Level Activity Mobility Predictor (CHAMP): A Performance-Based Measure of Functional Ability of People with Lower Limb Loss" (paper presented at the American Academy of Orthotists & Prosthetists 37th Academy Annual Meeting and Scientific Symposium, Orlando, FL, 16–19 March 2011).

9   K. Kiesel, P. J. Plisky, and M. L. Voight, "Can Serious Injury in Professional Football Be Predicted by a Preseason Functional Movement Screen?," *North American Journal of Sport Physical Therapy* 2, no. 3 (August 2007): 147–58; W. F. Peate, G. Bates, K. Lunda, S. Francis, and K. Bellamy, "Core Strength: A New Model for Injury Prediction and Prevention," *Journal of Occupational Medicine and Toxicology* 2 (April 2007): 3, doi:10.1186/1745-6673-2-3; Kate I. Minick, K. B. Kiesel, L. Burton, A. Taylor, P. Plisky, and R. J. Butler, "Interrater Reliability of the Functional Movement Screen," *Journal of Strength and Conditioning Research* 24, no. 2 (February 2010): 479–86, doi:10.1519/JSC.0b013e3181c09c04.

10 J. Latimer, C. G. Maher, K. Refshauge, and I. Colaco, "The Reliability and Validity of the Biering-Sorensen Test in Asymptomatic Subjects and Subjects Reporting Current or Previous Nonspecific Low Back Pain," *Spine* 24, no. 20 (October 1999): 2085–9, discussion 2090.

11 S. Nadeau, L. J. Hébert, A. Brière, M. Perron, and D. Gravel, "Quantification of the Levels of Effort at the Lower Limb during the Weight Load March in the Canadian Military Population" (paper presented at the 14th biennial conference for the Canadian Society of Biomechanics, Waterloo, ON, August 2006).

12 Ibid.

13 M. Horvat, B. G. McManis, and F. E. Seagraves, "Reliability and Objectivity of the Nicholas Manual Muscle Tester with Children," *Isokinetic and Exercise Science* 2, no. 4 (1992): 175–81; Frank E. Seagraves and Michael Horvat, "Comparison of Isometric Test Procedures to Assess Muscular Strength in Elementary School Girls," *Pediatric Exercise Science* 7, no. 1 (February 1995): 61–8; C. Hill, R. Croce, J. Miller, and F. Cleland, "Muscle Torque Relationships between Hand-Held

Dynamometry and Isokinetic Measurements in Children Aged 9 to 11," *Journal of Strength and Conditioning Research* 10, no. 2 (1996): 77–82; E. A. C. Beenakker, J. H. van der Hoeven, J. M. Fock, and N. M. Maurits, "Reference Values of Maximum Isometric Muscle Force Obtained in 270 Children Aged 4–16 Years by Hand-Held Dynamometry," *Neuromuscular Disorder* 11, no. 5 (July 2001): 441–6; Nicholas F. Taylor, Karen J. Dodd, and H. Kerr Graham, "Test-Retest Reliability of Hand-Held Dynamometric Strength Testing in Young People with Cerebral Palsy," *Archives Physical Medicine Rehabilitation* 85, no. 1 (January 2004): 77–80; Luc J. Hébert, J. F. Remec, J. Saulnier, C. Vial, and J. Puymirat, "The Assessment of Muscle Strength with Hand Held Dynamometers in Myotonic Dystrophy Type 1 Patient: A Non-Invasive Discriminative Biological Marker to Use in Multi-Centre Studies," *BMC Musculo-Skeletal Disorders* 11, no. 72 (2010): 1–9; Jill E. Mayhew, J. M. Florence, T. P. Mayhew, E. K. Henricson, R. T. Leshner, R. J. McCarter, and D. M. Escolar, "Reliable Surrogate Outcome Measures in Multicenter Clinical Trials of Duchenne Muscular Dystrophy," *Muscle Nerve* 35, no. 1 (January 2007): 36–42; Kate Mahony, A. Hunt, D. Daley, S. Sims, and R. Adams, "Inter-Tester Reliability and Precision of Manual Muscle Testing and Hand-Held Dynamometry in Lower Limb Muscles of Children with Spina Bifida," *Physical & Occupational Therapy in Pediatrics* 29, no. 1 (2009): 44–59, doi:10.1080/01942630802574858.

14 Heidi Nadollek, Sandra Brauer, and Rosemary Isles, "Outcomes after Trans-Tibial Amputation: The Relationship between Quiet Stance Ability, Strength of Hip Abductor Muscles and Gait," *Physiotherapy Research International* 7, no. 4 (November 2002): 203–14, doi:10.1002/pri.260; C. Grumillier, N. Martinet, J. Paysant, J. M. André, and C. Beyaert, "Compensatory Mechanism Involving the Hip Joint of the Intact Limb during Gait in Unilateral Trans-Tibial Amputees," *Journal of Biomechanics* 41, no. 14 (October 2008): 2926–31, doi:10.1016/j.jbiomech.2008.07.018; C. H. Lloyd, S. J. Stanhope, I. S. Davis, and T. D. Royer, "Strength Asymmetry and Osteoarthritis Risk Factors in Unilateral Trans-Tibial, Amputee Gait," *Gait Posture* 32, no. 3 (July 2010): 296–300, doi:10.1016/j.gaitpost.2010.05.003; Natalie Vanicek, S. Strike, L. McNaughton, and R. Polman, "Gait Patterns in Trans-Tibial Amputee Fallers vs Non-Fallers: Biomechanical Differences during Level Walking," *Gait Posture* 29, no. 3 (April 2009): 415–20, doi:10.1016/j.gaitpost.2008.10.062.

15 Lynda Elaine Powell and Anita M. Myers, "The Activities-Specific Balance Confidence (ABC) Scale," *Journals of Gerontology Series A: Biological Sciences and Medical Sciences* 50A, no. 1 (January 1995): M28–34, doi:10.1093/gerona/50A.1.M28; William C. Miller, A. B. Deathe, M. Speechley, and J. Koval, "The Influence of Falling, Fear of Falling, and Balance Confidence on Prosthetic Mobility and Social Activity among Individuals with a Lower Extremity Amputation," *Archives of Physical Medicine and Rehabilitation* 82, no. 9 (September 2001): 1238–44; William C. Miller, Mark Speechley, and A. Barry Deathe, "Balance Confidence among People with Lower-Limb Amputations," *Physical Therapy* 82, no. 9 (September 2002): 856–65.

16 Michael Devlin, T. Pauley, K. Head, and S. Garfinkel, "Houghton Scale of Prosthetic Use in People with Lower-Extremity Amputations: Reliability, Validity, and Responsiveness to Change," *Archives of Physical Medicine and Rehabilitation* 85, no. 8 (August 2004): 1339–44; William C. Miller, A. Barry Deathe, and Mark Speechley, "Psychometric Properties of the Activities-Specific Balance Confidence Scale among

Individuals with a Lower-Limb Amputation," *Archives of Physical Medicine and Rehabilitation* 84, no. 5 (May 2003): 656–61.

17 J. Hebert, literature review for Canadian Forces Expert Advisory Panel Focus Group for CAREN, Ottawa, ON, 9–10 May 2012.

18 Jason M. Wilken, K. M. Rodriguez, M. Brawner, and B. J. Darter, "Reliability and Minimal Detectible Change Values for Gait Kinematics and Kinetics in Healthy Adults," *Gait Posture* 35, no. 2 (February 2012): 301–7, doi:10.1016/j.gaitpost.2011. 09.105.

19 Ronald C. Kessler, "Post Traumatic Stress Disorder in the National Comorbidity Survey," *Archives of General Psychiatry* 52, no. 12 (December 1995): 1048–60.

20 Ibid.

21 M. J. Lambert, N. B. Hansen, V. Umphress, K. Lunnen, J. Okiishi, G. M. Burlingame, and C. W. Reisenger "Administration and Scoring Manual for the Outcome Questionnaire (OQ 45.2) Stevenson," MD: *American Professional Credentialing Services LCC* (1996).

22 Edward B. Blanchard, J. Jones-Alexander, T. C. Buckley, and C. A. Forneris, "Psychometric Properties of the PTSD Checklist (PCL)," *Behaviour Research and Therapy* 34, no. 8 (August 1996): 669–73; Kenneth J. Ruggiero, K. Del Ben, J. R. Scotti, and A. E. Rabalais, "Psychometric Properties of the PTSD Checklist – Civilian Version," *Journal of Traumatic Stress* 16, no. 5 (October 2003): 495–502, doi:10.1023/A:1025714729117.

23 J. P. Allen, R. Z. Litten, J. B. Fertig, and T. Babor, "A Review of Research on the Alcohol Use Disorders Identification Test (AUDIT)," *Alcoholism: Clinical and Experimental Research* 21, no. 4 (June 1997), 613–19; Cheryl J. Cherpitel, "Analysis of Cut Points for Screening Instruments for Alcohol Problems in the Emergency Room," *Journal of Studies on Alcohol* 56, no. 6 (November 1995): 695–700; Katherine M. Conigrave, Wayne D. Hall, and John B. Saunders, "The AUDIT Questionnaire: Choosing a Cut-off Score," *Addiction* 90, no. 10 (October 1995): 1349–56; Mariana Cremonte, Rubén Daniel Ledesma, Cheryl J. Cherpitel, and Guilherme Borges, "Psychometric Properties of Alcohol Screening Tests in the Emergency Department in Argentina, Mexico and the United States," *Addictive Behaviors* 35, no. 9 (2010): 818–25.

24 Paul Richter, J. Werner, A. Heerlein, A. Kraus, and H. Sauer, "On the Validity of the Beck Depression Inventory: A Review," *Psychopathology* 31, no. 3 (1998): 160–8, doi:10.1159/000066239.

5

Essential Task Identification for Military Occupations Using the TRIAGE Technique

PAIGE MATTIE, MIKE SPIVOCK, AND DANIEL THÉORET

Abstract

Health and fitness research in the Canadian Forces (CF) often requires the opinions of subject matter experts. The process of integrating diverging views to obtain a group consensus can pose a challenge to researchers. The Technique for Research of Information by Animation of a Group of Experts (TRIAGE) is a method of data collection based on the attainment of group consensus.[1] The TRIAGE technique has been employed by this research group in various qualitative reviews as a group consultation technique involving military personnel. This methodology has allowed for an efficient and economical review of extensive volumes of material without requiring complex and lengthy data analyses. The successful application of TRIAGE in research requiring consensus by groups of military personnel, as well as the versatility of this technique in health and fitness research in the CF, is discussed.

Introduction

Research in the areas of health, fitness, and occupational requirements in the Canadian Forces (CF) often requires the researcher to draw on the experience and opinions of subject matter experts (SMEs). The Human Performance Research & Development (HP R&D) cell, within the Directorate of Fitness, has relied on expert opinion throughout several recent initiatives in the physical and occupational fitness standards. In order to draw on the expert advice of SMEs thoroughly and efficiently, HP R&D sought out a scientific methodology that would satisfy four requirements:

1   The research method employed must be based on the achievement of group consensus to ensure validity and legal defensibility of the end product.

2 Input from SMEs must be gathered in such a way that complex and lengthy analyses following data collection is not required.
3 The resources required to effectively apply the methodology must be consistent with available personnel and financial resources.
4 The technique can be consistently applied in several diverse projects conducted by our research group.

This paper discusses one such technique, which has been adapted from the literature in order to satisfy the requirements of attaining expert consensus in personnel research.

Various group consultation techniques are available that solicit the opinions and experiences from SMEs within a group. Of these, the Delphi technique, the Nominal Group Technique, and the traditional focus group may be the most well known. While these methods offer individual strengths and are effective in other contexts, each fails to accommodate all four criteria. The Technique for Research of Information by Animation of a Group of Experts (TRIAGE)[2] is a methodology that is gaining recognition in various domains, including health program evaluation and in the development of measurement instruments. TRIAGE is a method of data collection based on the attainment of group consensus, which seeks to enable group decision-making in an organized and efficient manner. This method was first employed by our research group in the early phases of Project Fitness for Operational Requirements of CF Employment (FORCE): the initiative that developed a new baseline physical fitness standard for all CF personnel. TRIAGE was used to identify essential tasks that all CF personnel can be called to perform, regardless of occupation, rank, or environment.[3] The technique is a valuable component of the research methodology applied in the Occupational Fitness Standards (OFS) Project.[4] This initiative examines all trades in the CF in order to identify lists of essential occupational tasks along with corresponding task demands, for use primarily by medical officers in assessing job suitability. OFS is conducting individualized TRIAGE groups for each of the approximately 100 CF occupations.

The Classic TRIAGE Process

The TRIAGE technique is a structured, inductive form of data collection that comprises three formal and distinct steps.[5] The first step, *preparation*, involves the articulation of the research question of interest and the recruitment of appropriate SMEs for the topic. Included in this stage is the compilation and distribution of all relevant materials for preliminary review by the SMEs. The second step, *individual production*, begins once the participants have received the documents. All SMEs are asked to provide responses, or *indicators*, to the research question and to return their contribution to the evaluator or research team. The compilation of information received from the SMEs represents the construction of the *dynamic memory* used in a later step. In the third and final phase, *interaction production*,

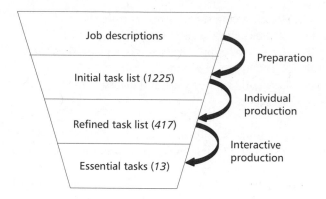

Figure 5.1 | Phases of TRIAGE applied in the OFS Project for the AWS TECH occupation

participants are brought together with the research team. At this stage, through facilitated discussion and group decision-making, the SMEs are required to reach consensus on each piece of material within the *dynamic memory*. The researcher assumes the role of group facilitator and leads the discussion according to a structured process until consensus is reached on each *indicator* or item of interest.

Applications to Personnel Research

The TRIAGE technique has been adapted by HP R&D to meet the unique demands of various initiatives and to achieve a product requested by the client, the CF. In the first of three phases of Project FORCE,[6] TRIAGE was applied in its more traditional form, with SMEs contributing information developed from their own opinions and experience and presented in their own wording. Conversely, the process applied in OFS begins with large volumes of information (integrated job descriptions containing as many as 2,000 tasks) that are distilled to more manageable, concise lists of relevant data through evaluation of the information by SMEs throughout multiple stages of TRIAGE. Either approach begins with assembly of relevant materials by the research team, followed by evaluation and contribution by participants individually, and ending with interactive group consultation. An example of the complete refinement of information through the TRIAGE stages for the air weapons systems technician (AWS TECH) occupation is shown in figure 5.1.

Phase 1: Preparation

In this phase, CF members are selected on the basis of their expertise in the area of interest and their potential to make a strong and valuable contribution on the specific material being evaluated. In selecting SMEs, HP R&D seeks to include participants with a moderate range in rank, years of service, degree of training, and/ or practical experience in the area of interest. Achieving this range in experience

Table 5.1 | SME profiles for MARS OFF occupation

Rank	Years in CF	Years in trade
Lieutenant (N)	37	2
Commander	37	37
Acting sub-lieutenant	4	1
Lieutenant (N)	12	12
Lieutenant-commander	25	25

and training aims to ensure that a broad scope of detail on the criterion of interest is captured. For instance, in examination of such things as essential task lists and occupational demands, the higher-ranking SMEs provide expertise in the trends and activities relevant to the trade over past years or decades, while lower-ranking SMEs offer insight into current occupational demands and training. It is essential that all participants have the experience and knowledge in the area to qualify as experts, therefore a specified range of ranking is typically requested during the selection of participants. An example of the range in rank and years of service for the maritime surface and subsurface officer (MARS OFF) occupation is depicted in table 5.1.

Preparation of documents for distribution to the SMEs also occurs in this initial stage. In the OFS Project, these documents included an overview of OFS, a legal definition of *essential* as it pertains to occupational tasks, and instructions on how to indicate their responses and return their contribution to the research team.

Phase 2: Individual Production

In this second phase, the prepared documents are distributed to the SMEs for preliminary review and analysis. In HP R&D initiatives employing this technique, participants have been asked to either develop *indicators* or statements reflecting the requested criteria based on their individual experience[7] or to review a list of items, identifying from this list the information they view as most relevant to the research question.[8] Any information produced or selected by SMEs is returned to the research team, which is then organized for use in the ensuing stage. Importantly, the information received from participants is not analyzed or modified by the research team in any way at this stage.

Phase 3: Interactive Production

In this final phase, the group of experts is invited to attend a one-day TRIAGE session. While the SMEs typically vary in rank level and years of service, introduction

of all participants seeks not to highlight the rank or accomplishments of participants but to establish a casual, informal, and welcoming environment for all members present. The SMEs are briefed on the objectives, procedures, and end-use of
the project, as well as on the expectation of participant involvement throughout
the session. Several important definitions are provided to participants to ensure
an equivalent comprehension of key terms. In order to facilitate systematic and
efficient progression through the information, it is recommended that a visual aid
be used.[9] Traditionally, this visual supplement has been physical material, such as
flip charts, onto which information is directed from one category to another as it
is discussed. The members of HP R&D felt that this supplement could be enhanced
to enable easier management by the facilitator as well as to allow more efficient
progression from one item of material to the next. As such, a visual tool was designed that was specific to the nature and requirements of HP R&D projects and
was simple for the facilitator to incorporate. This advanced visual aid is an interactive platform developed on the Microsoft ACCESS® platform and is considered
by HP R&D to be a significant improvement upon the previous method. This new
tool allows one to insert extensive quantities of information, such as detailed occupational task lists, into the interactive platform prior to commencement of the
TRIAGE session. Further, one can easily direct information from one category to
another as decisions are made on that item. Importantly, as the new visual aid is
operated by computer platform with no use of physical materials, the potential for
the facilitator and/or the SMEs to become distracted by the aid itself is minimized.

In order to address each item of material sequentially, sections are presented on
the visual display to organize the progression through material and to categorize
each item into one of five outcomes. The layout of these various sections for the
infantry occupation (INF) is shown in figure 5.2. All tasks begin in the *dynamic
memory* or unprocessed category and are sequentially moved into the *grouping* or
combination separation box. Here, the SMEs are guided by a series of questions on
the nature and meaning of the item, the relation of that item to others on the list,
and whether the item meets the criteria being evaluated. In this stage for Project
FORCE, the facilitator encouraged discussion amongst the SMEs by asking questions such as "Does this task meet the definition of essential?" and "Do other tasks
on the list represent the same construct?" SMEs can select one item that best represents several original points and retain what offers the most accurate or reflective
wording to encompass all ideas. SMEs are also provided with the option of creating
a new statement that better encompasses a combination of similar items. Additionally, if an item contains more than one general idea, participants may divide
the statement into several statements that reflect only one concept each. Once a
group consensus and decision is achieved on the relevance of each point, that particular item is directed to the Selection, Garbage, Refrigerator, or Veto location. If
the SMEs believe an item is irrelevant or unnecessary, it is immediately moved to
Garbage and will no longer be discussed or revisited. Should the group feel unable

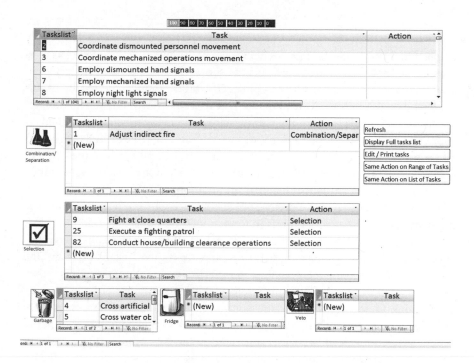

Figure 5.2 | Interactive visual aid developed for application of TRIAGE by HP & RD

to reach consensus on a topic during initial discussion and would prefer to return to that idea later, that item is directed to Refrigerator, where it is stored for further evaluation. The Veto box is used if, after further discussion, the group remains unable to reach consensus and prefers to direct that item to an outside group or individual who will make a final judgment. In Project FORCE, items were placed in this box when it was known that planned but unconfirmed changes in future operations would lead to differences in how tasks were performed. In general the inclusion of this option ensures that the SMEs will never feel forced to make an uninformed decision, should the group feel they lack the necessary expertise on a particular topic. The most critical box, labelled Selection, will contain items determined by group consensus to meet the criteria of interest and that best represent a statement or collection of statements. SMEs are permitted and encouraged to return to the Selection box at any time to review and revise items in it. Once all points have been discussed through this process, the final output, as determined by group consensus, is listed in the Selection box and constitute the product of the TRIAGE session. This list forms the basis for further detailed content validation in the following stages of HP R&D projects.

Discussion

Applied in several aspects of personnel research, the TRIAGE technique has consistently yielded concise data sets, such as short lists of common physically demanding tasks or essential occupation-specific tasks. Though the results of this technique do not necessarily lend themselves to traditional validation studies, efforts have been made to assess the representativeness of the task lists generated. In Project FORCE, where this technique was used to identify an essential task list for all CF personnel, this list was deemed representative by all levels of the chain of command up to and including the chief of the defence staff and all Level 1 branch commanders at Armed Forces Council. In addition, since two distinct TRIAGE groups were conducted in this project, one involving experts in planning domestic missions and the other with experts in foreign missions, one can glean indicators of concurrent validity. Though the two task lists did contain significant differences – with the foreign missions focusing more on combat-related tasks and the domestic ones involving more support to other government organizations – they also contained expected similarities. Both yielded very similar tasks in casualty evacuations, protection of high-value assets, and general military duties, as these tasks are performed similarly, both domestically and in an expeditionary scenario. In the occupation-specific task lists generated in the OFS project, they have been accepted and approved by occupational authorities at the upper echelon of the CF chain of command as well. Furthermore, in terms of discriminant validity, the lists generated for each occupation are indeed unique.

The TRIAGE process has been employed by HP R&D since 2010 in the OFS Project, as well as in early stages of development of several other research initiatives requiring group consensus by SMEs, such as Project FORCE and in establishing essential, common tasks for close protection operators. In the scope of these projects, this technique appears to be a highly effective group consultation technique in research requiring consensus by groups comprising military personnel.

As outlined previously, HP R&D required a scientific methodology that would achieve several specific requirements, all of which we believe have been accommodated by a modified version of the TRIAGE technique. First, a qualitative technique that focused on the achievement of group consensus was necessary to ensure validity and legal defensibility of the end product. TRIAGE, being an inherently consensus-based consultation technique, indeed operates on the basis of group decision-making, as opposed to an aggregation of individual participant contributions. Second, a methodology that did not involve a complex and time-consuming form of analysis was required, as projects such as OFS would comprise over 100 independent group consultations, each involving the evaluation of substantial quantities of information. TRIAGE has repeatedly allowed for the organization of extensive volumes of information into concise task lists during group consultations lasting only several hours, with the greatest volume of information assessed, in one TRIAGE session exceeding 2,000 unique items. At completion of the *interactive productive* phase, the product is achieved, with no further qualitative analyses necessary. A third requirement was that the methodology would accommodate both the financial and personnel resources available to HP R&D. In line with this, some of the specific strengths of TRIAGE are that the technique is highly economical and can be applied using minimal material and personnel resources. Finally, a technique was sought that could be applied in multiple research initiatives. TRIAGE has been employed by HP R&D in a variety of reviews with diverse groups of SMEs, each time yielding the intended outcome of a consensus-based and defensible end product.

An additional function of TRIAGE observed in its application by HP R&D is a capacity to work well with small groups of participants. While it is suggested that the technique is appropriate for use with small or large groups ranging from five to over forty participants,[10] our experience with the technique in the OFS Project lends further support for its utility with smaller working groups, provided that all aspects of the occupation are represented (e.g., training, operations, different platforms where relevant). The design and development of a visual aid specific to the needs of HP R&D appeared to enhance the efficiency with which the group can progress through material. This may be related to the ease with which the evaluator can direct items around the visual board or can quickly return to any previously selected or eliminated tasks. Certainly, our revised visual aid appeared to effectively capture and maintain the attention of all participants, allowing SMEs to remain engaged in the discussion as reference to the item of interest was constantly available to them.

It has been the experience of HP R&D that facilitating group consensus and decision making may be influenced by several factors. First, group interaction and active participation by group members is imperative. It is therefore vital that the facilitator ensure that all SMEs are contributing to the discussion and subsequent decision making. Second, as recommended,[11] the TRIAGE group must be managed by a group facilitator who is competent in group dynamics and group management. Specifically, the facilitator must be able to remain flexible throughout the discussion, accommodating the needs of individuals and adapting his or her communication style to engage or manage varying types of personalities. He or she must ensure equal participation by all members of the group, minimizing the potential for one member to assume an assertive role and attempt to exert stronger influence than the others in the decision making. Further, the facilitator must be able to engage in conflict management and to stimulate discussion when involvement by the group is lacking. It is essential that the facilitator continuously ask relevant, guiding questions to facilitate group decision making, while ensuring that any questions or instructions do not unduly influence the outcome of the process.

We have also observed that the organization of information received from SMEs is valuable in rendering the TRIAGE process more efficient. In the individual production phase, the responses provided by SMEs are organized according to the frequency with which each item or idea was selected by the SMEs as relevant to the research question. As a result, the most popular responses are then reviewed first in the ensuing *interactive production* phase. In our experience, the organization of material in this manner appears to assist SMEs in understanding the process, while also increasing the speed of progression through the material.

As with any qualitative methodology, there are several limitations to the TRIAGE technique.

The quality of information obtained through this process will depend directly on the quality of the initial list of indicators, as well as on the participants' competency and expertise. As such, care must be taken in the recruitment of SMEs of a particular topic. It is also recommended that a researcher be cautious about the breadth of themes covered within a single TRIAGE session,[12] as efforts to cover too great a number of broad areas can jeopardize results and risk the SMEs becoming disengaged. Further, if a TRIAGE session continues for an extended time, participants may find the process tiring. As a result, their degree of interest in the session or level of concentration may waiver. It is therefore suggested that a single session last no longer than three hours.[13] Finally, in most cases the results obtained through this process are usable only within the context of that particular study. However, in projects undertaken by HP R&D, the resulting outputs from the TRIAGE process have provided a suitable basis from which to pursue further content validation by alternative methods.

In addition to these limitations, HP R&D has observed several caveats in the implementation of TRIAGE. Given the requirement that our enhanced visual aid be managed by an additional member of the research team, it is necessary that at least two HP R&D personnel who are comfortable with the session content and are experienced in the process be present for each TRIAGE session. Also, at the *individual production* stage, we have typically received contributions from several but not all of the SMEs. As the order of information presented in the following stage is meant to reflect the information viewed as most relevant by all participants, not receiving input from several participants may delay the progression of the session while those participants who are less familiar with the material reach an understanding of the nature and objective of the process. We have consistently observed that, following discussion of approximately twenty items, the SMEs will reach a point at which the process is well understood, discussion flows easily, and participants engage in effective decision making. However, the time required to reach this state will inevitably depend on the expertise of the SMEs, the degree of preparation by the SMEs, the level of engagement of participants during the TRIAGE session, and the capabilities of the facilitator.

Conclusion

TRIAGE is a group consultation process that provides readily usable data in a relatively short session. The applicability of this process not only to program evaluation but also to personnel research, particularly in the identification of essential tasks within occupations or across the Canadian Forces, has been demonstrated.

Notes

1 Marie Gervais and Genevieve Pépin, "TRIAGE: A New Group Technique Gaining Recognition in Evaluation," *Evaluation Journal of Australasia* 2 (2002): 46.
2 Ibid., 45.
3 Michael Spivak, Tara Reilly, Philip Newton, Rachel Blacklock, and Suzanne Jansen, *Project FORCE Phase 1 Report: Identification of Common, Essential, Physically Demanding Tasks in the CF* (Ottawa: Department of National Defence, 2011), 17.
4 Daniel Théoret, Christopher Driscoll, Laura McRae, Assane Niang, Andrea Karam, Michael Spivak, and Patrick Gagnon, "A Systematic Approach for the Development of Occupation Specific Fitness Standards in the Canadian Forces" (paper presented at 2nd International Congress on Soldiers' Physical Performance, Jyväskylä, Finland, 2011).
5 Gervais and Pépin, "TRIAGE," 46.
6 Spivock et al., *Project FORCE Phase 1 Report*, 30.
7 Ibid., 31.
8 Théoret et al., *Systematic Approach*.
9 Gervais and Pépin, "TRIAGE," 47.
10 Ibid.
11 Ibid., 48.
12 Ibid.
13 Ibid.

6

Life Satisfaction among Canadian Forces Members

ALLA SKOMOROVSKY, AMANDA THOMPSON,
AND KARLA EMENO

Abstract

The present study examines the sources of life satisfaction among Canadian Forces members (N = 633). Multiple regression analyses showed that six out of seven domains – material well-being, physical health, psychological distress, satisfaction with military life, relationship satisfaction, and social support – were correlated with life satisfaction and served as unique predictors when others were statistically controlled for. Another domain – community safety – was not correlated with life satisfaction. Sequential cluster analysis showed that these six domains differentiated between military personnel with high and low life satisfaction, suggesting the presence of the multi-dimensional model of life satisfaction. The proposed life satisfaction model offers a useful approach for improving support services tailored to enhancing life satisfaction in the military context.

Life Satisfaction among Canadian Forces Members

Military jobs are more physically and psychologically demanding than most civilian jobs, involving high levels of fear, sensory overload, sensory deprivation, a constantly changing environment, and exposure to climatic changes, as well as stressors, such as deployment and prolonged periods of time away from home.[1] The stressors that military personnel encounter may lead to poorer well-being.[2] Moreover, low life-satisfaction was found to be associated with mental health problems, including suicide ideation[3] and turnover intentions.[4] For example, high occupational stress and work–family conflicts were predictive of poorer life satisfaction, which, in turn, were associated with turnover intentions.[5] Some evidence suggests that Regular Force military personnel are more dissatisfied with their lives than reservists and civilian workers.[6] The high demands of military life may have a negative impact on the overall life satisfaction of military personnel, which, in turn, may lead to attrition and psychological health problems. Therefore, it is important to identify the main factors that predict life satisfaction among military personnel.

Life Satisfaction

Generally, life satisfaction is a subjective evaluation of the quality of one's life as a whole.[7] According to Diener, Suh, Lucas, and Smith,[8] overall life satisfaction represents the cognitive (i.e., judgmental) component of subjective well-being, or happiness, and has been found to predict mental health outcomes.[9] For example, those high in life satisfaction are less likely to attempt suicide[10] or become depressed.[11] Similarly, low life-satisfaction has been linked to many negative work-related outcomes, such as increased intention to leave.[12] Although life satisfaction is often measured on a single scale (e.g., "How satisfied are you with your life as a whole?"), research indicates that it is a more complex construct and should be viewed as the result, in part, of satisfaction with various life domains.[13] This view of life satisfaction is based on the assumption that individuals evaluate the details of their experience when making overall satisfaction judgments[14] using a "bottom-up" approach.[15]

Although some research has examined a multi-dimensional life satisfaction model among civilians,[16] very limited research has been conducted using a similar life satisfaction model among military personnel. Accordingly, the present study examined the sources of life satisfaction among Canadian Forces (CF) personnel and evaluated a life satisfaction model comprising the seven main sources of life satisfaction identified in previous research: material well-being, physical health, psychological distress, occupational satisfaction (i.e., satisfaction with military life), relationship satisfaction, perceptions of safety, and perceptions of social support. These seven domains are discussed in detail below.

Material Well-being

The relationship between material well-being and subjective well-being has been the subject of disagreement in the literature. Although some studies have found that low income contributes to lowered subjective well-being,[17] other studies have not found such a relationship.[18] Recent research, however, has begun to draw a more consistent connection between material well-being and overall subjective well-being. Nevertheless, as Cummins[19] has pointed out, the exact link between material well-being and subjective well-being remains difficult to determine because of potential confounding factors, such as unemployment and health. Nickerson, Schwarz, and Diener,[20] for example, found a positive association between financial success and life satisfaction. In addition, Cummins, Eckersley, Pallant, Van Vugt, and Misajon[21] found that standard of living made the single largest contribution to a personal index that predicted overall life satisfaction, explaining a considerable amount of unique variance. The researchers concluded that material well-being is an important domain to consider.

Physical Health

An extensive literature has documented the importance of the relationship between individual health and quality of life.[22] However, the nature of the relationship between physical health and subjective well-being is not necessarily straightforward. In general, researchers do not dispute the important role of physical health in overall life satisfaction; however, it has been argued that the causal relationship between health behaviours and overall well-being may be bidirectional.[23]

Psychological Well-being / Psychological Distress

Psychological well-being is also thought to play an essential role in quality of life.[24] The concept denotes optimal psychological functioning.[25] A recent study showed that even mild symptoms of psychological distress (e.g., depression) are associated with substantial reductions in overall quality of life and well-being.[26] Furthermore, it is now generally accepted that elevated levels of stress are associated with negative health outcomes and decreased well-being.[27]

Occupational Satisfaction

The work environment is believed to be one of the major sources of life satisfaction for most adults,[28] and research has revealed a relatively strong and significant relationship between occupational (i.e., job) satisfaction and life satisfaction.[29] For example, Hart[30] examined life satisfaction among police officers and found job satisfaction to be a significant contributor to overall life satisfaction. Similarly, meta-analyses by Tait, Padgett, and Baldwin,[31] as well as Bowling, Eschleman, and Wang[32] found average correlations of .35 and .40 (respectively) between job satisfaction and life satisfaction. In addition, military family research has shown that spouses of military personnel who were underemployed, overqualified, or unemployed (i.e., those with presumably lower levels of job satisfaction) had significantly lower levels of psychological well-being and life satisfaction.[33] Occupational research in military and civilian work environments has also shown that job-related stress is associated with decreased well-being, including psychological strain[34] and health complaints.[35]

Relationship Satisfaction

Evidence suggests that having close relationships is an important determinant of overall subjective well-being.[36] For example, individuals who reported higher-quality relationships were found to report higher levels of well-being.[37] In particular, support from one's spouse has been found to have a direct and positive effect on general well-being.[38] In contrast, individuals who experience higher work–family conflict have been shown to report lower levels of general well-being.[39] Similarly, military research has shown that satisfaction with one's marriage and family life is a major component of overall well-being and life satisfaction among U.S. military wives,[40] and perceived support from the military spouse has been associated with greater life satisfaction.[41]

Perceptions of Safety

Research suggests that the relationship between perceptions of safety and life satisfaction is not a straightforward one. Whorton and Moore[42] included concern for crime in their measure of well-being. Cummins, Eckersley et al.[43] also included concern for crime and perceptions of safety in their community wellness model. However, their results showed that safety did not explain any variance in satisfaction with life as a whole. More recently, Jackson and Stafford's[44] longitudinal cohort study showed that worry about crime had a robust and negative statistical effect on well-being. In tracking 10,308 British civil servants, the authors found that fear of crime at baseline was prospectively associated with lower quality of life, as well as poorer mental health and reduced physical functioning on objective and subjective indicators. The findings of this study reinforce recent evidence that fear of crime at baseline harms public health at a later period.[45]

Perceptions of Social Support

Perceiving relationships as supportive has been found to enhance individuals' overall well-being.[46] Perceptions of social support were found to be associated with overall well-being both directly and indirectly.[47] Specifically, some researchers have found significant main effects between low perceived social support and psychological distress,[48] whereas other researchers have found that social support plays a stress-buffering role.[49] Moreover, in military research, social support was found to protect military members and their families against the development of depressive symptoms as a function stressors related to military life.[50]

Aim

The present study examined the sources of life satisfaction among CF members across seven domains that have been previously found to play an important role in life satisfaction: material well-being, physical health, psychological distress, occupational satisfaction (i.e., satisfaction with military life), relationship satisfaction, perceptions of safety, and perceptions of social support. It was hypothesized that these seven domains jointly predict life satisfaction among military members.

Methods

Participants

An electronic survey was sent to 4,700 randomly selected Regular Force CF members at three military bases (Petawawa, ON; Halifax, NS; and Cold Lake, AB) in January 2011. A total of 935 responses were received, indicating an overall adjusted response rate of 21.3%. However, given that one of the variables of interest was relationship satisfaction, only CF members who reported to be in an intimate relationship (spouse or partner) were retained for final analyses. In addition, cluster analysis cannot be run with missing data, so only participants who completed the indicators of life satisfaction were included in the final sample.[51] This resulted in a final sample of 633 CF members.

Out of those participants who provided their descriptive information, 504 (79.6%) were male and 129 (20.4%) female; 533 (84.2%) anglophone and 95 (15.0%) francophone; 485 (76.6%) were non-commissioned members and 148 (23.4%) officers. In addition, the distribution of military personnel across the three stationed bases was as follows: 121 (19.2%) participants from Cold Lake, 309 (48.8%) from Halifax, and 203 (32.1%) from Petawawa.

Measures

Material Well-being

Material well-being was assessed by self-reported standard of living. Two questions were adapted from the 2008 Canadian Community Health Survey[52] to measure standard of living: (1) "Overall, how would you rate your current standard of living?" Responses were measured on a five-point scale (1 = very low; 5 = very high). Responses marked "Don't know" were recoded as missing. Higher scores indicate higher levels of perceived standard of living. (2) "Overall, how satisfied are you with your current standard of living?" Responses were measured on a five-point scale (1 = very dissatisfied; 5 = very satisfied). Responses marked "Don't know" were recoded as missing. Higher scores indicate higher levels of satisfaction with standard of living (table 6.1).

Physical Health

Physical health was assessed using one question adapted from the twelve-item Short-Form Health Survey.[53] Respondents used a five-point rating scale (1 = excel-

Table 6.1 | Descriptive characteristics of CF candidates on life satisfaction indicators and inter-item reliability

Descriptive characteristics	Possible range	Mean	SD	Cronbach alpha
Material well-being	1–5	3.52	.79	.78
Physical health	1–5	3.39	.90	n/a
Psychological distress	1–4	1.64	.66	.92
Satisfaction with military life	1–7	4.59	1.15	.93
Relationship satisfaction	1–5	4.17	.99	.98
Community safety	1–5	4.05	.72	.84
Social support	1–5	4.02	.90	.98
Life satisfaction	1–5	3.81	.59	.86

lent; 5 = poor) to rate their general health. The items were recoded so that higher scores on this scale indicate higher levels of perceived general health (table 6.1).

Psychological Distress

Psychological distress was assessed using the nine-item Center for Epidemiologic Studies Depression Scale.[54] Respondents used a four-point rating scale (1 = rarely or none of the time; 4 = most or all of the time) to indicate how often each of a series of events has occurred over the previous week (e.g., "I felt depressed," "I had trouble keeping my mind on what I was doing"). Two positively worded items ("I felt happy," "I enjoyed life") were recoded, so that higher scores on this scale indicate higher levels of psychological distress (table 6.1).

Occupational Satisfaction

Occupational satisfaction was measured by assessing satisfaction with military life. Overall satisfaction with aspects of military life was assessed using thirteen items developed for this survey. Using a seven-point rating scale (1 = completely unsatisfied; 7 = completely satisfied), respondents indicated their degree of satisfaction with career progression, working hours, opportunities for professional development, and posting frequency. Higher scores indicate higher levels of satisfaction with military service (table 6.1).

Relationship Satisfaction

Quality of relationships with partners was assessed using six items from the Quality Marriage Index.[55] Using a five-point rating scale (1 = strongly disagree; 5 =

strongly agree), respondents indicated the extent to which they were happy with their relationships (e.g., "I think we have a good relationship," "I think our relationship is strong," "My relationship with my partner makes me happy"). Higher scores indicate more positive attitudes toward the relationship (table 6.1).

Community Safety

Perceived neighbourhood safety was assessed using four items developed for this survey. Using a five-point scale (1 = strongly disagree; 5 = strongly agree), respondents indicated the extent to which they perceived their neighbourhood to be safe (e.g., "It is safe to be at home during the night in my neighbourhood," "It is safe to leave a car in the street at night in my neighbourhood"). Higher scores indicate higher perceptions of a safe neighbourhood (table 6.1).

Social Support

Social support was measured using the nineteen-item Social Support Scale.[56] Using a five-point scale (1 = none of the time; 5 = all of the time), respondents indicated the extent to which different types of support were available (e.g., emotional, instrumental, and informational). Higher scores indicate higher levels of perceived support (table 6.1).

Life Satisfaction

The Satisfaction with Life Scale is adapted from the Canadian Community Health Survey.[57] An additional item "How satisfied are you with your life in general?" was added. Including this additional item, ten domains of life satisfaction were measured using a five-point Likert scale (1 = very satisfied; 5 = very dissatisfied). The items were recoded so that higher scores on this scale indicate higher levels of life satisfaction (table 6.1).

Results

Preliminary analyses involved examining the relationships between the sources of life satisfaction. For these purposes, zero-order correlations were calculated. Examination of the Pearson correlations demonstrated that there were significant correlations between the sources of life satisfaction (table 6.2). Most coefficients demonstrated minor or moderate correlations between the domains. For example, occupational satisfaction and social support had moderate negative correlations with psychological distress, suggesting that military members who had greater satisfaction with the military way of life or greater social support had lower depressive symptomatology. In addition, social support had a moderate positive

Table 6.2 | Sources of life satisfaction: Pearson correlations between variables

	1	2	3	4	5	6	7	8
1 Material well-being	–							
2 Physical health	.25***	–						
3 Psychological distress	-.23***	-.37***	–					
4 Satisfaction with military life	.33***	.38***	-.46***	–				
5 Relationship satisfaction	.13***	.21***	-.28***	.16**	–			
6 Community safety	.16***	.13***	-.03	.12**	.08*	–		
7 Social support	.17***	.26***	-.44***	.31***	.42***	.13*	–	
8 Life satisfaction	.50***	.51***	-.55***	.53***	.35***	.18***	.44***	–

$* p < .05; ** p < .01; *** p < .001$

correlation with relationship satisfaction, suggesting that the two domains share a considerable amount of variance.

The main analyses involved three steps. First, a multiple regression analysis was conducted to assess which sources independently predicted life satisfaction. All the sources were simultaneously entered in the regression predicting life satisfaction. Only those accounting for a unique variance in life satisfaction were retained for further analyses. The second step involved a two-step cluster analysis performed using the sources of life satisfaction identified in the previous step. The aim of this step was to determine whether different groups of personnel with distinct profiles of life satisfaction could be identified. Two-step cluster analysis was chosen in this study because the sample size in this study was moderate to large and no a priori hypotheses were made pertaining to the number or nature of the clusters in this study. This method relies on a sequential clustering approach and uses the distancing criteria to find the optimal number of clusters.[58] The validity of the profiles was then tested using a series of post hoc analysis of variance (ANOVA) tests to assess mean differences in the indicators of life satisfaction across the clusters with Bonferonni corrections applied.[59] Finally, the potential role of age and sex in life satisfaction were examined with regression and chi square analyses to determine whether cluster membership was related to age and/or sex.

Multiple regression analyses showed that the variables of interest significantly predicted life satisfaction, $R^2 = .568$, $F(7, 611) = 115.07$, $p < .001$, accounting for almost 60% of the variance (table 6.3). All seven domains were correlated with life satisfaction. Specifically, higher material well-being, physical health, satisfaction with military life, relationship satisfaction, perceptions of community safety, and social support were associated with greater life satisfaction among military personnel. Greater psychological distress was associated with lower life satisfaction. In addition, six out of seven domains – material well-being, physical health,

Table 6.3 | Multiple regression analyses assessing the sources of life satisfaction

	Pearson r	β	R^2
			.568***
Material well-being	.50***	.33***	
Physical health	.51***	.21***	
Depression	-.55***	-.28***	
Satisfaction with military life	.53***	.22***	
Relationship satisfaction	.35***	.13***	
Community safety	.18***	.07	
Social support	.44***	.13***	

*** $p < .001$

Table 6.4 | Testing validity of life satisfaction clusters across sources of life satisfaction

	Low life satisfaction mean (SD)	*High life satisfaction mean* (SD)	*ANOVA* F *test*
Material well-being	3.24 (.79)	3.67 (.74)	65.64***
Physical health	2.99 (.96)	3.60 (.79)	75.28***
Psychological distress	2.24 (.73)	1.31 (.40)	366.25***
Satisfaction with military life	3.90 (1.10)	4.97 (1.01)	141.93***
Relationship satisfaction	3.38 (1.17)	4.59 (.54)	357.45***
Social support	3.28 (.93)	4.42 (.54)	443.36***

*** $p < .001$

psychological distress, satisfaction with military life, relationship satisfaction, and social support – served as unique predictors of life satisfaction when other domains were statistically controlled for. Satisfaction with community safety was not correlated with life satisfaction.

The results of the two-step cluster analysis using the standardized values of the six sources of life satisfaction (material well-being, physical health, occupational satisfaction, relationship satisfaction, psychological well-being, and social support) suggested the suitability of a two-cluster solution (ΔBIC = -401.25). Specifically, 204 participants were classified as belonging to a low life-satisfaction profile and compared to 429 participants who were classified as members of a high life-satisfaction profile. Further, the results of the six ANOVA tests showed that mean scores in all six domains of life satisfaction were significantly lower in the low life-satisfaction profile compared to the mean scores in the high life-satisfaction profile using the Bonferonni correction (table 6.4). Finally, differences in cluster membership were examined to rule out age and gender as confounding variables in the analysis. Results of an ANOVA revealed that the age of individuals ($F(1, 630)$ = .752, β = .04, ns) in each cluster was not significantly different, and the chi square test showed that the proportions of males and females in each cluster were not significantly different ($\chi^2 (1)$ = .91, ns).

Discussion

Previous literature suggested that poor life satisfaction is predictive of mental health problems[60] and negative work-related outcomes, such as turnover intentions.[61] In light of the highly stressful and unique physical and psychological demands associated with military jobs,[62] it was therefore vital to identify the main sources of life satisfaction among military personnel. As predicted, most of the domains examined played an important role in the life satisfaction of military personnel. Specifically, the results revealed that material well-being, physical health, psychological well-being (assessed by depressive symptoms), satisfaction with military life, relationship satisfaction, and perceptions of social support were important and unique predictors of life satisfaction among CF members. Furthermore, the results showed the suitability of a two-cluster solution, where these six domains differentiated between military personnel with high and low life satisfaction. These findings suggest the presence of a multi-dimensional model of life satisfaction among military personnel.

This multi-dimensional model of life satisfaction is consistent with the models of overall wellness and life satisfaction proposed in previous research.[63] Like the model developed by Cummins and his colleagues,[64] the proposed life-satisfaction model affirms that overall life satisfaction comprises both hedonic aspects (concerned with enjoyment and pleasure, e.g., material well-being) and eudemonic aspects (concerned with the realization of individual potential, e.g., occupational satisfaction). A comprehensive model of life satisfaction should integrate both aspects, which is an approach consistent with previous research, such as the Well-Being Module developed for the European Social Survey.[65]

The dimensions identified in this study also overlap with the dimensions presented in the Comprehensive Quality of Life Scale:[66] emotional well-being, physical health, intimacy (measured as relationship satisfaction in this study), material well-being, productivity (measured as occupational satisfaction in this study), safety, and community (measured as social support in this study).

Although most of the findings in this study were consistent with the model developed by Cummins and his colleagues, the main inconsistency was found to be related to the role of community safety in life satisfaction. Community safety in this study was not uniquely predicting life satisfaction among military personnel.

Although this finding seems to be inconsistent with the model developed by Cummins McCabe, Gullone et al.[67] and with the findings obtained by Jackson and Stafford,[68] the lack of the significant contribution to life-satisfaction variance by the safety domain has been noted earlier by Cummins, Eckersley et al.[69]

The inconsistency in the findings regarding the role of perceptions of safety in overall life satisfaction suggests that the role of perceptions of safety is not straightforward and may depend on multiple confounding factors. For example, the importance of safety for overall life satisfaction may greatly depend on the location (i.e., community) where the data were collected. The data for this study were collected at three military-based locations, where the community safety may not be a concern. Indeed, the levels of perceived safety were found to be very high at all three locations.

Another confounding variable can be the personal characteristics of the study participants. Some evidence suggests that community safety is more important for females than for males. For instance, it is a well-documented finding that males are more likely to exhibit risk-taking behaviour than females,[70] which could imply that they place less emphasis on safety in general. In another study, Bennett et al.[71] found that women who rated the night-time safety of their neighbourhood more highly were more likely to be physically active (i.e., walk more steps) than women who rated perceived night-time neighbourhood safety lower. This effect was not found for men, which could suggest that women are more influenced than men by perceived community safety. Given that there were four times more male than female participants in the present study, the importance of community safety in life satisfaction might have been diminished for the study participants overall. It is also possible that the role of community safety is less important for military personnel. Given the constant safety concerns associated with military life and especially with the combat deployments,[72] military personnel may be less likely to emphasize community-related safety.

The role of age and gender in the clusters of life satisfaction was examined in order to detect their potential effects as confounding variables. Results revealed that cluster membership was not related to age, which is consistent with previous research showing that life satisfaction does not decline with age.[73] In studies where life satisfaction was found to decrease with age, the variations were usually small and disappeared once confounding variables (e.g., income) were statistically controlled for.[74] The present study also found that life satisfaction cluster membership was unrelated to gender. This finding is again consistent with the subjective well-being literature.[75] Although some studies found significant gender differences in subjective well-being, with females typically reporting higher subjective well-being than males, these differences often disappeared when other demographic variables are controlled for.[76] Therefore, age and gender should be examined in future research as covariates of life satisfaction of military personnel.

The model in this study differed from that of Cummins et al. in the organization of some of the domains of life satisfaction. In the model of Cummins and his colleagues,[77] for example, the emotional well-being domain contains spiritual well-being and leisure satisfaction components, which were not examined in this study. In addition, perceptions of social support are an integral part of overall community satisfaction in their model; and they included additional components related to community life – such as community connectedness and satisfaction with various community services – which were not examined in the present study. Thus, the life-satisfaction model of Cummins and his colleagues has a broader variety of domains than the model examined in this study. In light of this, it would be useful to include in future life-satisfaction model development research some of the main components of the domains identified in previous research that were not examined in this study – in particular, spiritual well-being, leisure satisfaction, and satisfaction with community services.

The proposed model of life satisfaction offers a useful approach for improving support services tailored to enhancing the life satisfaction of military members, while distinguishing each of the key sources of life satisfaction. Specifically, findings from the present study suggest that interventions should target physical health maintenance and improvement practices (e.g., promoting physical exercise and proper diet), spousal support building (helping military couples strengthen their relationships), and financial counselling (helping military members reduce stress associated with budget planning). For example, the study's findings emphasize the importance of bringing an individual's health to the forefront; thus an educational component could be incorporated into the regularly scheduled training days, to enhance the general awareness of good physical health practices and stress-management techniques. Furthermore, given that coping has been found to be directly and indirectly associated with psychological distress of military personnel,[78] it may be beneficial to consider providing coping training (e.g., coping skills techniques), including approaches that focus on reducing stress related to the military way of life. Consistent with this suggestion, it has already been recommended that the CF provide coping training to military personnel.[79] However, future research should consider and examine the best coping training method that may reduce psychological distress among military personnel. For example, future research should examine whether the intervention should focus on helping individuals to choose effective coping strategies or to increase the effectiveness of the coping strategies they already employ.[80]

Limitations

Several limitations should be borne in mind when interpreting the results of this study. First, the methodological constraints of the current study may negatively affect the generalizability of the results. Only three bases were included in the sample, meaning that the conclusions are base-specific and are not generalizable to the whole military organization. The second limitation concerns data quality. Specific issues involve scale construction, potential respondent fatigue, non-normality, and missing data. For example, the survey required approximately one hour to complete, and it is possible that respondent fatigue influenced the results, limiting the validity of conclusions based on these data. Similarly, inconsistent scale construction might have also influenced the results. Different scales on the survey had different numbers of Likert points, which required participants to continually adjust and re-evaluate their responses. Although the implications of mixing scale formats in this way have not received extensive research, some findings show that the numbering and labelling of scales has a significant impact on survey results.[81]

Third, it is important to take into account the operationalization of the main sources of life satisfaction. Although the survey included key variables for each construct, several additional constructs could be included in future refinements. Specifically, psychological well-being was measured by depressive symptoms only, and the indicators of positive well-being were not included. However, current psychology research has broadened the definition of well-being to include not only the absence of negative life and health indicators, but also the presence of positive life and health indicators.[82] Similarly, the current study assessed perception of availability of social support (i.e., the support we receive from others), but not the social contribution (i.e., how we give to others). The omission of social contribution may be relevant because evidence suggests that volunteering or doing things for others may contribute to general well-being to a greater extent than the support we receive from others.[83]

The final limitation concerns the data analysis. Regression and cluster analyses were conducted to examine the roles of various domains in life satisfaction. However, hierarchical confirmatory structure analyses would be a valuable tool for identifying which domains contribute the most to CF personnel's ratings of life satisfaction. Accordingly, future research should incorporate a structural equation analysis in order to further examine and confirm the model of life satisfaction among military personnel.

Conclusion

Despite its limitations, this study has several important implications. The overall goal of this study was to examine life satisfaction among CF personnel and identify its key sources. The results showed that material well-being, physical health, psychological distress, occupational satisfaction, relationship satisfaction, and social support are important predictors of life satisfaction among military personnel. The proposed model offers a useful approach for improving support services tailored to enhancing life satisfaction in a military context.

Notes

1 G. P. Krueger, "Military Psychology: United States," *International Encyclopedia of the Social & Behavioral Sciences*, ed. N. J. Smelser and P. B. Baltes (2001): 9868–73, http://www.sciencedirect.com/science/article/pii/B0080430767014285.

2 G. L. Bowen and J. A. Martin, "The Resiliency Model of Role Performance for Service Members, Veterans, and Their Families: A Focus on Social Connections and Individual Assets," *Journal of Human Behavior in the Social Environment* 21 (2011): 162–78; B. M. Bray, J. A. Fairbank, and M. E. Marsden, "Stress and Substance Use among Military Women and Men," *American Journal of Drug and Alcohol Abuse* 25 (1999): 239–56.

3 I. Bray and D. Gunnell, "Suicide Rates, Life Satisfaction and Happiness as Markers for Population Mental Health," *Social Psychiatry and Psychiatric Epidemiology* 41 (2006): 333–7.

4 E. G. Lambert, N. L. Hogan, E. A. Paoline, and D. N. Baker, "The Good Life: The Impact of Job Satisfaction and Occupational Stressors on Correctional Staff Life Satisfaction – An Exploratory Study," *Journal of Crime and Justice* 28 (2005): 1–26.

5 J. C. Rode, M. T. Rehg, J. P. Near, and J. R. Underhill, "The Effect of Work/Family Conflict on Intention to Quit: The Mediating Roles of Job and Life Satisfaction," *Applied Research in Quality of Life* 2 (2007): 65–82.

6 J. Park, "A Profile of the Canadian Forces: Statistics Canada," *Perspectives* (July 2008): 17–30, http://www.statcan.gc.ca/pub/75-001-x/2008107/pdf/10657-eng.pdf.

7 L. Sousa and S. Lyubomirsky, "Life Satisfaction," in *Encyclopedia of Women and Gender: Sex Similarities and Differences and the Impact of Society on Gender*, ed. J. Worell (San Diego, CA: Academic, 2001), 2:667–76.

8 E. Diener, E. M. Suh, R. E. Lucas, and H. L. Smith, "Subjective Well-being: Three Decades of Progress," *Psychological Bulletin* 125 (1999): 276–302.

9 W. Pavot and E. Diener, "The Satisfaction with Life Scale and the Emerging Construct of Life Satisfaction," *Journal of Positive Psychology* 3 (2008): 137–52.

10 T. Moum, "Subjective Well-being as a Short- and Long-Term Predictor of Suicide in the General Population" (paper presented at the World Conference on Quality of Life, Prince George, BC, August 1996).

11 M. B. Frisch, "Improving Mental and Physical Health Care through Quality of Life Therapy and Assessment," in *Advances in Quality of Life Theory and Research*, ed. E. Diener, 207–41 (Dordrecht, Netherlands: Kluwer, 2000).

12 R. F. Ghiselli, J. M. La Lopa, and B. Bai, "Job Satisfaction, Life Satisfaction, and Turnover Intent among Food-Service Managers," *Cornell Hotel and Restaurant Administration Quarterly* 42 (2001): 28–37.

13 R. A. Cummins, "The Domains of Life Satisfaction: An Attempt to Order Chaos," *Social Indicators Research* 38 (1996): 303–28; Rode et al., "Effect of Work/Family Conflict."

14 R. W. Rice, D. B. McFarlin, R. G. Hunt, and J. P. Near, "Organizational Work and the Perceived Quality of Life: Toward a Conceptual Model," *Academy of Management Review* 10 (1985): 296–310.

15 A. P. Brief, A. H. Butcher, J. M. George, and K. E. Link, "Integrating Bottom-Up and Top-Down Theories of Subjective Well-being: The Case of Health," *Journal of Personality and Social Psychology* 64 (1993): 646–53.

16 R. A. Cummins, M. McCabe, E. Gullone, and Y. Romeo, "The Comprehensive Quality of Life Scale (ComQol): Instrument Development and Psychometric Evaluation on College Staff and Students," *Educational and Psychological Measurement* 54 (1994): 372–82; R. A. Cummins, M. P. McCabe, Y. Romeo, S. Reid, and L. Waters, "An Initial Evaluation of the Comprehensive Quality of Life Scale – Intellectual Disability," *International Journal of Disability, Development and Education* 44 (1997): 7–19; F. A. Huppert, N. Marks, A. Clark, J. Siegrist, A. Stutzer, J. Vittersø, and M. Wahrendorf, "Measuring Well-being across Europe: Description of the ESS Well-being Module and Preliminary Findings," *Social Indicators Research* 91 (2008): 301–15; J. Jackson and M. Stafford, "Public Health and Fear of Crime: A Prospective Cohort Study," *British Journal of Criminology* 49 (2009): 832–47.

17 K. Kokko and L. Pulkkinen, "Unemployment and Psychological Distress: Mediator Effects," *Journal of Adult Development* 5 (1998): 205–17.

18 R. Schulz and S. Decker, "Long-term Adjustment to Physical Disability: The Role of Social Support, Perceived Control, and Self-Blame," *Journal of Personality and Social Psychology* 48 (1985): 1162–72.

19 R. A. Cummins, "Objective and Subjective Quality of Life: An Interactive Model," *Social Indicators Research* 52 (2000): 55–72.

20 C. Nickerson, N. Schwarz, and E. Diener, "Financial Aspirations, Financial Success, and Overall Life Satisfaction: Who? and How?," *Journal of Happiness Studies* 8 (2007): 467–515.

21 R. A. Cummins, R. Eckersley, J. Pallant, J. Van Vugt, and R. Misajon, "Developing a National Index of Subjective Wellbeing: The Australian Unity Wellbeing Index," *Social Indicators Research* 64 (2003): 159–90.

22 For a review, see M. Rapley, *Quality of Life Research* (London: Sage Publications, 2003).

23 J. K. Boehm and L. D. Kubzansky, "The Heart's Content: The Association between Positive Psychological Well-being and Cardiovascular Health," *Psychological Bulletin* 138 (2012): 655–91.

24 Rapley, *Quality of Life Research*.

25 R. M. Ryan and E. L. Deci, "On Happiness and Human Potentials: A Review of Research on Hedonic and Eudaimonic Well-being," *Annual Review of Psychology* 52 (2001): 141–66.

26 A. A. Nierenberg, M. Rapaport, P. J. Schettler, R. H. Howland, J. A. Smith, D. Edwards, and D. Mischoulon, "Deficits in Psychological Well-being and Quality-of-Life in Minor Depression: Implications for DSM–V," *CNS Neuroscience & Therapeutics* 16 (2010): 208–16.

27 P. D. Bliese and C. A. Castro, "Role Clarity, Work Overload and Organizational Support: Multilevel Evidence of the Importance of Support," *Work and Stress* 14 (2000): 65–73; S. Johnson, C. Cooper, S. Cartwright, I. Donald, P. Taylor, and C. Millet, "The Experience of Work-Related Stress across Occupations," *Journal of Managerial Psychology* 20 (2005): 178–87; S. E. Pflanz and A. D. Ogle, "Job Stress,

Depression, Work Performance, and Perceptions of Supervisors in Military Personnel," *Military Medicine* 171 (2006): 861–5.

28 Lambert et al., "The Good Life."

29 T. A. Judge and S. Watanabe, "Another Look at the Job Satisfaction–Life Satisfaction Relationship," *Journal of Applied Psychology* 6 (2003): 939–48; M. Tait, M. Y. Padgett, and T. T. Baldwin, "Job and Life Satisfaction: A Reevaluation of the Strength of the Relationship and Gender Effects as a Function of the Date of the Study," *Journal of Applied Psychology* 74 (1989): 502–7.

30 P. M. Hart, "Predicting Employee Life Satisfaction: A Coherent Model of Personality, Work, and Nonwork Experiences, and Domain Satisfactions," *Journal of Applied Psychology* 84 (1999): 564–84.

31 Tait, Padgett, and Baldwin, "Job and Life Satisfaction."

32 N. A. Bowling, K. J. Eschleman, and Q. Wang, "A Meta-Analytic Examination of the Relationship between Job Satisfaction and Subjective Well-being," *Journal of Occupational and Organizational Psychology* 83 (2010): 915–34.

33 S. Dursun and K. Sudom, *Impacts of Military Life on Families: Results from the Perstempo Survey of Canadian Forces Spouses*, DGMPRA TR 2009-001 (Ottawa: Director General Military Personnel Research and Analysis, 2009).

34 P. D. Bliese and C. A. Castro, "Role Clarity, Work Overload and Organizational Support: Multilevel Evidence of the Importance of Support," *Work and Stress* 14 (2000): 65–73.

35 R. L. Repetti, "Short-term Effects of Occupational Stressors on Daily Mood and Health Complaints," *Health Psychology* 12 (1993): 125–31.

36 For a review, see Ryan and Deci, "On Happiness and Human Potentials."

37 H. T. Reis, W. A. Collins, and E. Berscheid, "The Relationship Context of Human Behaviour and Development," *Psychological Bulletin* 126 (2000): 844–72.

38 C. Dehle, D. Larsen, and J. E. Landers, "Social Support in Marriage," *American Journal of Family Therapy* 29 (2001): 307–24.

39 S. Aryee, "Antecedents and Outcomes of Work–Family Conflict among Married Professional Women: Evidence from Singapore," *Human Relations* 45 (1992): 813–37; M. R. Frone, "Work–Family Conflict and Employee Psychiatric Disorders: The National Co-morbidity Survey," *Journal of Applied Psychology* 85 (2000): 888–95; L. T. Thomas and D. C. Ganster, "Impact of Family-Supportive Work Variables on Work–Family Conflict and Strain: A Control Perspective," *Journal of Applied Psychology* 80 (1995): 6–15.

40 L. N. Rosen and L. Z. Moghadam, "Matching the Support to the Stressor: Implications for the Buffering Hypothesis," *Military Psychology* 2 (1990): 193–204.

41 Dursun and Sudom, *Impacts of Military Life on Families*.

42 J. W. Whorton and A. B. Moore, "Summative Scales for Measuring Community Satisfaction," *Social Indicators Research* 15 (1984): 297–307.

43 Cummins, Eckersley et al., "Developing a National Index of Subjective Wellbeing."

44 J. Jackson and M. Stafford, "Public Health and Fear of Crime: A Prospective Cohort Study," *British Journal of Criminology* 49 (2009): 832–47.

45 M. Stafford, T. Chandola, and M. Marmot, "Association between Fear of Crime and Mental Health and Physical Functioning," *American Journal of Public Health* 97 (2007): 2076–81.

46 S. Cohen and G. McKay, "Social Support, Stress and the Buffering Hypothesis: A
    Theoretical Analysis," in *Handbook of Psychology and Health*, ed. A. Baum, S. E.
    Taylor, and J. E. Singer, 253–67 (Hillsdale, NJ: Lawrence Erlbaum, 1984); S. Cohen
    and T. A. Wills, "Stress, Social Support, and the Buffering Hypothesis," *Psychological
    Bulletin* 98 (1985): 310–57; E. S. Zhou, F. J. Penedo, N. E. Bustillo, C. Benedict, M.
    Rasheed, S. Lechner, M. Soloway, B. R. Kava, N. Schneiderman, and M. H. Antoni,
    "Longitudinal Effects of Social Support and Adaptive Coping on the Emotional Well-
    being of Survivors of Localized Prostate Cancer," *Journal of Supportive Oncology* 8
    (2010): 196–201.

47 B. Lakey and E. Orehek, "Relational Regulation Theory: A New Approach to Explain
    the Link between Perceived Social Support and Mental Health," *Psychological Review*
    118 (2011): 482–95; L. N. Rosen, and L. Z. Moghadam, "Social Support, Family
    Separation, and Well-being among Military Wives," *Behavioral Medicine* 14 (1988):
    64–70.

48 B. Lakey and A. Cronin, "Low Social Support and Major Depression: Research,
    Theory and Methodological Issues," in *Risk Factors for Depression*, ed. K. S. Dobson
    and D. Dozois, 385–408 (San Diego, CA: Academic, 2008).

49 Cohen and Wills, "Stress, Social Support, and the Buffering Hypothesis"; K. Rigby,
    "Effects of Peer Victimization in Schools and Perceived Social Support on Adolescent
    Well-being," *Journal of Adolescence* 23 (2000): 57–68; D. J. Terry, M. Nielsen, and L.
    Perchard, "Effects of Work Stress on Psychological Well-being and Job Satisfaction:
    The Stress-Buffering Role of Social Support," *Australian Journal of Psychology* 45
    (1993): 168–75.

50 R. H. Pietrzak, D. C. Johnson, M. B. Goldstein, J. C. Malley, and S. M. Southwick,
    "Psychological Resilience and Postdeployment Social Support Protect against
    Traumatic Stress and Depressive Symptoms in Soldiers Returning from Operations
    Enduring Freedom and Iraqi Freedom," *Depression and Anxiety* 26 (2009): 745–51;
    X. S. Ren, K. Skinner, and A. Lee, "Social Support, Social Selection and Self-Assessed
    Health Status: Results from the Veterans Health Study in the United States," *Social
    Science & Medicine* 48 (1999): 1721–34; L. N. Rosen, and L. Z. Moghadam, "Social
    Support, Family Separation, and Well-being among Military Wives," *Behavioral
    Medicine* 14 (1988): 64–70.

51 S. Theodoridis and K. Koutroumbas, *Pattern Recognition* (San Diego, CA: Academic,
    1999).

52 Statistics Canada, "Canadian Community Health Survey – Annual Component
    (CCHS)" (2008), http://www23.statcan.gc.ca/imdb/p2SV.pl?Function=getSurvey&SD
    DS=3226&lang=en&db=imdb&adm=8&dis=2.

53 J. E. Ware, M. Kosinski, and S. D. Keller, "A 12 Item Short Form Health Survey:
    Construction of Scales and Preliminary Tests of Reliability and Validity," *Medical
    Care* 34 (1996): 220–33.

54 L. S. Radloff, "The CES-D Scale: A Self-Report Depression Scale for Research in the
    General Population," *Applied Psychological Measurement* 1 (1977): 385–401.

55 R. Norton, "Measuring Marital Quality: A Critical Look at the Dependent Variable,"
    Journal of Marriage and the Family 45 (1983): 141–51.

56 C. D. Sherbourne and A. L. Stewart, "The MOS Social Support Survey," *Social Science
    & Medicine* 32 (1991): 705–14.

57 Statistics Canada, "Canadian Community Health Survey."

58 Theodoridis and Koutroumbas, *Pattern Recognition*.

59 M. S. Aldenderfer, R. K. Blashfield, "Cluster Analysis," Sage University paper series on quantitative applications in the social sciences (series no. 07-044) (Beverly Hills, CA: Sage, 1984).

60 Frisch, "Improving Mental and Physical Health Care"; Moum, "Subjective Well-being"; W. Pavot and E. Diener, "The Satisfaction with Life Scale and the Emerging Construct of Life Satisfaction," *Journal of Positive Psychology* 3 (2008): 137–52.

61 Ghiselli, La Lopa, and Bai, "Job Satisfaction, Life Satisfaction, and Turnover Intent"; Lambert et al., "The Good Life"; Rode et al., "Effect of Work/Family Conflict."

62 Krueger, "Military Psychology: United States."

63 Cummins, "Domains of Life Satisfaction"; Cummins, McCabe, Gullone et al., "Comprehensive Quality of Life Scale (ComQol)"; Cummins, McCabe, Romeo et al., "An Initial Evaluation of the Comprehensive Quality of Life Scale – Intellectual Disability."

64 Cummins, "Domains of Life Satisfaction"; Cummins, McCabe, Romeo et al., "An Initial Evaluation of the Comprehensive Quality of Life Scale – Intellectual Disability."

65 Huppert et al., "Measuring Well-being across Europe."

66 Cummins, "Domains of Life Satisfaction."

67 Cummins, McCabe, Gullone et al., "Comprehensive Quality of Life Scale"; Cummins, McCabe, Romeo et al., "An Initial Evaluation of the Comprehensive Quality of Life Scale – Intellectual Disability."

68 J. Jackson and M. Stafford, "Public Health and Fear of Crime: A Prospective Cohort Study," *British Journal of Criminology* 49 (2009): 832–47.

69 Cummins, Eckersley et al., "Developing a National Index of Subjective Wellbeing."

70 J. P. Byrnes, D. C. Miller, and W. D. Schafer, "Gender Differences in Risk Taking: A Meta-analysis," *Psychological Bulletin* 125 (1999): 367–83.

71 G. G. Bennett, L. H. McNeill, K. Y. Wolin, D. T. Duncan, E. Puleo, and K. M. Emmons, "Safe to Walk? Neighborhood Safety and Physical Activity among Public Housing Residents," *PLOS Medicine* 4 (2007): 1599–607.

72 K. Sudom, *Quality of Life among Military Families: Results from the 2008/9 Survey of Canadian Forces Spouses* (Technical Report) (Ottawa: Director General Military Personnel Research and Analysis, 2010).

73 D. S. Butt and M. Beiser, "Successful Aging: A Theme for International Psychology," *Psychology and Aging* 2 (1987): 87–94; E. Diener and E. Suh, "Age and Subjective Well-being: An International Analysis," *Annual Review of Gerontology and Geriatrics* 17 (1998): 304–24; R. Inglehart, *Culture Shift in Advanced Industrial Society* (Princeton, NJ: Princeton University Press, 1990).

74 D. Shmotkin, "Subjective Well-being as a Function of Age and Gender: A Multivariate Look for Differentiated Trends," *Social Indicators Research* 23 (1990): 201–30.

75 E. Diener, E. M. Suh, R. E. Lucas, and H. L. Smith, "Subjective Well-being: Three Decades of Progress," *Psychological Bulletin* 125 (1999): 276–302.

76 R. Inglehart, *Culture Shift in Advanced Industrial Society* (Princeton, NJ: Princeton University Press, 1990); P. Warr and R. Payne, "Experience of Strain and Pleasure

among British Adults," *Social Science and Medicine* 16 (1982): 1691–7; J. M. White, "Marital Status and Well-being in Canada," *Journal of Family Issues* 13 (1992): 390–409.

77 Cummins, McCabe, Gullone et al., "Comprehensive Quality of Life Scale (ComQol)"; Cummins, McCabe, Romeo et al., "Initial Evaluation of the Comprehensive Quality of Life Scale – Intellectual Disability."

78 A. L. Day and H. Livingstone, "Chronic and Acute Stressors among Military Personnel: Do Coping Styles Buffer Their Negative Impact on Health?," *Journal of Occupational Health Psychology* 6 (2001): 348–60; R. E. Mitchell and C. A. Hodson, "Coping with Domestic Violence: Social Support and Psychological Health among Battered Women," *American Journal of Community Psychology* 11 (1983): 629–54.

79 D. E. Jones, K. Perkins, J. H. Cook, and A. L. Ong, "Intensive Coping Skills Training to Reduce Anxiety and Depression for Forward-Deployed Troops," *Military Medicine* 173 (2008): 241–6; G. Larsson, "Personality, Appraisal and Cognitive Processes, and Performance during Various Conditions of Stress," *Military Psychology* 1 (1989): 167–82.

80 N. Bolger and A. Zuckerman, "A Framework for Studying Personality in the Stress Process," *Journal of Personality and Social Psychology* 69 (1995): 890–902.

81 J. Hartley and L.R. Betts, "Four Layouts and a Finding: The Effects of Changes in the Order of the Verbal Labels and Numerical Values on Likert-Type Scales," *International Journal of Social Research Methodology: Theory & Practice* 13 (2010): 17–27.

82 Boehm and Kubzansky, "The Heart's Content."

83 S. L. Brown, R. M. Nesse, A. D. Vinokur, and D. M. Smith, "Providing Social Support May Be More Beneficial Than Receiving It: Results from a Prospective Study of Mortality," *Psychological Science* 14 (2003): 320–7; S. Meier and A. Stutzer, "Is Volunteering Rewarding in Itself?," *Economica* 75 (2008): 39–59; S. Post, "Altruism, Happiness, and Health: It's Good to Be Good," *International Journal of Behavioral Medicine* 12 (2005): 66–77.

7

Public Opinion and Soldier Identity: Tensions and Resolutions[1]

STÉPHANIE A. H. BÉLANGER AND MICHELLE MOORE

Abstract

Testimonies from CF members in combat arms who have been deployed on multiple occasions allow the exploration of new issues surrounding soldiers' identities (core soldiering values and well-being) and training in its full spectrum: from buildup (pre-deployment training) to reintegration, and buildup again. This paper analyzes which factors influence the way these military personnel justify their mission in Afghanistan, and more precisely, how they argue that the recourse to violence is the core of their mission and of their job. These factors, identified through a discourse analysis of warrior identity and of its questioning after multiple exposures to combat arms, are of critical importance to better understand the transforming military ethics, as well as the relationship of the soldier identity with the warrior culture in postmodern military warfare.

Introduction

The transformation of military culture[2] in modern warfare has affected how soldiers perceive their soldier identity and how this identity is constructed and reinforced throughout indoctrination, as well as during operations and post-deployment.[3] The relationship between the military culture and the soldier identity and the impact of this relationship, often lived as a tension, on soldiers' well-being,[4] can be explored through the discourse analysis of soldiers who have experienced these policy changes in combat. The sense of belonging to a social group, or social identity, is felt intensively in the everyday relationship of a soldier with the organizational culture (its regiment, peers, instructors, and superiors) and has a profound impact on the soldiers' well-being. The impact of the policy shift from peacekeeping[5] missions to peace-building[6] missions, or "counterinsurgency wars,"[7] and vice versa, has made a significant, but contradictory, impact on the civilian and military populations. There seems to be a distinction between the civilian population's apparent desire to be perceived as peacekeepers[8] and the soldiers' expressed desire to make a positive contribution to the international fight.

On the one hand, most surveys tend to show that the majority of the Canadian population (63%) "identify peacekeeping as a role of the Canadian Forces in the International Scene," with a decrease from 70% since they withdrew from Afghanistan.[9] The fact that this decrease seems imputable to an increase in the categories "Supporting reconstruction" and "Help civilians in unstable countries" stresses the importance of the Canadian Forces' (CF) role according to the Canadian population: peacekeeping, humanitarian assistance, and protection of civilians. In that line of thought, it is not random that the Canadian population's positive opinion of the Forces increased considerably in 2012 (86%) compared with 2008 (78%),[10] given that the redirection of the Afghanistan mission to training and education has become better aligned with what seems to be the imputed role of the soldiers.

On the other hand, as the ambassadors of these political decisions abroad, many soldiers (sixty-two out of the seventy-seven interviewed)[11] in combat arms recently interviewed in three different Canadian Forces Bases expressed a need to master a professional standard of recourse to force above that of their international counterparts. This soldier identity, linked to an emphasis on the importance of maintaining ethical behaviour, widely expressed in the vast majority of these seventy-seven interviews, was also expressed positively by the vast majority of soldiers surveyed in a research project that assessed the attitudes and opinions of 1,027 CF Regular Force personnel. This larger-scale study revealed that two-thirds of respondents believed that succeeding in the CF depended on their ability to fulfil their roles ethically.[12] Ethical behaviour is a particularly important aspect of the recourse to force to be perceived abroad as a professional organization. This necessary aspect of the soldier identity, recourse to force, is threatened with the notion of becoming a "useless" military instrument unable to engage an adversary.[13] In this context, soldiers tend to distinguish themselves from the most published discourse, the one of the "civilians," to find their own language through which they can describe their unique war experiences. This paper, based mainly on interviews with seventy-seven service members,[14] analyzes the impact of these tensions between the military culture of peacekeeping and the soldier's identity – which goes from peace building to combat – on the soldier's well-being as self-disclosed through soldiers' discourse. It explores which factors influence the way these military personnel justify their mission in Afghanistan, and more precisely, how they argue that the recourse to violence is the core of their mission and their job in a militray culture that embraces peacekeeping. These factors, exploratory here,[15] are of critical importance to better understand the transforming military ethics in modern warfare, as well as the relationship of the soldier identity with the warrior culture in postmodern international politics. Although academics have been collecting abundant data on the relationship between public opinion and decision making in international politics,[16] few have explored the role of the principal actors of international politics when diplomatic routes are not sufficient: the men and women in uniform, and the impact of these politics on their social identities and well-being.

Warrior Spirit

A socio-historical and discursive analysis of the origins of the Canadian military official discourse has been explained in the collective *Expériences de guerres: Regards, témoignages, récits*;[17] an updated analysis is briefly explored here. In the national literature, Canadian heroes are most often represented as sympathetic, strong, courageous, and especially hospitable. Examples of bonhomie, virility, courage, and hospitability are abundant in Canadian novels, legends, and songs: the adventurous explorers, the intrepid pioneers, the fur traders, the lumberjacks, the coureurs des bois all braved winter storms, built and lived in the most rustic shacks, and never refused a drink and a bowl of soup to a pilgrim or a wanderer at the door in a cold winter night.[18] These qualities, which we could call, without exaggeration, commonplace, can also be attributed to contemporary heroes: Canadian soldiers.

The first time that Canadian soldiers were attributed with characteristics similar to those of the coureurs des bois was during the Second World War. Jean Vaillancourt, in his novel *Les Canadiens errants* [The Wandering Canadians], compared his hero to those wandering Canadians who were "vigorous" and always ready to defend the values of their country.[19] Rusticity, good-hearted confidence in brothers in arms, tireless bravery under fire – all the qualities used to describe his hero – give the impression that he is describing Jos Montferrand's life, an intrepid adventurer and invincible fighter, faithful to the ones he loves. These commonplaces cross the Canadian production into warfare. For instance, Lieutenant-Colonel Ian Hope told of his experience as commander of Operational Force Orion in Afghanistan in *Dancing with the Dushman* (2008), where he employed the same stereotypes of bravery in war, confidence in the brothers in arms, and respect for doctrinal values.[20] Descriptions of heroism – the adventurous, the explorer, the coureur des bois – haven't been modified since the nineteenth century. Similarly, Master Corporal (retired) Paul Franklin is portrayed in Faulder's *A Long Walk Home* (2007) as an adventurous, courageous, and strong soldier, while he is conducting a mountain patrol on a small peak a few kilometres outside Kandahar: "It was in many ways a perfect day for climbing, cool and fresh in the morning with temperatures just above freezing. Though exhilarating, it was a tough climb … While scaling upwards, Paul spied caves on this mountain and others nearby that Taliban and al Qaeda fighters had once lived in, and maybe still did. He hiked past the grey cinders of leftover fires."[21] The evocation of climbing in a snowy environment (as portrayed in photographs included in the book), the emphasis on the strength of the soldier carrying not only his military gear, but his medical instruments as well, makes his courage not destructive, but magnanimous.[22]

Moreover, identical qualities are applied to the Afghan population: if the Jamaican rum or beer has been replaced by tea and the shack or the trenches by a cave, the bearded men in Afghanistan have the same rusticity, the same courage in a hostile environment, and the same marginal and extraordinary life far from the capitalist world. How the Afghan culture has been portrayed throughout Canadian literature plays an important role in how Afghan society is analyzed by writers who promulgate the doctrine and by soldiers. Canadian literature on war commonly portrays Afghans as non-threatening, courageous, and particularly hospitable.[23] The popular invention of a rustic wanderer, always willing to communicate, displaying a laidback attitude, yet trusting and respectful of ancient values, is often found in modern descriptions of Afghans. When the enemy is embedded in this same hospitable and sympathetic culture, doctrine and policy writers cannot entirely avoid the influence of this admiration for the culture. These ancient values of rusticity, relentless courage, and trust in one's comrades as factors of heroism fall in line with Canadian depictions of the warrior spirit,[24] these same values shared by Canadian soldiers.

Warriors' Experiences

However, this ancient discourse does not coincide with the realities of the modern world and the current situation in Afghanistan. Canada's unique experiences in Afghanistan require a new discourse that can challenge official and public opinions, and present the current realities of war. Men and women who enter the CF with the warrior spirit of heroism have difficulty reconciling these ancient motivations with the new reality in the war theatre.[25] Training manuals and military publications have recently started to portray the Canadian soldier in line with this shift in operations, displaying images of both the heavily armed soldier and the friendly, soft soldier, demonstrating his versatility to reconstruct villages while defending the people using lethal force.[26] The discrepancies in the official discourse, the doxa, are gradually being confronted, while also revealing the struggle to generate a consistent language to define this new warrior identity. Numerous researchers have turned a suspicious eye to how the change from peacekeeping missions to peace-building missions or "counterinsurgency wars" has had a negative impact on the troops.[27]

Moreover, studies show that Canadian opinion tends to become unified (as opposed to finding regional distinctions among the provinces) when there are higher casualties: "The Canadians' long-standing and widespread support of peacekeeping, as well as the Canadian elite's justification of the use of military force in casting it in peacekeeping terms, highlights the prevalence of this postmodernist strategic culture."[28] But this creates a cleavage between the civilian population and the soldiers in uniform. Evermore so, it creates a cleavage between the soldiers in uniform, who are the ambassadors of political decisions on the international scene,[29] and the decision-makers in Ottawa. For instance, Senator Hugh Segal argued for a winding down of the Canadian intervention on the international scene in the face of economic constraints as early as 2002, before the shift in military intervention from support to elections (2004) to the military push in Kandahar (2006); this argument was made before Canada even deployed its troops in support of the mission in Afghanistan.[30] The financial argument serves public opinion well, as Canadians prefer to portray themselves on the international scene only in peacekeeping missions: "We want to be safe and rich, and we want to be seen as virtuous."[31]

This theory, if widespread, is not supported by soldiers' experiences. One must not blur the fundamental difference between a soldier in uniform who has been deployed and public opinion: "Some other people will ask me, 'Hey, we hope that you will not be obliged to go outside, you know.' So I tell them that I have been over there twice. 'Twice?' OK, OK, once can be accepted, but twice, it's like, 'Ah!'"[32] (F33). The interviewee used nonverbal language to complete his answer, twisting his hand beside his head, meaning that "they" – the civilians asking him questions about his singular job – thought he lost his mind for having gone to Afghanistan twice. For soldiers, there is a clear distinction between their role as a soldier – "It's our job, you know"[33] (F33) – and the perception of the Canadian population, the "civilians" with whom they have conversations about the mission in Afghanistan – conversations all of them try to avoid as much as possible: "They don't understand" is the general reaction of the CF members.[34]

Often soldiers returning from Afghanistan describe the reality of their experiences as quite different from that in official statements. For example, a soldier was proudly saying, given the diversity of the army (changing from training in deserts of snow to deserts of sand), "Canadians are recognized to do good work"[35] (F30). "The Canadian Army is better trained, better prepared, has a better ethics code" (F34). In a detailed analysis, F35 explained the impact of combat missions on the pride that Canadian soldiers gain from doing their job; this pride provides the motivation to submit a request for another mission and even to enrol in the CF. F15 brags about the professionalism of soldiers, even while under extreme conditions: "We have a high reputation, a high reputation because we're known as professional soldiers. A lot of the other militaries have a lot of extra kit that I guess you could say that they rely on, where we rely on skills that we're trained, as opposed to machinery that can do the job for us. So they have a high regard for us" (F15).

Combat, and the extent of their combat-related knowledge and professionalism, became the primary distinction of CF members. They take pride in "doing their job well," and when asked, "What is your job?," the vast majority answer, "To help the people by eliminating the enemy." They insist on the tension between their positive experience, related to victories and increased self-confidence, and their fear of not being able to do their job right, to be a soldier: "Because I came home, I had to leave my friends at war. I didn't get to finish the tour myself, which was a lifelong dream. I actually started drinking pretty heavily … because I didn't, I didn't care anymore. I was just, I got home and I, there was no option to go back and it looked like the tour was winding down. So I had a lot of issues" (F15).

After a combat-related injury forced this soldier to come home prematurely, not being able to return to combat left him with feelings of guilt and uselessness that had a substantial impact on his identity as a soldier and on his mental health.

Furthermore, soldiers who face this tension between the public understanding of a humanitarian mission and their personal experiences of a combat mission often look for public outlets to express their confusion and address the disparities. Blogs, video posts, autobiographies, and responses to articles and media publications are filled with a range of soldier's tales, from simple personal accounts of how they felt or what they did, to stories laced with heavily ideological vocabulary. These soldiers share a common target in their mass communication responses: the references to Afghanistan as a humanitarian effort. The soldiers are portrayed to the public as professional models of Canada's exemplary military values, but these soldiers argue the necessity of armed conflict for mission success.

Bosnia[36] and Rwanda[37] are often used as examples of the failure of missions based on humanitarian objectives. General Dallaire, commander in chief of UN forces in Rwanda and a high-ranking officer with the experience and power necessary to succeed in his occupation, admits that he too was part of the idealistic population who believed good intentions could win over humanitarian disasters: "Nous étions à la veille d'un cataclysme et qu'une fois enclenché, aucun moyen ne permettrait de le contrôler."[38] General Dallaire's testimony on the failure of a combat-free peacekeeping effort brought reality to a population who believed that the Canadian military could save the world with their good intentions. A similar answer, articulated differently, can be found in a soldier's confrontation with his core role and identity: "Afghanistan has revived our country's pride in its military. Also, it was the reminder we soldiers needed. We remembered that we were soldiers, meant to fight wars and not dig Toronto out of a snowbank or just watch as dozens of civilians are butchered while we can't do anything about it because the UN wouldn't let us (Rwanda, anyone?)."[39] Rwanda is used as the prime example of employing soldiers without giving them the authority to fight back in a doomed employment of the CF. This member stresses the importance of combat in the soldier's identity: fighting natural disasters is a petty task for a soldier trained to fight a targetable enemy. By stripping soldiers of their ability to fight, they are left unable to fulfil the values that comprise their identity as a soldier.[40]

The transition mission in Afghanistan was an important part of the soldiers' positive image as contributors on the international scene.[41] This point of view is shared by all soldiers I interviewed and reveals the impact of these changes from the perspective of the troops in the battlefield. The changes in foreign policy objectives have dramatic and direct impact on soldiers' identity. Although most analysts stress the impact on the troops of losses in personnel and monetary costs, the soldiers interviewed do not seem to view this as a loss. They seem to see a greater loss in doing peacekeeping than peace building, as "war-fighting": "No Canadian can be expected to die on behalf of peace for some foreign country whose citizens don't want it kept. Therefore, by changing the essential purpose of the CF from war-fighting to peacekeeping, the discipline and teamwork that makes the CF such a useful instrument for peacekeeping is undermined."[42] This point of view is of the soldiers who are fighting out there. When asked, "What is the CF reputation on the international scene?," they all answer that when they are not allowed to engage, "The guys are useless" (F4).

From War to Peace: Conclusion

If the most common source of self-gratification is the ability to do their job, to do what they are trained for, to fight under fire,[43] soldiers insisted on accomplishing this duty professionally. In their eyes, professionalism distinguishes them on the international scene among their allies. While using slightly different words, all interviewees discussed the professionalism of their troops under fire, often by comparing themselves to other allies who are "cowboys" (F29). They thought it gave them an "excellent reputation" (F40), a feeling of competence, of control over the situation. This expresses a shift in paradigm: the more they enter combat, the more they show professionalism. To be a good ambassador to the world, to do their job well, to help with the reconstruction of Afghanistan, to be the perfect representative of Canadian politics, the troops feel they must have recourse to force in a way that is equal to no other army. This is the source of their pride; this is what gives them importance, hence, a better chance to impose themselves and win the war – in the broad sense of the term: to win the hearts of Afghans and to hunt down the insurgents. If Canadians wish to impose themselves on the international scene, they must find occasions similar to the 2006 military push in Kandahar, according to the troops. This is where they will find their motivation, this is where they will do their job, and this is where they will be in full alignment with international politics without jeopardizing their soldier identity, hence, their own well-being.

International politics are often based on public opinion that sees political failure in recourse to violence: for postmodern states, war is a "sign of political failure,"[44] meaning that the more peaceful communicative approach has failed. "Canadians' long-standing and widespread support of peacekeeping, as well as the Canadian elite's justification of the use of military force in casting it in peacekeeping terms, highlights the prevalence of this postmodernist strategic culture."[45] Where the population and the policy-makers express a sense of failure, the Canadian Forces soldiers express a sense of success. One soldier explained that it is easier to get along and to share with other men in uniform, even from another country, because it feels "like if we have known each other for years" (F1), rather than with civilians from their own village. For these soldiers, there is no doubt that the war in Afghanistan enhanced the reputation of the Canadian population among the allies and finally put the country in the game of international politics. They feel they had a role to play in this, and they played it well; the word "proud" in English and "fiers" in French emerged in the vast majority of the interviews.

Conclusion

The international politics changed and the soldiers expressed their worry to be tasked, in the future, to participate in peacekeeping missions: "We are the children of Afghanistan" (F36),[46] one said. Another soldier perceived the peacekeeping missions as being put in a position "where the actions that I know would be right … would be not allowed" (F10). The hesitation in this soldier's answer shows his fear of offending the interviewers' sensitivity. It shows a self-consciousness about thinking differently from the others: the mask, the soldier identity, has stuck to his face and he can no longer remove it. This core soldier identity takes over civilian identity. It looks as if the Land Forces are halfway along the full spectrum of training for the "Army of tomorrow," if the aim is to allow soldiers to be physically and mentally "ready and able to undertake operations along a continuum that encompasses offensive, defensive and stability operations conducted along the entire spectrum of conflict."[47] If they express a sense of satisfaction with the way they are trained, if they feel ready to participate in a full spectrum of operations, from humanitarian to combat missions, Canadian Forces soldiers, when interviewed, tend to fear or despise any operations that take advantage only of their "sympathetic, strong, courageous, and especially hospitable" character; they also want to be portrayed as armed soldiers, and align their personal success with mission success, which they measure with effective recourse to force.

Notes

1 This paper analyzes public surveys and testimonies, as well as interviews from a database of seventy-seven testimonies of service members in the combat arms who deployed to Afghanistan between 2002 and 2010, collected on three different military bases across Canada between 2010 and 2011 under a collective agreement between the Royal Military College of Canada and the chief of land staff. To insure confidentiality, the testimonies quoted from this research project are named by the letter F (for file) followed by the interview number (from 1 to 77). The opinions expressed in this article reflect the research of the author and do not necessarily represent the opinion of the Canadian Army, the Canadian Forces, or the Department of National Defence. This chapter would not have been possible without the precious help of Jean-Simon Demers, research assistant.

2 A. D. English, *Understanding Military Culture: A Canadian Perspective* (Montreal and Kingston: McGill-Queen's University Press, 2003), 5.

3 P. A. Keats, "Soldiers Working Internationally: Impacts of Masculinity, Military Culture, and Operational Stress on Cross-Cultural Adaptation," *International Journal for the Advancement of Counselling* 32, no. 4 (2010): 290–303; K. Haitiner and G. Kummel, "The Hybrid Soldier: Identity Changes in the Military," in *Armed Forces, Soldiers and Civil-Military Relations: Essays in Honor of Jürgen Kuhlmann*, ed. J. Kuhlmann and Gerhard Kümmel, 7:75–82 (Wiesbaden: VS Verlag für Sozialwissenschaften, 2009).

4 H. Tajfel, *Human Groups and Social Categories* (Cambridge, UK: Cambridge University Press, 1981); S. A. Haslam, J. Jetten, T. Postmes, and C. Haslam, "Social Identity, Health and Well-being: An Emerging Agenda for Applied Psychology," *Applied Psychology: An International Review* 58, no. 1 (2009): 1–23.

5 United Nations Association in Canada, "UN Peacekeeping," http://www.unac.org/peacekeeping/en/un-peacekeeping/definition/.

6 Ibid.

7 R. W. Murray and J. McCoy, "From Middle Power to Peacebuilder: The Use of the Canadian Forces in Modern Canadian Foreign Policy," *American Review of Canadian Studies* 40, no. 2 (2010): 177.

8 D. Stairs, "Myths, Morals, and Reality in Canadian Foreign Policy," *International Journal* 58, no. 2 (2003): 239–56.

9 Ekos Research Associates, *Canadians' Views of the Canadian Forces and Its Elements – 2012*, Final Report (Ottawa: Ekos Research Associates, March 2012), 27.

10 Ibid., 27.

11 Based on the sample described in note 1.

12 G. T. Howell and Martin Yelle, eds., *Your Say: Spring 2009 Core Section Results* (Ottawa: Director General Military Personnel Research and Analysis, 2011).

13 L. Windsor, D. Charters, and B. Wilson, *Kandahar Tour: The Turning Point in Canada's Afghan Mission* (Mississauga, ON: Wiley & Sons, 2008), 265, 20, 21, 214; R. McCutcheon and J. Derksen, "Canada's Role in Afghanistan: Submissions to the Manley Panel," *Peace Research* 39, no. 1 (2007): 94–149: V. J. Curtis, "Human Security and the Canadian Armed Forces [National Defence vs Foreign Affairs: Culture Clash in Canada's International Security Policy?]," *International Journal* 60, no. 1 (2005): 275.

14 Although this sample described in note 1 does not pretend to be representative, it offers insights on the way that the soldier identity is being constructed and modulated through self-disclosure in the context of the discourse analysis of testimonies of war.

15 A. Ledger, "Exploring Multiple Identities as Health Care Ethnographer," *International Institute for Qualitative Methodology* 9, no. 3 (2010): 303; F. Rapport, "Summative Analysis: A Qualitative Method of Social Science and Health Research," *International Journal of Qualitative Method* 9, no. 3 (2010): 288.

16 S. Roussel and C. Robichaud, "L'état postmoderne par excellence? Internationalisme et promotion de l'identité internationale du Canada," *Études internationales* 35, no. 1 (2004): 149–70; S. Roussel and D. Morin, "Les multiples incarnations de la culture stratégique et les débats qu'elles suscitent," in *Culture stratégique et poli-*

tique de défense: L'expérience canadienne, ed. Stéphane Roussel, 17–42 (Outremont: Athéna, 2007); R. Rempel, *Dreamland: How Canada's Pretend Foreign Policy Has Undermined Sovereignty* (Montreal and Kingston: McGill-Queen's University Press, 2006); J. L. Granatstein, *Whose War Is It? How Canada Can Survive in the Post-9/11 World* (Toronto: HarperCollins, 2007); P. Lagassé and J. Massie, "Canadian Security Policy: New Perspectives and Debates," *International Journal* 64, no. 3 (2009): 601; J. McCormick, "Democratizing Canadian Foreign Policy," *Canadian Foreign Policy Journal* 13, no. 1 (2006): 113–31.

17 S. A. H. Bélanger, "Regards canadiens sur la guerre d'Afghanistan," in *Expériences de guerres: Regards, témoignages, récits*, ed. Renée Dickason, 67–86 (Paris: Éditions Mare et Martin, 2012).

18 L. Hémon, *Maria Chapdeleine* (1916; Montreal: BQ, 1990), 203; H. Beaugrand, *La Chasse-galerie* (1900; Montreal: BQ, 1998), 105; J. Vaillancourt, *Les Canadiens errants* (Montreal: Cercle du livre de France, 1954), 250; G. Guèvremont, *Le Survenant* (1945; Montreal: Fides, 2004), 238.

19 Vaillancourt, *Les Canadiens errants*, 90.

20 I. Hope, *Dancing with the Dushman* (Winnipeg: Canadian Defence Academy Press, 2008), 3: "With these competent and hardened soldiers, together with supporting artillery, we could do it."

21 P. Franklin, *A Long Walk Home* (Victoria, BC: Brindle and Glass, 2007), 59.

22 Stéphanie A. H. Bélanger, "The Testimony of a War Amputee from Afghanistan: Discursive Myths and Realities," in *Shaping the Future: Military and Veteran Health Research*, ed. A. B. Aiken and S. A. H. Bélanger, 255–68 (Winnipeg: Canadian Academy Press, 2011).

23 R. Kilburn, "Afghanistan Update," *Canadian Military Journal* 9, no. 4 (2009): 106.

24 Vaillancourt, *Les Canadiens errants*, 250.

25 M. Goodspeed, "Canada and New Paradigms of War," *Canadian Military Journal* 9, no. 1 (2009): 113.

26 R. J. Walker, *Duty with Discernment: CLS Guidance on Ethics in Operations* (Kingston, ON: Directorate of Land Concepts and Design, 2009); M. Goodspeed, "Canada and New Paradigms of War," 113.

27 Murray and McCoy, "From Middle Power to Peacebuilder," 171–7; See also Windsor, Charters, and Wilson, *Kandahar Tour*, 214.

28 J. Massie, "Regional Strategic Subcultures: Canadians and the Use of Force in Afghanistan and Iraq," *Canadian Foreign Policy Journal* 14, no. 2 (2008): 23.

29 Curtis, "Human Security and the Canadian Armed Forces," 274.

30 H. Segal, "Canadian Foreign Policy and the International Environment," *Canadian Speeches* 16, no. 3 (2002): 41.

31 Stairs, *Myths, Morals, and Reality*, 239.

32 Our English translation from the French: "Y'en a d'autres qui vont me demander 'Aye on espère que tu seras pas pris pour aller à l'extérieur là,' Fait que là j'leur dit comme quoi que ça fait deux fois j'y vas ben là-bas, deux fois? OK, OK, une fois des, t'sé ça peut passer, deux fois c'est comme 'Ah?'" (F37).

33 Our English translation from the French: "C'est not' job, là" (F37).

34 It was the case of twenty-two out of thirty in this study; the other ones simply did not mention this tension, but none said it did not exist.

35 Our English translation from the French: "Les Canadiens n'ont pas une grosse armée mais elle est multifonctionnelle. À cause de la diversité des climats au Canada, l'armée doit être capable d'être déployée dans n'importe quelle condition, du désert de sable au désert de neige. Elle est donc une des plus polyvalentes et mieux équipées pour faire face à toutes sortes de situations. Les soldats Canadiens aussi sont reconnus pour faire du bon travail" (F30).

36 A. Loyd, *My War Gone By, I Miss It So* (New York: Atlantic Monthly, 2000); B. Stewart, *Broken Lives: A Personal View of the Bosnian Conflict* (London: Harper-Collins 1993); F. Doucette, *Empty Casing: A Soldier's Memoir of Sarajevo under Siege* (Vancouver: Douglas & McIntyre, 2008); R. Richardson, D. Verweij, and D. Winslow, "Moral Fitness for Peace Operations," *Journal of Political and Military Sociology* 32 (2004): 99–113.

37 M. Berdal, "The United Nations, Peacebuilding, and the Genocide in Rwanda," *Global Governance* 11 (2005): 115–30; P. Kerstens, "'Voice and Give Voice': Dialectics between Fiction and History in Narratives on the Rwandan Genocide," *International Journal of Francophone Studies* 9 (2006): 93–110; M. Enright, "Lost Mission to Rwanda: An Interview with General Romeo Dallaire," *Queen's Quarterly* 107 (2000): 412–25.

38 R. Dallaire, *J'ai serré la main du diable* (Outremont, QC: Libre-Expression, 2000), 278–9; J. Castonguay, *Rwanda: Souvenirs, témoignages, réflexions* (Montreal: Art Global 2005); G. Courtemanche, *Un dimanche à la piscine à Kigali* (Montreal: Boréal 2000); R. Lemarchand, "Power and Stratification in Rwanda: A Reconsideration," *Cahiers d'études africaines* 6, no. 24 (1966): 592–610; P. Uvin, "Ethnicity and Power in Burundi and Rwanda: Different Paths to Mass Violence," *Comparative Politics* 31, no. 3 (April 1999): 253–71; P. Verwimp, "Machetes and Firearms: The Organization of Massacres in Rwanda," *Journal of Peace Research* 43, no. 1 (January 2006): 5–22.

39 D. Patrick, "5 Canadians Killed in Afghanistan, Roadside Bomb Hits Armoured Vehicle," *CBC News*, 30 December 2009.

40 R. Dallaire, "Soldier, Senator, Humanitarian," interview, *Interculture Magazine* 2, no. 3 (2009): 2; Parrainé par le Gouvernement du Canada (Affaires étrangères et commerce international).

41 Hope, *Dancing with the Dushman*, 47.

42 Curtis, "Human Security and the Canadian Armed Forces," 275.

43 S. A. H. Bélanger, *A New Coalition for a Challenging Battlefield* (Kingston, ON: CDA, 2012).

44 P. Vennesson, "Les États-Unis et l'Europe face à la guerre: Perceptions et divergences dans l'emploi de la force armée," *Études internationales* 36, no. 4 (2005): 541.

45 C. Létourneau and J. Massie, "Un symbole à bout de souffle? Le maintien de la paix dans la culture stratégique canadienne," *Études internationales* 37, no. 4 (2006): 572.

46 Our English translation from the French: "On est les enfants d'Afghanistan" (F36).

47 A. B. Godefroy, ed., *Land Operations 2021 Adaptive Dispersed Operations: The Force Employment Concept for Canada's Army of Tomorrow* (Kingston, ON: Directorate of Land Concepts and Design, 2007).

8

Health-Care Management in the Canadian Forces Health Services: A Comparative Study on Military and Civilian Health Leadership Skills

BRENDA GAMBLE, OLENA KAPRAL, AND PAUL YIELDER

Abstract

Three national surveys of Canadian health-care leaders were conducted to determine the views on the leadership skills necessary to lead in the hospital and community/home-care setting. The electronic questionnaire distributed to members of the Canadian College of Health Leaders ($N = 513$), Canadian Home Care Association ($N = 109$), and Canadian Forces Health Services Group ($N = 94$) between 2010 and 2012 included items on demographic and employment characteristics and on leadership competencies. Competencies identified by all three groups were related to the concept of emotional intelligence. EI as a psychodynamic tool provides the skills for health-care managers who lead integrated teams to provide an environment that ensures that each profession has an opportunity to contribute to its fullest capabilities.

Introduction

During the last fifteen years the concept of emotional intelligence (EI) has garnered much attention in leadership circles as an important interactive psychodynamic tool that contributes to successful leadership in the workplace.[1] EI is the capacity to recognize our own feelings and those of others, as a motivational complex, and also to recognize and manage emotions in both ourselves and in others.[2] EI is a combination of interpersonal (i.e., social awareness and relationship management) and intrapersonal (i.e., self-awareness and self-management) skills that are learnt and developed throughout one's life in a maturational continuum that fundamentally supports intrinsic self-awareness and the capacity for relatedness to others.[3] Many observers believe that these skills provide leaders with the capacity to understand and motivate their teams. The importance and the usefulness of EI have been further highlighted in the health-care leadership literature[4] associated with the leadership and development of integrated teams.[5] EI is also reported to be a useful tool to deal with conflict by enhancing communication insight and awareness among team members, thereby enabling discrimination and enhancing choice in complex situations.[6]

Our team conducted three national surveys of Canadian health-care leaders from both the military and civilian sectors to determine views on the leadership skills necessary to lead in the hospital and community/home-care setting. The skills identified are closely aligned to the concept of emotional intelligence (EI). In light of the policy direction that supports inter-professional collaborative practice (IPCP) (i.e., integrated teamwork), the recognition of these skills by health-care leaders is timely.

Results from the national study are presented, and a discussion follows on the implications of the results for EI and IPCP. Results are relevant to both civilian and military health-care leaders in light of the fact that many members of the Canadian Forces Health Services Group (CFHSvcsGp) work in the civilian sector and will do so after retirement from the Canadian Forces. In addition, veterans who access care in the civilian sector will also potentially benefit from an approach of care that supports EI and IPCP.

National Surveys of Military and Civilian Health-Care Leaders

Objective of the Study

The national surveys were completed in partnership with the CFHSvcsGp, the Canadian Home Care Association (CHCA), and the Canadian College of Health Leaders (CCHL). The overall purpose of this study was to determine the employment and practice patterns of Canadian health-care service leaders across the civilian and military sectors, the work they do, and the perceptions of the skills needed to fulfil their duties. In addition, as indicated, the survey was also intended to identify the skills and competencies needed for successful health-care leadership.

Methods

Data were collected using a self-administered electronic questionnaire distributed to members of the CFHSvcsGp, CCHL, and the CHCA. The questionnaire items were the same for each group, with minor changes made to the demographic items to appropriately describe each sample. For example, CFHSvcsGp members were asked to identify what part of the Canadian Forces they served in. The questionnaire included variables related to demographics (e.g., Are you Regular Forces, Reserve Forces, Cadet, Other?), educational background (e.g., What type of clinical/technical training do you have?), employment history (e.g., Which of the following types of organizations best describes the health-care sector in which you currently work [or most recently worked in?]), and previous experience in the health-care system (e.g., In your current position, do you directly manage health-care workers who provide direct patient services [e.g., assessment, monitoring, treatment]?). Respondents were asked a series of questions to determine their views on the skills and competencies needed to lead in health care today (e.g., The skills/competencies required to lead/manage in the community are the same as the skills/competencies required to lead/manage in hospitals). Once results were collected, the data cleaning and descriptive analysis was completed using Statistical Analysis Software (SAS). Responses to the question, "What do you feel are the top five skills/competencies needed to lead/manage successfully within the next five to ten years?" were mapped against the National Centre for Healthcare Leadership (NCHL) Competencies Framework,[7] which identifies the competencies for health-care leadership now and in the future. Broad-base trends were identified and results were aggregated into five categories.

Results

Table 8.1 provides an overview of the number of responses for each group and the dates the questionnaire was administered.

This next section provides information on the employment characteristics for the CFHSvcs, the CHCA, and the CCHL.

Military Sector

CFHSvcs: The majority of those who responded identified working in the Canadian Army (71.4%). Overall 72.4% are commissioned officers; 87% work in health services with 55.4% indicating that they work in Canadian Forces clinics; 22.3% provide direct patient care, 27.6% identified their role as a manager, and 5.0% as a director, while 11.7% identified the role of professional practice leader or program coordinator.

Civilian Sector

CCHL: The majority of respondents work in the hospital and institutional sector (41.4%), 20.9% in government, 11.0% in consulting, 8.2% in the community sector, and 18.5% indicating the category other. Respondents were asked to select a title that best described their current, or most current, position in health care. The majority of respondents (77.2%) selected a management title, with 60.8% identifying as a top-level manager. Responsibilities included management (21.7%), management and planning (20.9%), or clinical and management (29.2%).

Table 8.1 | Group and number of responses

Date	Group	Responses (N)
January–May 2010	Canadian College of Health Leaders	513
August–December 2010	Canadian Home Care Association	109
May–June 2011	Canadian Forces Health Services	94

CHCA: The majority of respondents work in the community sector (83.0%), while 12.8% work in government and 4.3% work in other sectors; 67% identified having a top-level manager title (president, vice-president, CEO, etc.); the majority of respondents (42.9%) had both clinical and managing responsibilities, 22.4% had both managing and planning responsibility, and 18.4% had only managing responsibilities.

The CCHL, CHCA, and the CFHSvcs members were asked to list the top five skills/competencies needed to successfully lead in the next five to ten years. The results from this question are illustrated in figure 8.1. Respondents identified interpersonal and intrapersonal skills that closely align with the concept of emotional intelligence.

Discussion

The importance and usefulness of EI is that it provides another insightful perspective into the dynamics of inter-professional collaborative practice (IPCP). IPCP is "an inter-professional process for communication and decision making that enables the knowledge and skills of care providers to synergistically influence the client/patient care provided."[8] IPCP is a policy direction supported by government, health-care providers, and patients to deliver safer and more efficient care.[9] Key to IPCP is the ability of health-care providers to work together in integrated health teams.[10] The implementation of IPCP is not without its challenges.

The lack of management support has been identified as a key barrier to the successful implementation of IPCP.[11] Leaders can play a pivotal role in breaking down a number of the barriers to IPCP by facilitating the opportunity for health-care providers to work collaboratively in an environment that supports mutual respect for the skills and knowledge of each health-care provider. For example, health-care leaders can support health-care providers from different professions who work together in integrated teams to communicate effectively.

Historically, training and educational models for the health professions have been designed to train each profession separately (i.e., uni-professional education or silo education). Each professional group is socialized into a particular area of

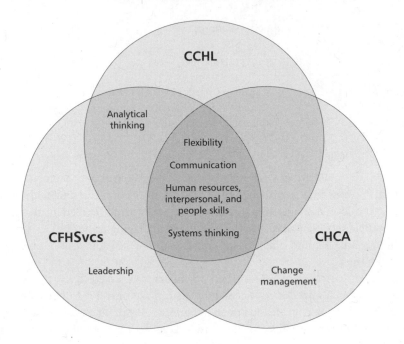

Figure 8.1 | A comparison of the skills/competencies needed to successfully lead in the civilian and military sector

expertise and knowledge and, to varying degrees, learns to protect its role as the result of conflict and miscommunication.[12] EI is a psychodynamic tool that provides the skills for health-care leaders (managers) who lead integrated teams to provide an environment that ensures that each profession has an opportunity to contribute to its fullest capabilities.

Studies have also demonstrated that those with little clinical experience (e.g., recent graduates, residents, etc.) are hesitant to fully communicate with the other team members to express their concerns or seek advice.[13] Clearly, social awareness could potentially provide a means of dealing with the emotions of the less experienced team members and assist them in recognizing the value they can bring to the team. Therefore EI is a valuable tool for health-care leaders who lead integrated teams to support effective communication and conflict resolution among team members.

Clearly those who responded are aware of the "emotion work" that it takes to lead. Previous research on "emotion work" has focused on the doctor–nurse relationship and little has been done to examine "emotion work" across other professional cultures (e.g., orthopedic surgeons and physiotherapists) and interprofessional settings (e.g., community/home and hospital).

Conclusion

Respondents in both the military and civilian sectors across the community/home and hospital settings all identified skills that align with the concept of EI. In light of the policy directions that support both IPCP and the shift of care from the hospital to the community/home, EI can be viewed as a useful concept for health-care leaders responsible for leading integrated teams to address conflict and miscommunication. Additional research is needed to examine the "emotion work" of diverse teams that include a variety of health-care workers to increase awareness of the usefulness of EI and to enhance team functioning and integration of the expertise of team members. The awareness of those health-care leaders who responded to our surveys of the importance of EI is a first step to implementing strategies to successfully lead integrated teams. The effectiveness of integrated teams is key to the delivery of safe and efficient care in the hospital and community/home. EI provides an additional skill set insight for military and civilian health-care leaders to enhance the delivery of care.

Notes

1 Daniel Goleman, Richard Boyatis, and Annie McKee, "Primal Leadership: The Hidden Driver of Great Performance," *Harvard Business Review* December (2001): 2–11; Goleman, *Working with Emotional Intelligence* (New York: Bantam Books, 2004).

2 Hay Group, "Emotional Intelligence … Because Being Clever Isn't Enough," http://www.haygroup.com/leadershipandtalentondemand/your-challenges/emotional-intelligence/index.aspx, accessed 6 November 2012.

3 S. I. Pfeiffer, "Emotional Intelligence: Popular But Elusive Construct," *Roeper Review* 23 (2011): 138–43; M. Jasper and M. Jumaa, "Leadership for Emotional Intelligence," in *Effective Healthcare Leadership,* ed. M. Jasper, and M. Jumaa, 138–43 (Oxford, UK: Blackwell Publishing, 2005).

4 Jasper and M. Jumaa, "Leadership for Emotional Intelligence"; Claudia S. P. Fernandez, Herbert B. Peterson, Shelly W. Holmström and AnnaMarie Connolly, "Developing Emotional Intelligence for Healthcare Leaders," in *New Perspectives and Applications,* ed. AnnaMaria Di Fabio (2012), doi:10.5772/31940; Susan H. Taft, "Emotionally Intelligent Leadership in Nursing and Health Care Organizations" (Jones & Bartlett Learning, 2012); Brenda Freshman and Louis Rubino, "Emotional Intelligence: A Core Competency for Health Care Administers," *Health Care Manager* 20, no. 4 (2002): 1–9.

5 A. McCallin and A. Bamford, "Interdisciplinary Teamwork: Is the Influence of Emotional Intelligence Fully Appreciated?," *Journal of Nursing Management* 15, no. 4 (2007): 386–91.

6 Jenny Godley and Shelly Russell-Mayhew, "Interprofessional Relationships in the Field of Obesity: Data from Canada," *Journal of Research in Interprofessional Practice and Education* 1, no. 2 (2010): 90–108; Juan-Jose Beunza, "Conflict Resolution

Techniques Applied to Interprofessional Collaborative Practice," *Journal of Interprofessional Care* 2 (2013): 110–2.

7 National Centre for Healthcare Leadership, "NCHL Health Leadership Competency Model," http://www.nchl.org/static.asp?path=2852,3238.

8 Daniel Way, Linda Jones, Bruce Baskerville, and Nick Busing, "Primary Health Care Services Provided by Nurse Practitioners and Family Physicians in Shared Practice," *Canadian Medical Association Journal* 165, no. 9 (2001): 1210–14.

9 World Health Organization, "Framework for Action on Interprofessional Education and Collaborative Practice," produced by Health Professions Networks Nursing and Midwifery Human Resources for Health (2010).

10 Beunza, "Conflict Resolution Techniques."

11 Charles Engel and Elin Gursky, "Management and Interprofessional Collaboration," in *Interprofessional Collaboration: From Policy to Practice in Health and Social Care*, ed. Audrey Leathard, 44–55 (New York: Brunner-Routledge, 2003).

12 Pippa Hall, "Interprofessional Teamwork: Professional Cultures as Barriers," *Journal of Interprofessional Care* 19, no. 1 (2005): S188–96.

13 Y. Kyratsis, R. Ahma, and A. Holmes. "Making Sense of Evidence in Management Decisions: The Role of Research-Based Knowledge on Innovation Adoption and Implementation in Healthcare," *Implementation Science* 7, no. 22 (2012), doi:10.1186/1748-5908-7-22; Debby Bright, Wendy Walker, and Julian Bion, "Clinical Review: Outreach – A Strategy for Improving the Care of the Acutely Ill Hospitalized Patient," *Critical Care* 8 (2004): 33–40.

9

Canadian Forces Nursing Officer Pediatric Clinical Preparedness

STEPHANIE MARIE SMITH

Abstract

Canadian Forces nursing officers (CFNOs) must be prepared to provide life-sustaining interventions for casualties on combat and humanitarian missions, delivered in austere environments with limited resources and staffing. This qualitative research project asked, "How clinically prepared are CFNOs to treat children in disasters?" I conducted twenty-two face-to-face interviews with CFNOs. Participants felt a lack of preparedness to treat children; they perceived clinical pediatric training, education, and experience before deployment to be insufficient and to receive an inadequate focus by Canadian Forces Health Services (CFHSvcs). Recommendations for CFNOs, the chief of nursing services, and the CFHSvcs to enforce clinical preparedness for deployments include affording CFNOs the opportunity to gain pediatric experience and having this experience continually supported during their careers, selecting clinical pediatric experts from interested CFNOs and supporting them within their role to maintain competency, reviewing and updating all deployable medical facility response plans, and conducting annual training exercises.

Introduction

The research question "Are Canadian Forces nursing officers adequately prepared to treat pediatric patients in disasters?" emerged from my experiences on past deployments. The purpose of the research question is to evaluate current training and preparedness among Canadian Forces nursing officers (CFNOs) and to provide recommendations to the CFHSvcs to ensure preparedness is achieved.

Literature Review

Incidence of Pediatric Trauma in Disasters

Over the last ten years, the CF has continually deployed nursing officers to human-made and natural disasters across the globe. Many CFNOs have deployed to Afghanistan and with the Disaster Assistance Response Team (DART). Over the last seven years, the DART has deployed three times. These deployments include the earthquake that caused a massive tsunami and subsequent floods in Sri Lanka on Operation Structure, the earthquake in Pakistan on Operation Plateau, and most recently the earthquake in Haiti, on Operation Hestia.[1] The proportion of pediatric victims treated on these deployments ranged from approximately 10% to 50% of the patient population. The incidence of pediatric victims in these natural disasters was much higher than the 10% to 28% seen in Afghanistan.[2] However, the literature indicates that children admitted to the military hospitals in Afghanistan remained there two to three times longer then the adult population.[3] In 2011, at least 800 pediatric patients were admitted with injuries caused by explosives devices, gunshots, motor vehicle crashes, and burns.[4]

The disasters in Afghanistan, Haiti, Pakistan, and Sri Lanka are unique, yet all have the reoccurring theme of pediatric casualties. Although the incidence of pediatric trauma was higher among the countries that saw natural disasters, the war victims in Afghanistan have presented devastating injuries, requiring specialized care.[5] It is therefore reasonable to assume that pediatric patients will compose a significant percentage of future disaster victims.

Preparedness Deficits

In a recent survey conducted at the Intensive Trauma Team Training Course in Vancouver, McLaughlin et al. found that 80% of the CF multidisciplinary team members did not feel confident applying knowledge and skills with pediatric trauma patients before the team members' deployment to Afghanistan.[6] Nurses must be afforded the opportunity to develop essential pediatric competencies to ensure they are equipped to apply the knowledge and skills required in complex disasters. Research evidence suggests a significant gap between nurses' knowledge and skill level working with children compared to the expected competence.[7]

Nurses who lack experience caring for pediatric casualties will not perform adequately in treating children in disasters, and therefore additional education and experience are required for nurses to develop effective pediatric communication and assessment skills. Nurses must also feel comfortable performing medication administration, managing pain, and conducting triage to recognize and prioritize serious injuries that are unique to children.[8] Medication dosages and intravenous fluids must be carefully calculated on the basis of the child's body weight to prevent overdose and to ensure fluid overload does not occur.[9] "It is critical that all health care workers be able to recognize unique signs and symptoms in children that may indicate a life-threatening situation, and then possess the experience and skills to intervene accordingly."[10] It is incumbent upon nurses to establish the knowledge and skills required to fulfil their role during a critical event to ensure children receive the care they deserve.[11]

Consequences of Preparedness Deficits

Children compose a significant portion of the population and are as likely as adults, if not more likely, to sustain serious injuries during disasters.[12] Ramenofsky and colleagues (as cited in the Committee on the Future of Emergency Care in the United States Health Care System [CFECUSHS]) completed a study of 100 pediatric trauma deaths and found that "53 could have survived if the EMS/ trauma system had functioned properly; errors were found in nearly 80 percent of those cases."[13] The literature has indicated that mortality rates among children are increased in disasters because health-care providers are not competent in treating this population and therefore overlook or ineffectively address pediatric needs.[14]

The stresses associated with providing care for injured children frequently place devastating impacts on the psychological well-being of a nurse and may lead to burnout, caregiver fatigue, vicarious traumatization, and post traumatic stress disorder (PTSD).[15] In addition, pediatric patients should not be considered "little adults," and the assumption that children can and should receive the same kind of care as adults must be dismantled if the provision of care during disasters is to be improved.[16]

Summary

Recognizing that disasters are increasing in frequency and severity,[17] improvements in pediatric nursing preparedness and training must be achieved to save lives. Nurses must develop the skills and competencies required to safely care for children in disasters and to promote the well-being of children and of the nurses providing care.[18] Children are more vulnerable than adults in disasters; however, a large majority of health-care providers, including nurses, have reported a lack of experience, resulting in a deficit of knowledge and skill required to safely provide care for this population.[19] Turale identified military nurses "as an untapped resource of expertise,"[20] signifying the importance of skill and knowledge development within all disaster areas among military nurses, who are expected to lead the field. Although deficits in training and experience are noted in the civilian and military nursing populations, it is clear that military nurses will be exposed to the pediatric population in their career. All health-care professionals expected to be proficient at treating children must seek out opportunities in pediatric education, training, and simulation to develop and maintain their competency.

Methodology

This study was conducted within an interpretative framework using a generic qualitative research method in an effort to describe and understand past clinical experiences treating children in disasters.[21] In addition to the qualitative data collected, many questions provided quantitative data that further developed a profile of the participants' deployment activities and experiences and training and education in pediatric treatment.

Participant Demographics

A letter of invitation was sent to all CFNOs through the chief of nursing services staff officer to solicit participation in the research study. Interested CFNOs were directed to contact the researcher directly to maintain confidentiality. Of the twenty-two participants, there were nineteen Regular Force nursing officers (full-time) and three Reserve Force nursing officers (part-time). There were nine generalist nursing officers (GNOs) and thirteen critical care nursing officers (CCNOs) interviewed. Participants' ages ranged from twenty-five to forty-six years old, with a mean of thirty-four years old. There were seven male participants and fifteen female, reflecting the approximate ratio of male to female nursing officers in the CF. All three elements – air, land, and navy – were represented among the participants. All participants completed a consent form before the interview.

Data Collection

Over a ten-week period, twenty-two face-to-face, structured interviews were conducted at bases in Borden, Halifax, Ottawa, Petawawa, and Trenton. A twelve-item questionnaire (see Appendix 9.1) was created by the researcher and was reviewed by four nursing officers for feedback. The questionnaire guided the structured interview. All participants were afforded opportunities to provide additional information or recommendations. The questions were grouped according to participant demographics, past pediatric clinical experience, pediatric education and training, exposure to the loss of a child, psychosocial implications, and training improvement recommendations. Transcripts were created from the audio files and used as tools to interpret what was said during the interviews.

Data Analysis

Content analysis of audio transcripts was conducted, and similar words and ideas were coded and linked from one transcript to another. "Codes are defined as tags or labels for assigned units of meaning to the descriptive or inferential information complied during a study."[22] The coding scheme emerged deductively from pre-existing ideas, questions, and assumptions and inductively from the data produced from the study.[23] Coding involved recognizing an important moment and encoding it as something important before interpreting it. Encoding data organizes the information so that themes or topics can be identified and developed.[24] The data were analyzed and organized into four themes.

Findings

I have categorized the results of the interviews into four themes based on the questions and responses:

1   Clinical pediatric experience before deployment
2   Deployment experience
3   Perceived level of preparedness to treat children
4   Recommended mandatory clinical pediatric training, education, and experience

Clinical Pediatric Experience before Deployment

Of the participants, 60% stated they had no clinical pediatric experience before their first deployment. Of the participants, 82% indicated that they did not anticipate treating children while on deployment and stated that they had been informed by senior medical personnel that they would treat adults only. These data also indicate that of the nineteen Regular Force CFNOs, only five (26%) had completed pediatric training before their first deployment. Of the thirteen participants who had no pediatric experience before their first deployment, three gained clinical pediatric experience before their second deployment as a result of personally requesting the experience.

Deployment Experience

The results associated with deployment experience have been further divided into five sections:

1   Deployment background

  2   Performing clinical pediatric skills
  3   Experiencing the loss of a child
  4   Coping mechanisms
  5   Psychological response to trauma

Deployment Background

Between 2002 and 2011, all participants had deployed to Afghanistan at least once, ten had deployed twice, and three had deployed on three occasions with an average tour length of six months. In addition, eleven participants deployed on humanitarian missions including Operation Structure in Sri Lanka in response to a catastrophic tsunami and subsequent earthquake in 2005, on the USNS *Mercy Ship* to the South Pacific between 2007 and 2009, and most recently on Operation Hestia in Haiti in response to a devastating earthquake in 2010. None of the participants had deployed on Operation Plateau in Pakistan in response to a disastrous earthquake in 2005.

All twenty-two participants affirmed that they treated a significant pediatric population on all deployments, whether in Afghanistan or on a humanitarian mission. Those who had deployed to Afghanistan estimated that 20–25% of the patients they treated were children. Those who had been involved in humanitarian missions estimated that this percentage increased to 30–50%.

Performing Clinical Pediatric Skills

Study participants identified varying levels of comfort with pediatric-related skills while on deployment. The level of comfort often related to the participants' prior training and experience in a clinical pediatric environment. Of the participants, two felt comfortable performing all pediatric skills, both of whom attribute their confidence to their six- to twelve-month employment in a pediatric intensive care unit. The remaining 91% felt uncomfortable performing one or more skills with the pediatric population. Of these participants, all indicated that they felt uncomfortable because they lacked practice conducting the skill, knowledge, or familiarity with specific pediatric equipment.

The majority of participants (85%) felt uncomfortable initiating intravenous and intra-osseous cannulation and collecting blood samples, with only one participant having attempted these procedures before deployment. Setting parameters, troubleshooting, and managing ventilators were procedures that almost half (45%) felt uncomfortable executing. As respiratory therapists control all ventilator changes in civilian hospitals, the participants had not been expected to manage ventilators before. In addition, of the participants who stated they were uncomfortable with ventilator management, none had used the specific type of ventilator before deployment. A further 27% of participants felt uncomfortable managing medication administration, 18% felt uncomfortable inserting urinary catheters,

Table 9.1 | Pediatric clinical skills participants felt uncomfortable performing (*n* = 20)

Pediatric skills	Uncomfortable	Never performed before
Initiating IVs, IOs, or blood collection	85%	79%
Setting parameters and troubleshooting ventilators	45%	45%
Managing medication administration	27%	27%
Inserting urinary catheters	18%	18%
Conducting inline suctioning	18%	18%

Note: IV = intravenous, IO = intraosseous

Table 9.2 | Loss of a child on deployment (*n* = 22)

Loss of a child	Yes	No	NA
Experienced the loss of a child on deployment	91%	9%	
First experience of the loss of a child was on deployment	82%	14%	4%

and 18% felt uncomfortable conducting inline suction, as they had never been trained in these skills before deployment. In addition, 45% of participants indicated that they experienced insufficient pediatric supplies frequently on deployment.

Experiencing the Loss of a Child

As shown in table 9.2, a significant number (*n* = 20; 91%) of the participants experienced the loss of a child under their care while on deployment. Of the two participants who did not experience the loss of a child directly under their care, both stated that many children died on their deployment. Of the participants who experienced this loss, for 82% it was their first experience. Before deployment, three participants, or 14%, had experienced pediatric deaths while in Canada. For one participant, it happened during her final three-month consolidation in university on a Pediatric Intensive Care Unit (PICU); two other participants were reserve nurses who had experienced numerous pediatric deaths during a six-month and one-year employment in a PICU. One participant had never directly experienced the loss of a child.

Of participants who experienced the loss of a child, all stated that it was an extremely emotional experience. A 75% majority stated that on deployment, the loss of a child was more traumatizing than the loss of an adult. The remaining 25%

Table 9.3 | Impact of experiencing the loss of a child on deployment (*n* = 20)

Response to loss of a child	Percentage
Feeling of being emotionally overwhelmed	100%
Internalizing emotions (avoiding discussions about loss)	85%
Externalizing emotions (crying, talking to others, angry outbursts)	15%
Vivid reoccurring images/dreams	10%

stated that the loss of a child was as traumatizing as the loss of an adult. All stated that they felt many of their peers were more traumatized by the loss of a child, especially those with children at home. All participants were asked to elaborate on their experience and how it affected their well-being. Table 9.3 indicates the impacts associated with experiencing the loss of a child.

As illustrated in table 9.3, all participants indicated that they felt emotionally overwhelmed by their experiences with pediatric deaths. Most participants (85%) internalized their emotions and avoided discussing their experiences because they had to "be tough" and continue doing their job. Only 15% externalized their emotions through uncontrolled expressions of crying or angry outbursts or controlled expressions through talking with coworkers, friends, or loved ones. Of the participants, 10% experienced vivid reoccurring thoughts and dreams associated with the death of children.

Coping Mechanisms

All participants used coping mechanisms to manage the stress associated with many traumatizing events that occur while on deployment. Located in a foreign and often dangerous country, and providing care to traumatically injured children, adults, and soldiers who frequently succumbed to their debilitating wounds imposed additional stress for all participants. The visual impact of witnessing the physical injuries caused by improvised explosive devices, bullets, mortars, falling buildings, and debris called upon strong coping mechanisms. Participants indicated the following as their primary coping mechanism: 41% spent time with friends and coworkers to whom they could relate, 32% wrote about their experiences in a journal, and 27% conducted physical fitness training to release negative energy.

Psychological Response to Trauma

Unfortunately in 32% of participants (*n* = 7), despite the use of these coping mechanisms, the stress associated with treating traumatically injured patients and wit-

Table 9.4 | Medical diagnosis of PTSD or compassion fatigue and burnout (*n* = 7)

Medical diagnosis	After first deployment (n = 2)	After third deployment (n = 5)
PTSD	0	2
Compassion fatigue/burnout	2	3

nessing death on numerous occasions exceeded the individual's capacity to cope with the stress. This led to the development of PTSD, compassion fatigue, or burnout, as shown in table 9.4.

Compassion fatigue and burnout were categorized together, as all participants were diagnosed with a component of both. Of these seven participants, two specifically attributed the medical diagnosis to the critical pediatric events they witnessed on deployment, and the remaining five attributed their medical diagnosis to constantly providing care to all traumatically injured patients.

Overall, 100% had treated the pediatric population while on deployment; 91% had felt uncomfortable performing one or more pediatric skills while on those deployments; 91% had experienced the loss of a child while on deployment; 100% coped with stress either by socializing with friends, writing in a journal, or working out; and 32% developed PTSD, compassion fatigue, or burnout related to trauma experiences.

Perceived Level of Preparedness to Treat Children

In relation to preparedness, all twenty-two participants were asked, "On deployment did you ever feel you were not adequately prepared to treat children because of a lack of experience working with the pediatric population?" Of the nineteen Regular Force CFNOs, only 11% felt adequately prepared to treat children. Of all participants, 23% indicated that they felt adequately prepared to treat pediatric patients. The remaining 77% felt unprepared to treat children on deployment. All indicated that a lack of knowledge and limited or no previous training or experience working with this population affected their pediatric preparedness. All participants stated there was a significant lack of awareness about the importance of pediatric experience.

The five participants who indicated they felt prepared stated this was as the result of having significant previous pediatric clinical training. All three reserve CFNOs felt prepared, and all have more than ten years' experience working full-time in critical care environments and conducting rural flight nursing, where they treated the pediatric population approximately 20% of the time. Only two of the nineteen Regular Force CFNOs felt prepared: one had completed final consolidation in a PICU and medical-surgical floor for three months and deployed as a

Table 9.5 | Amount of time required to develop confidence working with children
($n = 22$)

Amount of time required	Percentage of participants recommending the time amount
1 month	5%
1–3 months	36%
3–6 months	45%
6 months or more	14%

GNO; the other gained clinical pediatric experience through a four-month place-ment in a PICU on CCNO consolidation and deployed as a CCNO. This participant deployed with American clinicians, including a pediatric intensivist and multiple respiratory therapists, which he found beneficial, as he was not required to work outside his scope of practice. No other CCNOs who deployed before 2010 had access to these resources; all indicated specifically that ventilators were something they did not feel comfortable using and that having to do so caused a great deal of stress, as they were not prepared to manage this additional skill.

Recommended Mandatory Clinical Pediatric Training and Experience

On the basis of past deployment experience treating children, all participants were asked to recommend an amount of time they felt appropriate for mandatory clinical pediatric experience and preferences for pediatric emergency courses. As illustrated in table 9.5, 45% recommended three to six months' clinical pediatric ex-perience to develop confidence working with children, 36% recommended one to three months, 14% recommended six months or more, and 5% recommended one month. All participants felt that DART members should complete at least a one-month rotation in a pediatric environment to maintain their position annually.

Discussion

The literature indicated that many emergency health-care professionals who are expected to provide care to children are inadequately prepared to do so. This lack of preparedness is associated with deficits in education, training, experience, and awareness. In addition, the lack of organizational awareness significantly affects preparedness and the capacity to provide quality care when planning and policies overlook the pediatric population. It is imperative that hospital emergency depart-ments have the appropriate staff, equipment, supplies, and medications required to treat the pediatric population. Children deserve to receive the same quality care provided to adults; therefore, medical facilities and their staff must be sufficiently educated and trained to recognize the unique anatomical, developmental, and physiological characteristics among pediatric patients and possess the experience, skills, and knowledge to respond effectively.[25]

Children may be the direct, intentional targets in human-made disasters or inadvertent victims during natural disasters. Regardless, statistics from the past twenty years indicate that children are at greater risk during disasters than adults. In the war in Afghanistan, the earthquakes in Haiti and Pakistan, and the tsunami in Sri Lanka, children composed either a significant portion or the majority of people affected. "Children under 18 represented 39% of the overall population of the eight countries hardest hit by the December 2004 tsunami."[26] CFNOs have deployed to all of these disasters, treating many pediatric victims requiring medical attention. Learning from experiences and examining shortfalls are essential for ensuring that all staff are adequately prepared and the facility is adequately equipped to provide quality care to children on future missions.

On the Basis of Self-Perceived Readiness, How Clinically Prepared Are CFNOs to Treat Children in Disasters?

"Disaster preparedness is perhaps the single most important factor in disaster management. Planning and preparations involve countless hours of planning, practice and evaluation for the unexpected, as well as the expected, disaster."[27] It is one thing to be inadequately prepared for the unknown; however, it is naive and irresponsible not to prepare for the expected. The literature indicates that children are significantly affected by disasters, so there is no excuse for a lack of preparedness to provide essential medical care for them.

Although all CFNOs were expected to provide care to children when deployed to disasters, this study revealed that a minority, only 23% of the twenty-two CFNOs interviewed, felt adequately prepared to treat children. Of these, all three Reserve Force CFNOs indicated that they felt prepared because of their experience while employed in a pediatric environment. This finding indicates that clinical pediatric experience leads to confidence and a feeling of preparedness when treating children. Reserve Force CFNOs are expected to work for a minimum of ten days a year for the CF, while the remainder of their time is generally spent employed in a civilian hospital gaining valuable clinical experience. Of the nineteen Regular Force CFNOs interviewed, only 11% felt adequately prepared. A study completed on CF clinicians during pre-deployment training in Victoria reflected this statistic: only 11.4% were "familiar" or "very familiar" with pediatric trauma knowledge and skills, and only 20% felt confident applying knowledge and skill components during pediatric trauma.[28] In addition, Claravall conducted a study with four senior nurses in the U.S. Air Force, who found that pediatric experience was severely lacking and that nurses were not adequately prepared to treat children.[29] Claravall's study recommended creating a pediatric trauma module that would "address pediatric medication doses, age-appropriate interventions, and other required pediatric-competent skills such as IV insertions."[30]

Of the CFNOs who did not feel competent providing care for children or performing numerous skills, all attributed this to a lack of training, education, and experience required to develop confidence with this population. The majority of participants (59%) had no clinical pediatric experience before deployment. Of these participants, thirteen had minimal or no pediatric education and clinical training in school or after graduation. Of the 41% who had pediatric experience before deployment, only five of the nineteen (26%) Regular Force CFNOs had previous experience, indicating that the CFHSvcs is not adequately preparing Regular Force CFNOs for deployment.

Overall, these findings suggest that the response capability of CFNOs to treat children safely is significantly impaired. Deficits in pediatric training, education, and exposure are not only a significant concern for CF clinicians; this issue also plagues the majority of civilian clinicians employed in adult-centric medical facilities across North America.[31] "The majority of our health care clinicians are unprepared to provide the necessary clinical support for children in the event of a disaster."[32] A substantial proportion of the emergency physicians, nurses, and paramedics called upon to provide care in a disaster lack the pediatric clinical skills and knowledge required to function optimally when caring for and treating traumatically injured children.[33] More than 90% of children receive emergency care in a non-children's hospital or non-trauma centre, yet the majority of the professionals employed in these facilities and pre-hospital emergency-care providers feel unprepared to treat the pediatric population, because of inadequate exposure to critically ill or injured children.[34]

On the basis of the incidence of pediatric traumas treated on deployments in Afghanistan, Haiti, Pakistan, and Sri Lanka, it is reasonable to conclude that CFNOs must be prepared to provide care to children. Understanding the unique anatomical, physiological, and developmental characteristics of children is essential if errors are to be prevented and optimal care provided. The CFECUSHS[35] has published dramatic study statistics that indicated more than half of 100 pediatric deaths could have been prevented if medical professionals had performed procedures properly. It is unfortunate when children die because of influences that cannot be controlled, yet it is inexcusable when children die because of influences that should and could have been avoided. The perpetual cycle of inadequate preparation could eventually lead to CFNOs providing inappropriate and potentially dangerous care. It is incumbent upon the CFHSvcs to prepare all CFNOs to treat this special population adequately through education, training, and experience. Otherwise, accidental clinical mistakes may lead to fatal impacts.

What Are the Psychological Impacts Associated with Treating Traumatically Injured Children in Disasters?

Disaster nurses are not immune to the psychological and physical stress that accompanies a major traumatic incident, and they certainly "see their share of death, severe injury, desperation, and destruction."[36] Health-care professionals who treat children in disasters will likely witness numerous disturbing critical incidents and emotionally overwhelming tragedies. "A critical incident is a traumatic event of sufficient magnitude to overwhelm the usually effective coping skills of health care or emergency services personnel."[37] The multitude of stressful events that occur on deployment lead to psychological impacts, saturate caregiver coping mechanisms, and mirror what is seen in disaster victims. Everyone responds and copes differently, as "reactions to a disaster are as varied as the individuals that experience them."[38]

As indicated in the findings, the study participants employed coping mechanisms such as socializing and spending time with friends and coworkers, writing in a journal, and conducting physical fitness training to release negative energy. The literature has indicated that nurses who experience overwhelming stress in disasters must seek support from peers, socialize with others, participate in activities that provide a sense of purpose, and attend to personal needs in an attempt to maintain balance.[39] Therefore, I deduce that the majority of CFNOs are using effective techniques to minimize the likelihood of developing medical conditions such as compassion fatigue and burnout. It is incumbent upon supervisors to ensure that nurses are supported in all efforts of maintaining personal well-being.

A significant number (77%) of participants attributed substantial stress to feeling unprepared. This data are relevant, as the literature indicates that a perceived inability to meet patient needs is a significant source of stress for nurses. Unrealistic workloads coupled with insufficient clinical experience, knowledge, and training leads to ineffective patient care. This stress may lead to the development of psychological medical conditions.[40] In addition, the intensity of caring for physically injured trauma victims may alone contribute to nurses' personal stress and lead to developing medical conditions, including burnout, compassion fatigue, or PTSD. Therefore, the additional stress associated with feeling unprepared may precipitate the likelihood of developing these conditions when caring for traumatically injured patients.

Recommendations

On the basis of this discussion, six recommendations are provided:

1 CFNOs must be afforded the opportunity to gain pediatric experience immediately after graduation and have this experience continually supported during their careers.
2 Include the Emergency Nursing Pediatric Courses (ENPC) as a prerequisite for all GNOs, and include the ENPC and Pediatric Advanced Life Support course as a prerequisite for all CCNOs, as these courses provide valuable assessment and treatment strategies for nurses treating the pediatric population.

3   Educate all health services officers on the importance of conducting and supporting subordinates' clinical pediatric training.

4   CFNOs must advocate for clinical pediatric placements, and senior practice leaders must support these requests to ensure that pediatric competency is maintained.

5   Clinical pediatric experts should be selected from interested CFNOs and supported within their role to maintain competency and to mentor CF practitioners.

6   Review and update all deployable CF medical facility response plans to include pediatric equipment and pediatric clinical training.

7   Conduct annual training exercises with DART and Advanced Medical Surgical Capability members to ensure preparedness in dealing with pediatric casualties in disasters.

Appendix 9.1 | Structured Questionnaire for Interviews

1   Please specify on which deployments you treated the pediatric population (e.g., Afghanistan, Haiti, etc.).

2   Did you complete a pediatric placement while training to become a nursing officer (i.e., Consolidation)? If yes, please clarify specific area and length of time.

3   Have you ever completed a pediatric placement while doing Maintenance of Clinical Readiness Program? If yes, please clarify specific area and length of time.

4   Have you taken the Pediatric Advanced Life Support Course or the Emergency Nursing Pediatric Course? If yes, did you find this knowledge valuable while on deployment?

5   Did you feel clinically prepared to treat children while on deployment(s)? If yes, please clarify why you felt prepared. If no, please clarify why you did not feel prepared.

6   Were there specific clinical skills that you did not feel comfortable performing? If yes, please clarify and indicate if you had ever completed these skills before deployment (e.g., IVs, IOs, catheter insertion, med administration/calculations).

7   At any time while on deployment did you feel you were not adequately prepared to treat children because of a lack of experience working with the pediatric population? If yes, please explain what that felt like.

8   Did you experience the loss of a child while on deployment? If yes, please indicate what that experience was like. Was this your first experience of the loss of a child while on deployment?

9 How many months working in a pediatric environment do you feel you would require to develop confidence working with children?
    a One month
    b One to three months
    c Three to six months
    d More than six months

10 Do you think a pediatric component should be encompassed in the Maintenance of Clinical Readiness Program? Please explain why you stated "yes" or "no."

11 Do you feel the Canadian Forces Health Services place an adequate focus on developing clinical skills with the pediatric population? Please explain why you stated "yes" or "no."

12 Would you like to add any other information at this time?

Notes

1 Department of National Defence, "Disaster Assistance Response Team," http://www.cjoc-coic.forces.gc.ca/exp/hestia/index-eng.asp; Y. Kreiss, O. Merin, K. Peleg, G. Levy, S. Vinker, R. Sagi, A. Abargel, C. Bartal, G. Lin, A. Bar, E. Bar-On, M. Schwaber, and N. Ash, "Early Disaster Response in Haiti: The Israeli Field Hospital Experience," *Annals of Internal Medicine* 153, no. 1 (2010): 45–50, http://www.annals.org/article. aspx?articleid=745865; Y. H. Kwak, S. D. Shin, K. S. Kim, W. Y. Kwon, and G. J. Suh, "Experience of Korean Disaster Medical Assistance Team in Sri Lanka after the South Asia Tsunami," *Journal of Korean Medical Science* 21, no. 1 (2006): 143–50, doi:10.3346/jkms.2006.21.1.143; F. Sami, F. Ali, S. H. H. Zaidi, H. Rehman, T. Ahmad, and M. I. Siddiqui, "The October 2005 Earthquake in Northern Pakistan: Pattern of Injuries in Victims Brought to the Emergency Relief Hospital in Doraha, Mansehra," *Prehospital and Disaster Medicine* 24, no. 6 (2009): 535–39, http://annals.org/article.aspx?articleid=745865.

2 A. Beitler, G. W. Wortmann, L. J. Hofmann, and J. M. Goff, "Operation Enduring Freedom: The 48th Combat Support Hospital in Afghanistan," *Military Medicine* 171, no. 3 (2006): 189–93, http://www.ingentaconnect.com/content/amsus/zmm; M. W. Burnett, P. C. Spinella, K. S. Azarow, and C. W. Callahan, "Pediatric Care as Part of the US Army Medical Mission in the Global War on Terrorism in Afghanistan and Iraq, December 2001 to December 2004," *Pediatrics* 121, no. 2 (2008): 261–65, doi:10.1542/peds.2006-3666; K. M. Creamer, M. J. Edwards, C. H. Shields, M. W. Thompson, C. E. Yu, and W. Adelman, "Pediatric Wartime Admissions to US Military Combat Support Hospitals in Afghanistan and Iraq: Learning from the First 2,000 Admissions," *Journal of Trauma, Injury, Infection and Critical Care* 67, no. 4 (2009): 762–68, doi:10.1097/TA.0b013e31818ble15; E. Ginzburg, W. O'Neill, P. Goldschmidt-Clermont, E. de Marchena, D. Pust, and B. Green, "Rapid Medical Relief: Project Medishare and the Haitian Earthquake," *New England Journal of Medicine* 31 (2010): 1–3, doi:10.1056/nejmp1002026; "Half of Haiti Quake Injured Could Be Children,"

Daily Star, 29 January 2010, http://www.thedailystar.net/; K. Shah, S. Pirie, L. Compton, V. McAlister, B. Church, and R. Kao, "Utilization Profile of the Trauma Intensive Care Unit at the Role 3 Multinational Medical Unit at Kandahar Airfield between May 1 and Oct. 15, 2009," *Canadian Journal of Surgery* 54 (2011): S130–34, doi:10.1503/cjs.006611.

3   M. Fuenfer, P. Spinella, A. Naclerio, and K. Creamer, "The U.S. Military Wartime Pediatric Trauma Mission: How Surgeons and Pediatricians Are Adapting the System to Address the Need," *Military Medicine* 174, no. 9 (2009): 887–91, http://www.ingentaconnect.com/content/amsus/zmm.

4   M. Borgmann, R. Matos, L. Blackbourne, and P. Spinella, "Ten Years of Military Pediatric Care in Afghanistan and Iraq," *Journal of Trauma Acute Care Surgery* 73, no. 6 (2012): S509–13, doi:10.1097/TA.0b013e318275477c.

5   Creamer et al., "Pediatric Wartime Admissions."

6   T. McLaughlin, P. Hennecke, N. R. Garraway, D. C. Evans, M. Hameed, R. K. Simons, and J. Doucet, "A Predeployment Trauma Team Training Course Creates Confidence on Teamwork and Clinical Skills: A Post-Afghanistan Deployment Validation Study of Canadian Forces Health Care Personnel," *Journal of Trauma, Injury, Infection and Critical Care* 71, no. 5 (2011): S487–92, doi:10.1097/TA.0b013e318232e9e7.

7   Committee on the Future of Emergency Care in the United States Health System, "Arming the Emergency Care Workforce with Pediatric Knowledge and Skills," in *Emergency Care for Children: Growing Pains*, 151–86 (Washington, DC: National Academies, 2007), http://www.nap.edu/openbook.php?record_id=11655&page=151.

8   Ibid.; Emergency Nurses Association, *Emergency Nursing Pediatric Course Provider Manual*, 3rd ed. (Des Plaines, IL: Emergency Nurses Association, 2004); National Commission on Children and Disasters, *2010 Report to the President and Congress*, AHRQ publication no. 10-M037) (Rockville, MD: Agency for Healthcare Research and Quality, 2010), http://www.childrenanddisasters.acf.hhs.gov/.

9   Illinois Emergency Medical Services for Children, "Pediatric Disaster Preparedness Guidelines," 2005, 3, http://www.luhs.org/depts/emsc/peddisasterguide.pdf.

10 S. Krug, "Testimony of Steven Krug, MD, FAAP on Behalf of the American Academy of Pediatrics," in *Homeland Security Subcommittee on Emergency Preparedness, Science and Technology's Emergency Care Crisis: A Nation Unprepared for Public Health Disasters* (2006), http://www.aap.org/sections/pem/er_readiness_testimony final.pdf.

11 E. B. Hsu, T. L. Thomas, E. B. Bass, D. Whyne, G. D. Kelen, and G. B. Green, "Healthcare Worker Competencies for Disaster Training," *BioMed Central Medical Education* 6, no. 19 (2006): 1–8, doi:10.1186/1472-6920-6-19; A. Penrose and M. Takaki, "Children's Right in Emergencies and Disasters," *Lancet* 367 (2006): 698–9, http://www.thelancet.com.

12 National Commission on Children and Disasters, *2010 Report to the President*.

13 Committee on Future of Emergency Care in the United States Health System, "Arming the Emergency Care," 7.

14 Ibid.

15 M. K. Kearney, R. B. Weininger, and M. L. Vachon, "Self-Care of Physicians Caring for Patients at the End of Life: Being Connected … A Key to My Survival," *Journal of the American Medical Association* 301, no. 11 (2009): 1155–64, doi:10.1001/

jama.2009.352; B. Sabo, "Adverse Psychological Consequences: Compassion Fatigue, Burnout and Vicarious Traumatization; Are Nurses Who Provide Palliative and Hematological Cancer Care Vulnerable?," *Indian Journal of Palliative Care* 14, no. 1 (2008): 23–9, doi:10.4103/0973-1075.41929.

16   G. M. Allen, S. J. Parrillo, J. Will, and J. A. Mohr, "Principles of Disaster Planning for the Pediatric Population," *Prehospital and Disaster Medicine* 22, no. 6 (2007): 537–40, http://pdm.medicine.wisc.edu.

17   S. Briggs, "International Disaster Response," in *International Disaster Nursing*, ed. R. Powers and E. Daily, 351–63 (New York: Cambridge, 2010); M. Kingma, "International Council of Nurses: Disaster Nursing," *Prehospital and Disaster Medicine* 23, no. 1 (2008): 1–2, http://pdm.medicine.wisc.edu.

18   Allen et al., "Principles of Disaster Planning"; International Nursing Coalition for Mass Casualty Education, "Educational Competencies for Registered Nurses Responding to Mass Casualty Incidents," American Association of Colleges of Nursing, 2003, http://www .aacn.nche.edu/leading-initiatives/education-resources/ INCMCECompetencies.pdf.

19   Allen et al., "Principles of Disaster Planning"; Committee on Future of Emergency Care in the United States Health System, "Arming the Emergency Care."

20   S. Turale, "Nurses: Are We Ready for a Disaster?" *Journal of Nursing Science* 28, no. 1 (2010): 8–11, http://www.ns.mahidol.ac.th/english/journal_NS/pdf/vol28/issue1/ sue_turale.pdf.

21   K. Caelli, L. Ray, and J. Mill, "Clear as Mud: Toward Greater Clarity in Generic Qualitative Research," *International Journal of Qualitative Methods* 2, no. 2 (2003): 1–24, http://www.ualberta.ca/~iiqm/backissues/2_2/pdf/caellietal.pdf.

22   J. T. DeCuir-Gunby, P. L. Marshall, and A. W. McCulloch, "Developing and Using a Codebook for the Analysis of Interview Data: An Example from a Professional Development Research Project," *Field Methods* 23, no. 2 (2011): 136, doi:10.1177/1525822X10388468.

23   C. Seale, "Validity, Reliability and the Quality of Research," in *Researching Society and Culture*, ed. C. Seale, 2nd ed. (Thousand Oaks, CA: Sage, 2004), 313.

24   J. Fereday and E. Muir-Cochrane, "Demonstrating Rigor Using Thematic Analysis: A Hybrid Approach of Inductive and Deductive Coding and Theme Development," *International Journal of Qualitative Methods* 5, no. 1 (2006), 1–11, http://www.ualberta.ca/~iiqm/backissues/5_1/pdf/fereday.pdf.

25   Allen et al., "Principles of Disaster Planning"; American Academy of Pediatrics, Committee on Pediatric Emergency Medicine, & American College of Emergency Physicians, Pediatric Committee, "Care of Children in the Emergency Department: Guidelines for Preparedness," *Pediatrics* 107, no. 4 (2001): 777–81, http://pediatrics.aappublications.org/content/107/4/777.full.html; Committee on Future of Emergency Care in the United States Health System, "Arming the Emergency Care"; G. Foltin, M. Tunik, M. Treiber, and A. Cooper, *Pediatric Disaster Preparedness: A Resource for Planning, Management, and Provision of Out-of-hospital Emergency Care* (New York: Center for Pediatric Emergency Medicine, 2008), http://webdoc .nyumc.org/nyumc/files/cpem/u3/pediatric_disaster_ preparedness.pdf; Krug, "Testimony of Steven Krug."

26 J. DeVito and M. Godshall, "Special Populations in Disasters: The Child and Pregnant Woman," in *Disaster Nursing: A Handbook for Practice*, ed. D. S. Adelman and T. J. Legg (Sudbury, MA: Jones and Bartlett, 2009), 58.

27 S. Sonnier, "Communicating in a Disaster," in Adelman and Legg, *Disaster Nursing*, 138.

28 McLaughlin et al., "Predeployment Trauma Team."

29 L. Claravall, "Evaluating Air Force Expeditionary Nursing: Are We Prepared?" (master's thesis, Air War College, Maxwell AFB, AL, 2007), http://www.DTIc.mil/cgi-bin/GetTRDoc?AD=ADA489248.

30 Ibid., 12.

31 S. E. Mace and A. I. Bern, "Needs Assessment: Are Disaster Medical Assistance Teams Up for the Challenge of a Pediatric Disaster?," *American Journal of Emergency Medicine* 25, no. 7 (2007): 762–69, doi:10.1016/j.ajem.2006.12.011.

32 D. Siegal, K. Strauss-Riggs, and A. Costello, *Pediatric Disaster Preparedness Curriculum Development: Conference Report* (Rockville, MD: National Center for Disaster Medicine and Public Health, 2011), 2, http://www.chladisastercenter.org/atf/CF/%7B569B48DC-84E9-4870-8993-073DC4963E8F%7D/NCDMPH%20PEDS%20CONFERENCE%20REPORT_FINAL.pdf.

33 American Academy of Pediatrics, Committee on Pediatric Emergency Medicine, American College of Emergency Physicians, Pediatric Committee, & Emergency Nurses Association Pediatric Committee, "Joint Policy Statement: Guidelines for Care of Children in the Emergency Department," *Pediatrics* 24, no. 4 (2009): 1233–43, doi:10.1542/peds.2009-1807; P. Arbon, "Understanding and Preparing for Disasters and Catastrophic Emergencies," *Nursing and Health Sciences* 11, no. 4 (2009): 333–5, doi:10.1111/j.1442-2018.2009.00494_2.x; Siegal, Strauss-Riggs, and Costello, *Pediatric Disaster Preparedness Curriculum*.

34 M. Gausche-Hill, C. Schmitz, and R. J. Lewis, "Pediatric Preparedness of US Emergency Departments: A 2003 Survey," *Pediatrics* 120, no. 6 (2007): 1229–37, doi:10.1542/peds.2006-3780; Krug, "Testimony of Steven Krug."

35 Committee on Future of Emergency Care in the United States Health System, "Arming the Emergency Care."

36 C. Kleinman and J. Rubino, "The Psychology of Disasters," in Adelmam and Legg, *Disaster Nursing*, 127.

37 Emergency Nurses Association, *Emergency Nursing Pediatric*, 267.

38 Kleinman and Rubino, "Psychology of Disasters," 117.

39 Ibid.

40 R. J. Burke and E. R. Greenglass, "Hospital Restructuring, Work–Family Conflict and Psychological Burnout among Nursing Staff," *Psychology & Health* 16, no. 5 (2001): 583–94, doi:10.1080/08870440108405528; Kearney, Weininger, and Vachon, "Self-Care of Physicians Caring"; S. McNeely, "Stress and Coping Strategies in Nurses from Palliative, Psychiatric and General Nursing Areas," *Health Manpower Management* 22, no. 3 (1996): 10–12, doi:10.1108/EUM0000000004276; Sabo, "Adverse Psychological Consequences."

10

Group for Children and Families Having a Parent with an Operational Stress Injury

NADIA KOHLER AND REBECCA WIGFIELD

Abstract

$E = MC^3$ is a turnkey program for professionals. The therapeutic program focuses on children ages seven through twelve who live with a parent affected by operational stress injury (OSI). The overall purpose of the group intervention approach is to develop the strengths of each family member in order to improve well-being of the individual and of the family as a whole. The program's goal is to end family members' isolation, help children and parents to better understand OSIs and their effects on the family, promote communication within the family, improve relationships between parents and children, and help prevent mental health problems and family violence. At the end of the program, families reported that children expressed themselves more and felt less guilty, children had a better understanding of an OSI, communication within the family was improved, with the help of tools provided, it was still possible to have a good time as a family, parents were no longer isolated, and children realized that they could not cure their parent. Although the results are essentially qualitative, there is potential for researchers to evaluate the program with added psychometric tools. The $E = MC^3$ program was built to meet the needs of military families and has been offered twice to the community of the Canadian Forces Military Base in Valcartier, QC. It has since been nationalized so that all Military Family Resource Centres across Canada can offer the program as well. The two groups in Valcartier consisted of four families each. The first group had children aged nine to twelve and the second, children aged six to ten. The program has six workshops for children, three for parents, and two for the family as a whole. The $E = MC^3$ project is a therapeutic group intervention program for families living with an OSI-affected parent. It includes workshops for children aged seven to twelve, workshops for their parents, and workshops for the family as a whole.

The Story behind $E = MC^3$

The idea for $E = MC^3$ arose eight years ago when a group of partners noticed that several families were coping with an OSI and that there were no services tailored for children and their parents as a unit. In order to meet that need they worked together to develop a project that would offer three parallel support groups: one for CF members who had sustained an OSI, one for spouses, and one for children aged nine to eleven. Each group would address topics relevant to its participants and, on occasion, the groups would combine to discuss certain family aspects.

The project evolved until 2009, when the children's workshops were presented to the Directorate of Military Family Services (DMFS). As a result of that presentation, the Valcartier Family Centre (VFC) received funding to finalize the development of $E = MC^3$ and the tools necessary to offer it nationwide. The first group was offered in 2009 and the program nationalized in 2012 to allow all Military Family Resource Centres to offer it.

What Is $E = MC^3$?

The program name $E = MC^3$ stands for Ensemble pour Mieux Comprendre (Together to Better Understand). The 3 represents the child, father, and mother. The overall goal of the program is to develop each family member's strengths in order to improve the member's well-being as an individual and as part of the family. Specifically, the program works to help break the families' isolation and improve interactions within the family, despite the presence of the OSI. It does this by helping children and parents better understand OSIs and their effects on the family while promoting communication within the family. It can help prevent mental health problems and family violence. The $E = MC^3$ program helps families address OSIs with a family perspective, as opposed to an individual one within a therapeutic group. The themes are understanding operational stress injuries, the parent's role in the family, having fun as a family, discovering internal and external resources, identifying feelings and expressing emotions, and the child's needs and wishes in the family.

Steps to Forming a Group

The $E = MC^3$ program is offered within a group setting in several phases: recruitment (continuous promotion), pre-group interviews, workshops for children, parents, and families, mid-term assessment, post-group interviews, and follow-up support for the families if needed. The program is made up of eleven group meetings: six workshops for children, three for parents, and two for the family as a whole. The workshops welcome participants, discuss a new theory about the OSI, do an activity together, and conclude with an evaluation of the workshop. The family workshops enable each family to spend a good time together and with other families who are experiencing the same thing. The workshops last one to two hours.

Target Audience

The seven to twelve age group has been targeted because these children can read and write, have learned to work in a group, and can better understand abstract concepts, such as a psychological injury. Children under seven have a different level of understanding, while the maturity gap between seven-year-olds and those over twelve is already large, and the needs and language levels are very different for those under seven. If multiple children from the same family participate in the group, one must ensure that each one respects the others and is comfortable expressing an opinion.

Parents

It is critical that parents support the child from beginning to end, to ensure that the child does not feel that the responsibility for changing the family is his or hers. By attending parent and family workshops and continuing the discussion at home on topics addressed in the group, parents show their child that they are there for him or her and that the child can go to them to talk about feelings and ask questions. Through those actions, the parents also work toward the objective of the group, to improve family communication and well-being. With the new family realities, counsellors must adjust to family situations and remain flexible in their choices. For example, if the parents are separated, the reconstituted family may wish to take part in the group: the injured member, the new spouse, and the spouse's children. Participation and involvement of the member with the OSI is essential to the success of the group for the children and family.

Eligibility and Exclusion Criteria

The member with an OSI does not need a medical diagnosis to be eligible to join the group. Since the group addresses OSIs in general, a diagnosis of PTSD is not a selection criterion. What should be given greater consideration is the member's stability, to ensure that he or she will be able to be involved from beginning to end. The exclusion criterion for the group is violence in the family, which must be dealt with first in order to be able to work together as a family on strengthening family ties. Also, high levels of conflict in the parents' relationship or difficulties working in a group may warrant exclusion for the group process. Since active parent participation is strongly recommended, there must be an agreement between the parents, even if they are separated. Three workshops are for parents only and two for the whole family. If the parents' relationship is overly strained and only one parent takes part in the group, it is the child who will pay the price. For example, if the father participates, the child will be able to discuss the group with him; however, when the child is with the mother, the continuity will be broken, because the mother will be unaware of what has been discussed in the group. The child will therefore receive fewer benefits from the group than if both parents were involved.

One must always assess whether or not the child can work well in a group setting. For example, if a child has severe attention deficit hyperactivity disorder (ADHD) and is not taking medication or involved in therapy, it may be hard to take part in the group. However, some of the child's behaviour may be a result of the effects of the OSI. For example, some children may present signs of anxiety, depression, or behavioural problems. Counsellors can expect the group to consist of children affected to differing extents by their parent's OSI. Therefore, each child's ability to function in a group must be assessed accurately. As with children, the group may not be the best intervention option for some parents. For example, parents with alcohol or drug problems or a mental health condition may find it hard to take part in the group. If the group setting is not the ideal option for a child or a parent, the material can also be used to work with a single family in individual counselling sessions.

Literature Review

Effects on the Family

Studies show that mental health disorders in members of the military affect the functioning of the family and may hinder the adaptation and integration of the member within the family.[1] Most studies involve veterans with PTSD, and the literature provides scant useful data about the effects of OSI. However, on the basis of one study, it can be said that the type of mental illness is not a predictor of marked differences in family functioning.[2] Consequently, the effects of an OSI are comparable to the effects of PTSD. Since the term OSI is relatively new, there are several possible definitions. An OSI can be described as "any persistent psychological difficulty resulting from operational duties performed by a Canadian Forces member. The term OSI is used to describe a broad range of problems which usually result in impairment in functioning. OSIs include diagnosed medical conditions such as anxiety, depression, and post traumatic stress disorder (PTSD) as well as a range of less severe conditions, but the term OSI is not intended to be used in a medical or legal context."[3]

The effects of an OSI on family functioning vary from one family to another, but the most common effects are transformation of family roles and responsibilities, increased spousal and family conflict and difficulty resolving conflict, diminished communication and emotional expressiveness within the family, social isolation, and increased risk of secondary traumatic stress in family members. When a soldier has physical or psychological problems, the spouse can assume the role of head of the household and, in so doing, become overburdened with chores and parental responsibilities. The uneven distribution of work, which may be combined with the role of caregiver to the soldier and protector of the children, may cause fatigue, frustration, and anger in the spouse, as well as jeopardize the spouse's mental health.[4] This transformation of roles can sometimes result in children taking on the role of parents despite their young age, and this "parentification" makes them more likely to develop psychological distress and behavioural disorders.[5]

There can also be an increased level of spousal and family conflict as well as a difficulty in resolving conflicts.[6] According to the literature, returning soldiers use aggression more often when trying to resolve conflicts, so a high incidence of physical and psychological violence is reported.[7] The reason is that, since many soldiers draw on feelings of hostility and aggression to survive in combat, they tend to react angrily and violently in situations in which they feel helpless.[8] Such violence undermines family members' feelings of trust and security.[9]

Since emotional detachment and restricted range of affect are manifestations of OSI, it is common for soldiers to find it difficult to connect, express their emotions, and experience affection. Hence there can be a diminishment in communication and emotional expressiveness within the family. Social isolation is also a common trait in OSI-affected families. Since family members do not want to have to justify the soldier's reactions, or are afraid of the potential career consequences of his or her conduct, they withdraw from their social networks.[10] Social isolation is also a form of avoidance: to remain in his or her comfort zone, the soldier develops strategies to avoid leaving home or meeting other people. Moreover, the soldier's fragile health and unpredictable reactions can subject the family to failures (e.g., a cancelled outing). Consequently, family activities, which would normally be a pleasant time, can instead be a source of stress and conflict. Finally, family members can be more at risk of experiencing secondary traumatic stress. Secondary traumatic stress is trauma transmitted by another person.[11] Helping someone who has suffered psychological trauma means sharing stress or traumatizing events, and that can cause spouses and children to develop symptoms similar to the soldier's, such as depression, guilt, anxiety, and aggression.

Effects on the Children

Not all children with an OSI-affected parent will develop emotional problems or have more mental health issues than other children. However, a child's development can be affected by certain behaviours engaged in by the OSI-affected parent and by the type of relationship the parent has with the children. There are three behavioural patterns most often observed in children with an OSI-affected parent:

1　The children come to experience an emotional imbalance similar to that of the injured parent. They have trouble making friends and find it difficult to concentrate in school, because they are too concerned with their parent's well-being.

2　The children become parental "rescuers." They take on parental responsibilities, feel guilty about family problems, and blame themselves. They lose interest in activities typical for their age group.

3　The children become emotionally uninvolved with their family. They realize that their injured parent needs support, but they themselves receive very little support from their parents. To gain recognition, they might excel in some fields but exhibit anxious and depressive traits.[12]

Potential Feelings Common to Family Members

OSI-affected families will experience unpleasant emotions at times, but it is important to realize that these families also experience positive feelings like joy, pleasure, and pride. Each individual and family is unique: people's feelings vary and depend on several factors (manifestations of OSI, person's experiences prior to traumatizing event, family relationships prior to OSI, etc.), and some families adapt well, with little change to their lifestyle. Table 10.1 displays the potential feelings common to family members.[13]

Main Needs of Family Members

Primary needs of family members are information and education, psycho-education, psychotherapy, listening, and concrete assistance. Information and education are needed on OSI signs, preconceived notions and prejudices about OSIs, resources for injured individuals and their families, and symptoms of stress and burnout. Psycho-education is on topics such as stress management, meeting personal needs, crisis management, and communication. Psychotherapy helps to understand and explain the traumatizing event that the injured person experienced and the behaviours that have resulted. It also helps the injured person overcome difficulties as a member of the family. Listening legitimizes feelings, shares experiences, and reduces isolation. And concrete assistance will help the family adjust to the new situation (e.g., homework assistance for the children, respite, etc.).[14]

Theoretical Explanation for the Family Approach of $E = MC^3$

This section focuses on the theoretical aspects behind the $E = MC^3$ program, which helps families address OSIs with a family perspective, as opposed to an individual one. Systems theory helps explain how problems can develop in families of soldiers with an OSI. The theory views the family as an interactive unit

Table 10.1 | Feelings of OSI-affected families and their effects

Feelings	*Effects*
Guilt	Symptoms of stress and anxiety
Shame	Low self-esteem
Anger	Self-neglect
Fear (tense atmosphere, violence)	
Incomprehension (inability to "recognize" oneself or others, and trouble understanding and accepting the OSI)	
Sadness	
Loneliness (feeling of being different, the only person in that situation, and cut off from one's social network)	
Rejection (feeling unloved)	
Discouragement/overburdening (feeling of being overwhelmed by events and taxed beyond capacity by the events of daily life)	
Helplessness (inability to control the symptoms of the OSI or help others function better)	
Exhaustion	
Worry (about the family's future and the effects of the OSI on family members, especially the children)	

consisting of individuals with different functions operating according to a set of unifying principles. According to the theory, family ties are very strong and are the cause of many behaviours, feelings, values, and attitudes of the family members. Therefore, when one family member has problems, the functioning of the others is inevitably affected.[15] That is why the entire family system is affected when a soldier develops an OSI. Furthermore, PTSD and OSI studies show that these problems affect not only the soldier, but every family member. It is therefore essential to offer services not only to the soldiers, but also to their families, to help them adjust to the new situation and increase the likelihood that the treatment of the soldier will succeed.[16] In the same vein, the May 2006 Senate Committee report entitled *Out of the Shadows at Last,*[17] which examines the transformation of mental health services in Canada, states, "Where the family unit is dysfunctional it should be treated as a whole, with all family members provided the assistance they need." A central point in the literature is the importance of developing a holistic approach that works with the entire system, rather than each individual separately. It is to that end that $E = MC^3$ strives to provide support services to every member of the family coping with the repercussions of an OSI.

Interventions

Family Intervention

The most suitable intervention for some people will be family therapy, particularly where the injury directly affects relationships between family members. Family therapy addresses the interpersonal relationships, promotes effective communication, examines each person's roles, and teaches techniques to resolve problems and parenting skills tailored for the difficulties resulting from the injury. A few intervention models suggested include cognitive-behavioural therapy (CBT), the systemic approach, and the "systemic adaptation to trauma process model" for couples.[18]

Group-Based Intervention

For others, group-based intervention is the most appropriate. It ends the family's isolation, educates its members about the injuries, the symptoms, their effects, and the available resources, and helps them demystify the taboos associated with the injuries.[19]

"The overall purpose of group-based social work is to deal with the person and his environment. The objectives are personal development (the way the person relates to himself and to others and functions in society) and social change (Paré, 1971). The group format enables people with similar interests or common problems not only to help each other, but also to act collectively in order to produce social changes (Homes and Darveau-Fournier, 1980)."[20]

Accordingly, the $E = MC^3$ program uses family and group intervention to help families end their isolation and to share and normalize their experiences with people living in similar situations.

Participants' Expectations and Results

Expectations

Information and answers gathered from the children's and parents' questionnaire used in the pre-group interviews are summarized in the following paragraph. In addition, throughout the group process, parents and children shared their expectations about the group's impact on their families.

The parents expected to become OSI-literate and get tools to learn how to express themselves and tips on how to react to and work with their children. They also wanted tools to enable their children to understand why Dad or Mom is the way he or she is. Furthermore, they hoped to find solutions and tools to help their children be happy each day as well as help them realize that they are not the only ones going through their situation. By breaking their isolation, they expected to meet people who were going through the same experience. Meanwhile, the children expected to learn how to be nicer and not make their Dad or Mom angry while getting advice on how to act with their parents. They wanted to understand why their Mom or Dad gets angry so often. Moreover, the children wanted to make friends with others who were going through the same thing as they are. As you can see, the children's expectations were mostly about how to be a good child and not make their Dad or Mom angry. That shows the importance of addressing that issue with them within the group, so they understand that they are not responsible for their parent's behaviour (e.g., mood swings) and that the behaviour is a manifestation of their parent's OSI.

Results

The objectives for the post-group interviews were to see what the children had learned, review each participant's experience one month after the final workshop, and determine the need for individual or family follow-up support.

Parents reported that their children were expressing themselves more and feeling less guilty; the project had enabled their children to understand what an OSI is; communication within their family had improved; they came to realize that it was still possible to have a good time as a family (e.g., family meetings); they were no longer isolated, and they had met other people whose families were going through something similar. As for the children, they conveyed that they had learned what an OSI was and what its effects were. They had met other children whose father or mother had an OSI, and felt less alone. They related that they felt less guilty and that they now knew that they could not cure their Dad or Mom. They also described using their "feelings chart" with their family. Everyone reported that the group had improved their individual and family well-being.

Family Follow-up Support

While an $E = MC^3$ group is in progress, the families have access to counsellors if they wish to have a family review or discuss a specific situation. Once the group has wound down, some families may wish to receive follow-up support from a social worker. If that service is not available from the Military Family Resource Centre (MFRC) in which the group is located, families may be referred to an appropriate external resource.

Conclusion

OSIs and other mental health problems affect many military members and their families. The Canadian Forces are aware of this reality and are offering more and more services to prevent related difficulties. The Road to Mental Readiness program (R2MR), offered to soldiers during pre-deployment buildups, is an example of such a service. Moreover, the stigma of mental health problems continues to diminish, and soldiers are becoming less reluctant to ask for help. The belief that consulting a professional is a sign of weakness is fading. Naturally, there is still a lot of work to do in order to get people to seek help earlier and ensure that all family members can take advantage of psychosocial services that address OSIs systemically.

The main objective of $E = MC^3$ is to provide support to OSI-affected members and their families so they can lay taboos to rest and deal with the signs of OSIs and their effects on each family member. The first $E = MC^3$ group was a positive experience for participants and facilitators alike. The children and their parents said that they were delighted to have had the opportunity to participate. Their comments suggest that their participation had a positive impact on every family member. As for the facilitators, they were pleased with the way the first group turned out and were able to see real changes (e.g., in interaction and communication) in the families based on initial observations and post-group follow-up. This program is a complete turnkey program that can easily be transposed to different operational realities such as the police force, firefighters, and ambulance workers.

Notes

1   L. Evans, T. McHugh, M. Hopwood, and C. Watt. "Chronic Posttraumatic Stress Disorder and Family Functioning of Vietnam Veterans and Their Partners," *Australian and New Zealand Journal of Psychiatry* 37 (2003): 765–72; E. B. Foa, T. M. Keane, M. J. Friedman, and J. A. Cohen, eds., *Effective Treatments for PTSD: Practice Guidelines from the International Society for Traumatic Stress Studies*, 2nd ed. (New York: Guilford, 2000); H. Shroeder, *Effects of Post-Traumatic Stress Disorder on Military Families: A Qualitative Study on the Perspective of Females Whose Partners Have Been Diagnosed* (master's thesis, University of Manitoba, Winnipeg, 2006).

2   M. S. Friedmann, W. H. McDermut, D. A. Solomon, C. E. Ryan, G. I. Keitner, and I. W. Miller. "Functioning and Mental Illness: A Comparison of Psychiatric and Nonclinical Families," *Family Process* 36 (1997): 357–67; S. Adams, "Des esprits en conflits: Blessures de stress opérationnel," http://www.legionmagazine.com/fr/index.php/2009/11/des-esprits-en-conflit-blessures-de-stress-operationnel/#more-276.

3   Operational Stress Injury Social Support, "What Are Operational Stress Injuries?," http://www.osiss.ca/en/injured.html, accessed in 2010.

4   J. Westerink and L. Giarratano. "The Impact of Posttraumatic Stress Disorder on Partners and Children of Australian Vietnam Veterans," *Australian and New Zealand Journal of Psychiatry* 33 (1999): 841–7; D. Fikretoglu, "The Impact of Operational Stress Injuries on Veteran's Families: A Review of the Existing Research" (unpublished, Veterans Affairs Canada, 2008).

5   K. L. Hall. *Counseling Military Families: What Health Professionals Need to Know* (New York, Routledge Taylor and Francis, 2008).

6   Westerink and Giarratano, "Impact of Posttraumatic Stress Disorder."

7 B. K. Jordan, R. A. Kulka, C. R. Marmar, J. A. Fairbank, W. E. Schlenger, R. L. Hough, and D. S. Weiss, "Problems in Families of Male Vietnam Veterans with Posttraumatic Stress Disorder," *Journal of Consulting and Clinical Psychology* 60 (1990): 916–26.
8 J. Giroux, "Groupe d'éducation, de soutien et de croissance pour conjointes de militaires atteints par un syndrome de stress post-traumatique" (unpublished essay, Université Laval, Quebec, 2003).
9 Hall, *Counseling Military Families.*
10 Giroux, "Groupe d'éducation."
11 Shroeder, *Effects of Post-Traumatic Stress Disorder.*
12 L. Harkness, "The Effects of Combat-Related PTSD on Children," *PTSD Clinical Quarterly* 2 (1991): 1–16.
13 Valcartier Health Centre, *Groupe sur blessure de stress opérationnel (GBSO).* (Valcartier: Valcartier Health Centre, 2010).
14 Operational Stress Injury Social Support, *Rapport de l'analyse des besoins en soutien social auprès des proches de militaires et d'anciens combattants touchés d'une blessure de stress opérationnel* (Ottawa: Department of National Defence; Joint Speakers Bureau, 2009).
15 C. Figley, *Helping Traumatised Families* (San Francisco: Jossey-Bass, 1989).
16 Ibid.
17 Standing Senate Committee on Social Affairs, Science and Technology, *Out of the Shadows at Last: Transforming Mental Health, Mental Illness, and Addiction Services in Canada* (2006). http://www.parl.gc.ca/content/sen/committee/391/soci/rep/rep02may06-e.htm.
18 Evans et al. "Chronic Posttraumatic Stress Disorder," 765–72; C. C. Hendrix, A. P. Jurich and W. R. Schumm, "Long-Term Impact of Vietnam War Service on Family Environment and Satisfaction," *Families in Society* 76 (1995): 498–506; Jordan et al., "Problems in Families of Male Vietnam Veterans," 916–26; S. L. Sayers, V. A. Farrow, J. Ross, and D. W. Oslin, "Family Problems among Recently Returned Military Veterans Referred for a Mental Health Evaluation," *Journal of Clinical Psychiatry* 70 (2009): 163–70.
19 J. D. Ford, P. Chandler, B. Thacker, D. Greaves, D. Shaw, S. Seenhauser, and L. Schwartz, "Family Systems Therapy after Operation Desert Storm with European-Theater Veterans," *Journal of Marital and Family Therapy* 24 (1998): 243–50; Shroeder, *Effects of Post-Traumatic Stress Disorder.*
20 Giroux, "Groupe d'éducation," trans. Mac Wigfield; J. Isabelle, "L'état de stress post-traumatique et son impact sur la famille militaire" (MA thesis, University of Ottawa, 2000); D. Turcotte and J. Lindsay. *L'intervention sociale auprès des groupes* (Montreal: Gaëtan Morin Éditeur – Chenelière Éducation, 2002).

PART TWO

Veteran and Transition Health

11

Veterans' Health in Canada: A Scoping Review of the Literature

STEVEN ROSE, ALICE B. AIKEN, MARY ANN MCCOLL,
AND ALLIE CAREW

Abstract

The purpose of this project was to conduct a scoping review of the Canadian academic and government peer-reviewed literature to identify the major health concerns of Canadian veterans, and identify what is being done to address them. A scoping review of the literature was conducted and analyzed. The results yielded 227 publications, which were grouped by subject and graphed. Fully one-third of the articles pertained to PTSD, while the rest related to various health conditions and treatments. We were unable to answer our research questions because the literature was so thin, though some interesting trends were observed in the PTSD literature. The majority of articles have been published since 2009, perhaps indicating that there has been a renaissance in veterans' health research.

Introduction

Over the last decade, Canada has seen more people affected by military service-related injuries and illnesses than any time since the Korean War, yet Canada still lags behind its allies in research on military, veteran, and family health. As our military returns from Afghanistan, the time has never been better for a renaissance in military and veteran health research.

Worldwide interest in the unique health needs of military personnel, veterans, and their families increased following the 1991 Persian Gulf War, when military members from countries around the world returned home with health concerns. The Gulf War also marked the beginning of an era of difficult Canadian military operations and an accelerated tempo of deployments to the heart of many of the world's most complex conflicts, including Rwanda, Somalia, Kosovo, Afghanistan, Haiti, and Libya.

The project involved a scoping review of the Canadian academic and government peer-reviewed literature to identify the major health concerns of Canadian veterans, and identify what is being done to address these health concerns. In light of the global explosion of expert opinion and research findings on veterans' health, this study examines the extent of the literature in the Canadian context. This study thematically identifies the state of the literature in order to inform researchers on potential knowledge gaps, and to determine emerging research trends on veterans' health in Canada.

Methods

The study employs a scoping review approach to scan an extensive body of literature to determine how the research question is addressed in the literature. According to Arksey and O'Malley* and Levac, Colquhoun, and O'Brien** the scoping review unfolds in five stages:

1 Identify the research questions.
2 Identify relevant studies.
3 Determine and apply inclusion and exclusion criteria.
4 Chart the data.
5 Summarize and report the results.
    a Identify the research questions: What are the main health concerns of Canadian veterans, and what is being done to address these concerns?
    b Identify relevant studies:
       Articles were included if they
         ◆ Were published between 1980 and 2012
         ◆ Specifically had Canadian veterans as a study group

A database search was conducted in Embase, Medline, and Psycinfo using the following keywords: *veteran$, health, Canad$, post traumatic stress disorder, heart, pain, brain, trauma, limb, amputation, therapy, depression, suicide, transition, care,* and *injury.*

---

* Hilary Arksey and Lisa O'Malley, "Scoping Studies: Towards a Methodological Framework," *International Journal of Social Research Methodology* 8, no. 1 (February 2005): 19–32, http://www.tandfonline.com/doi/abs/10.1080/1364557032000119616.

** Danielle Levac, Heather Colquhoun, and Kelly K. O'Brien, "Scoping Studies: Advancing the Methodology," *Implementation Science* 5 (January 2010): 69, http://www.pubmedcentral.nih.gov/articlerender.fcgi?artid=2954944&tool=pm centrez&rendertype=abstract.

The keyword *Canad$* was included in each search since excluding it resulted in an overwhelming majority of the results being American studies. The dollar sign ($) is included since it represents alternate endings in database searches. This allows us to simultaneously search for *Canada, Canadian,* and *Canadians,* as well as *veteran* and *veterans.*

Inclusion criteria were applied by reading the title to determine its relevance to the study. If it was unclear, vague, or too general, we used the Find Tool (CTRL-F) to search the article for the use of *veteran* and *Canada* to determine whether the study included this specific population in its focus. Lastly, articles were screened for their date of publication. Articles published prior to 1980 were not included in the study. After these inclusion criteria were applied, we were left with ninety-eight articles: seventy-five from Embase, sixteen from Medline, and seven from Psychinfo.

In order to supplement our database search, we hand-searched the bibliography of each article. Ninety-three new articles were acquired through hand-searches of bibliographies.

Authors who appeared more than once in our study up to this point were then contacted to determine whether they had published any relevant articles we had yet to acquire. With a very high response rate, this step added fifty-three academic or non-academic sources. Most of the articles acquired in this step were peer-reviewed reports provided by Veteran Affairs Canada.

Determine and Apply Exclusion Criteria

In the charting process, seventeen articles found in the databases were eliminated for their irrelevance to the study, because their focus was not Canadian veterans specifically, or they did not deal with a health concern or care method. Therefore, a total of eighty-one articles were acquired from database searches.

All of the articles obtained through hand searching (ninety-three) and contacting authors (fifty-three) were entered into the study, as the exclusion criteria did not apply.

After completing these steps, this scoping study includes 227 peer-reviewed articles and reports on Canadian veterans' health.

Chart the Data

This process required reading through each article to determine the following pieces of information: author, year, title, health concern(s) studied, population(s) in study, methods used, results/conclusions, type of article/report, and name of journal/affiliation. Each article was charted on a spreadsheet with these criteria filled out. When charting the data, it was determined that eleven of the articles in the study do not focus on specific health concern or care/treatment concerns.

Although these articles do not present a central concern, they were deemed relevant to the study because of their general discussion of Canadian veterans' health. Since the tables below present specific themes in health issues and treatment methods, these eleven articles do not appear in this paper.

Summarize and Report the Results

In order to succinctly summarize this extensive body of data, articles were categorized according to

- type of publication (journal, report, or book chapter),
- date of publication,
- health concern(s) in focus, and
- treatment and care concerns.

Results

This study collected 227 publications: 144 journal articles, 55 reports, 13 theses, and 15 book chapters. Of these articles, 138 relate to health concerns and 78 to treatment programs, practices, or policies, and 11 spoke generally about the health of veterans but not on any topic specifically, thus are not represented graphically in the results.

The vast majority of publications were published from 2009 to 2012, the largest spike occurring in 2011, although 2012 data end at March 2012 so that is an incomplete data set. Figure 11.1 depicts the number of publications per year since 1992. Although data were collected from 1980, not enough reports were published annually to affect the graph, therefore they are not charted.

Tables 11.1 to 11.4 depict the type of health concerns studied. It is worth noting that roughly one-third of the publications collected focus on PTSD/psychological trauma. Of the 138, 93 relate to psychological health, 36 to physical health, and 9 to social health.

The health concerns are divided into three tables that explore three categories: psychological concerns, physical concerns, and social concerns.

The table on psychological concerns uses a matrix to represent overlaps in articles that discuss two or more concerns, whereas the other two sections do not use a matrix, since there is an insignificant number of overlapping publications.

Table 11.4 presents the publications focused on what is being done about veterans' health concerns. Of the seventy-eight, twelve speak about care needs; thirteen about services/programs and utilization; thirty-two about transition programs; six about psychological treatment, resilience, and adaptation; and twelve on health benefits, income concerns, and legislation. Specific health concerns are listed along the left column. Of these, eight publications pertain to a specific health concern, while seventy do not and instead speak about veterans' health concerns generally.

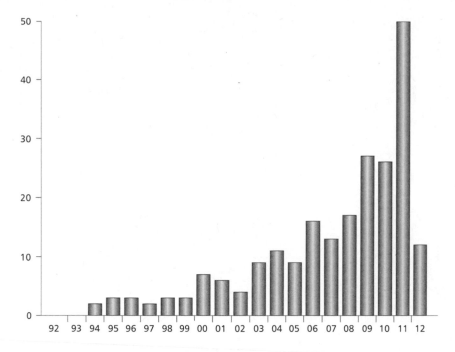

Figure 11.1 | Publications per year

Discussion

We were unable to answer our research questions on the main health concerns of Canadian veterans and what is being done to address these concerns, for lack of literature on Canadian veterans specifically.

Fully one-third of the literature, 76 of 227 articles, pertained to PTSD, with only 17 other articles on other mental health problems. Of the 76 articles that related to PTSD, 16 also studied other mental health conditions such as depression, suicide, substance abuse, and co-morbidity. A further 6 articles that focused primarily on depression or suicide also spoke of other problems such as substance abuse and co-morbidity. Only one article focused specifically on the care needs of veterans with PTSD, while 13 spoke of programs and utilization and 6 spoke of psychological treatment.

In physical health, there were five articles on falls in elderly veterans, but other than that, conditions were cited randomly in one or two articles, with no conclusions able to be drawn. We are aware that many advances have been made in the treatment of amputations since the war in Afghanistan; however, they are not reflected in the literature.

In social health concerns, only nine articles were found, mostly using the search term *transition* and had to do with problems after leaving service. In terms of

Table 11.1 | Number of articles about psychological health concerns (smaller, superscript numbers refer to the full citations provided in the endnotes of this chapter)

	PTSD / Psychological trauma	Depression	Suicide	Substance abuse	Co-morbidity	Psychological well-being	Intellectual development	Dementia	Social anxiety disorder
PTSD / Psychological trauma	1 2 3 4 5 6 7 8 9 10 11 12 13 14 15 16 17 18 19 20 21 22 23 24 25 26 27 28 29 30 31 32 33 34 35 36 37 38 39 40 41 42 43 44 45 46 47 48 49 50 51 52 53 54 55 56 57 58 59 60 61 62 63 64 65 66 67 68 69 70 71 72 73 74 75 76 76								
Depression	31 37 58 49 41 63 71 72 74 9	77 78 79 3							

Suicide — 8 31 59 74 : 4 | 31 74 : 2 | 80 81 82 83 84 : 5

Substance abuse — 35 65 : 2 | 58 71 72 : 3 | 0

Co-morbidity — 71 72 : 2 | 59 : 1 | 0

Psychological well-being — 34 : 1 | 85 86 : 2

Intellectual development — 87 88 89 90 : 4

Dementia — 91 92 : 2

Social anxiety disorder — 93 : 1

Table 11.2 | Number of articles about physical health concerns (smaller, superscript numbers refer to the full citations provided in the endnotes of this chapter)

Health concern	Article citation number
Amputation	1 [94]
Blindness	1 [95]
Cancer	2 [96 97]
Causes of death	1 [98]
Disability	2 [99 100]
Falls	5 [101 102 103 104 105]
Gulf War syndrome	2 [106 107]
Hearing loss	1 [108]
Infectious diseases	3 [109 110 111]
Musculoskeletal disorders + orthopedic injuries	1 [112]
Uranium and chemical illness / exposure	4 [113 114 115 116]
Nutrition/obesity	4 [117 118 119 120]
Physical pain	3 [121 122 123]
Polytrauma	1 [124]
Reproductive health	1 [125]
Road traffic accidents	1 [126]
Spinal cord injuries	1 [127]
Traumatic brain injury	2 [128 129]
Total	36

Table 11.3 | Number of articles about social health concerns (smaller, superscript numbers refer to the full citations provided in the endnotes of this chapter)

Health concern	Article citation number
Stigma / barriers to care	2 [130 131]
Gender discrimination	1 [132]
Intimate partner violence + family relationships	3 [133 134 135]
Homelessness	3 [136 137 138]
Total	9

Table 11.4. Number of articles about care/treatment concerns (smaller superscript numbers refer to the full citations provided in the endnotes of this chapter)

	Care needs	Care services / care programs / care utilization	Transition programs	Psychological treatment / resilience and adaption	Health benefits / pension / income / SES + legislation for veterans	Total
Disability	1 [139]				3 [140 141 142]	4
Family issues	1 [143]					1
Intellectual development			1 [144]			1
PTSD / psychological trauma	1 [145]					1
Suicide			1 [146]			1
Not associated with a specific health concern	147 148 149 150 151 152 153 154 9	155 156 157 158 159 160 161 162 163 164 165 166 167 13	168 169 170 171 172 173 174 175 176 177 178 179 180 181 182 183 184 185 186 187 188 189 190 191 192 193 194 195 196 197 30	198 199 200 201 202 203 6	204 205 206 207 208 209 210 211 212 9	70
Total	12	13	32	6	12	78

treatments, however, thirty-two articles have been published about transition programs; however, these review existing programs, rather than giving an overview of transition needs of veterans.

PTSD is the one area where reliable trends can be observed. Four articles on the subject attempt to define PTSD to more clearly understand the underlying mechanisms that contribute to the disorder. Naifeh et al. (2010) go beyond previous structurally homogenous models of PTSD in order to show the heterogeneity of PTSD's latent factor structure. Engdahl et al. (2011) test the factor structure of PTSD by studying previously deployed and non-deployed peacekeepers and suggest that the factor structure of PTSD may be different in the two groups. Whereas these studies take a broader approach to conceptualizing PTSD, Elhai et al. (2011) and Armour et al. (2012) look more specifically at the conceptual relationship between PTSD and depression. Elhai et al. (2011) explore the interrelationships between the factor structures of depression and PTSD's dysphonia factor structure. Armour et al. (2012) build on this work by considering whether the dysphoric arousal model of Elhai et al. is suitable for all trauma populations, particularly the external constructs of both depression and anxiety.

There is also a cluster of articles that discuss the association between PTSD and physical health, some also including co-morbid mental health conditions. The conditions studied in association with PTSD very widely between the studies, although there is some overlap. Pekevski (2011) and Poundja, Fikretoglu, and Brunet (2006) both assess the connection between PTSD symptoms and physical pain. Where they differ is in their focus on mediators between PTSD and physical pain: Pekevski looks at alcohol use, whereas Poundja et al. look at depression and focus more specifically on particular physical health conditions: gastrointestinal disorders, musculoskeletal problems, headaches, and cardiovascular problems. Lastly, Sareen et al. (2007) show the relation between PTSD and physical health conditions by showing its significant association to cardiovascular diseases, respiratory diseases, chronic pain conditions, gastrointestinal illnesses, cancer, suicide attempts, poor quality of life, and short- and long-term disability.

In terms of treatment for PTSD, in this area, two articles focus on drug treatments, two on counselling treatments, and two on treatment outcomes. In drug treatments, Fraser (2009) reports on clinical trials that test the usefulness of synthetic cannabinoid in the management of treatment-resistant nightmares in individuals with PTSD. Richardson et al. (2011) look at the effectiveness of the drug aripiprazole in the treatment of veterans with PTSD and co-morbid major depression. In terms of counselling treatments, Cave (2003), in a doctoral thesis, inquiries into the effectiveness of a group-based enactment-approach to therapy for traumatized soldiers, and Simms, O'Donnell, and Molyneaux, (2009) consider virtual reality exposure therapy as a treatment for PTSD. Richardson, Elhai, and Sarreen (2011) measure responses of various treatment approaches to PTSD and determine the long-term effectiveness of current PTSD treatments (including both counselling and drug therapies). Lastly, Ray (2009) looks at responses to treatment in terms of the lived-experience of peacekeeping veterans.

And in terms of seeking treatment, Richardson, Elhai, Pedlar (2006), Elhai, Don Richardson, Pedlar (2007), and Fikretetoglu et al. (2007) conducted studies inquiring as to whether persons who suffer trauma-related mental illness seek treatment. Their conclusions are similar since the studies show that there is an increased likelihood of treatment utilization in those suffering from PTSD. Although this is the case, Fikretoglu et al. (2007) state that one in three are not seeking treatment. Sareen et al. (2010) look at the perceived need for treatment when controlling for trauma-related mental illness. They conclude that a range of issues need to be considered beyond mental illness in screening programs, since "the strongest and most consistent correlates of perceived need were long-term restriction in activities, suicidal ideation, female gender, and regular service status."

For other health problems, the results are far less reportable as they pertain to Canadian veterans.

Conclusion

The results of this scoping review indicate that a paucity of literature pertains to Canadian veterans' health. While a good number of articles pertain to mental health issues – specifically PTSD – there are some problems with this approach. First, there are many mental health issues identified by military and veteran mental health practitioners that are not related to PTSD, such as depression, substance abuse, and suicide. From the literature, one would assume that this is all PTSD when in fact that may not be the case.

The paucity of literature on other health issues is concerning. Both the CF and VAC suggest that the majority of their expenses go to physical health problems, yet little is published in this regard. There have been many new treatment advances, for example in the treatment of upper and lower limb amputations that have arisen from the conflict in Afghanistan. It would be helpful if more were published in this regard.

One area that appears to be growing tremendously is that of transition research. It appears that it has been recognized as an area of research that pertains uniquely to veterans. It will be interesting to see the publications over the next several years about this topic.

The results of this study show that there are many gaps in the published and peer-reviewed literature that pertains to Canadian veteran health research. In order to develop appropriate knowledge mobilization tools, or to draw any conclusions we must still rely on the international literature. This can be helpful, but does not take into account the unique Canadian context of training, equipment, environment, resources for transition, or the Canadian health care system upon which the veteran must rely after release.

However, the spike in literature since 2009 can lead us to the conclusion that perhaps there has been a renaissance in literature pertaining to veterans' health. In all likelihood over the next few years, the growth will continue and conclusions about the health of Canadian veterans can be drawn, mobilized, and acted upon.

Notes

1   Cherie Armour, Jon D. Elhai, Don Richardson, Kendra Ractliffe, Li Wang, and Ask Elklit, "Assessing a Five Factor Model of PTSD: Is Dysphoric Arousal a Unique PTSD Construct Showing Differential Relationships with Anxiety and Depression?," *Journal of Anxiety Disorders* 26, no. 2 (March 2012): 368–76, http://www.ncbi.nlm.nih.gov/pubmed/22204787.

2   Gordon J. G. Asmundson, Murray B. Stein, and Donald R. McCreary, "Posttraumatic Stress Disorder Symptoms Influence Health Status of Deployed Peacekeepers and Nondeployed Military Personnel," *Journal of Nervous and Mental Disease* 190, no. 12 (December 2002): 807–15, http://www.ncbi.nlm.nih.gov/pubmed/12486368

3   Gordon J. G. Asmundson, Kristi D. Wright, Donald R. McCreary, and David Pedlar, "Post-traumatic Stress Disorder Symptoms in United Nations Peacekeepers: An Examination of Factor Structure in Peacekeepers with and without Chronic Pain," *Cognitive Behaviour Therapy* 32, no. 1 (January 2003): 26–37.

4   Gordon J. G. Asmundson, Kristi D. Wright, and Murray B. Stein, "Pain and PTS-DPTSD Symptoms in Female Veterans.," *European Journal of Pain* 8, no. 4 (August 2004): 345–50, http://www.ncbi.nlm.nih.gov/pubmed/15207515.

5   Al Beal, "Post-traumatic Stress Disorder in Prisoners of War and Combat Veterans of the Dieppe Raid: A 50-Year Follow-up," *Canadian Journal of Psychiatry* 40, no. 4 (1995): 177–84.

6   Shay-Lee Belik, Murray B. Stein, Gordon J. G. Asmundson, and Jitender Sareen, "Relation between Traumatic Events and Suicide Attempts in Canadian Military Personnel," *Canadian Journal of Psychiatry / Revue canadienne de psychiatrie* 54, no. 2 (February 2009): 93–104, http://www.ncbi.nlm.nih.gov/pubmed/19254440.

7   Tracey L. Biehn, Jon D. Elhai, Thomas H. Fine, Laura D. Seligman, and Don J. Richardson, "PTSD Factor Structure Differences between Veterans with and without a PTSD Diagnosis," *Journal of Anxiety Disorders* 26, no. 3 (April 2012): 480–5, http://linkinghub.elsevier.com/retrieve/pii/S0887618512000205.

8   R. Birenbaum, "Peacekeeping Stress Prompts New Approaches to Mental-Health Issues in Canadian Military," *Canadian Medical Association Journal / Journal de l'Association medicale canadienne* 151, no. 10 (15 November 1994): 1484–6, http://www.pubmedcentral.nih.gov/articlerender.fcgi?artid=1337422&tool=pm centrez&rendertype=abstract.

9   David Boulos, *Cumulative Incidence of PTSD and Other Mental Disorders in Canadian Forces Personnel Deployed in Support of the Mission in Afghanistan, 2001–2008* (Ottawa: Queen's Printer, 2008).

10 Douglas G. Cave, "Enacting Change: A Therapeutic Enactment Group-Based Program for Traumatized Soldiers" (PhD diss., University of British Columbia, 2003).

11 Erica Weir, "Veterans and Post-traumatic Stress Disorder," *Canadian Medical Association Journal* 163, no. 9 (2000): 1187.

12 R. Cossar, "Training Resilient Soldiers: Looking for Solutions to Operational Stress," *Canadian Army Journal* 13, no. 1 (2010): 85–103.

13 Heather J. NcCurag Edge and Gary W. Ivey, "Mediation of Cognitive Appraisal on Combat Exposure and Psychological Distress," *Military Psychology* 24, no. 1 (January 2012): 71–85,

14 Jon D. Elhai, Ateka A. Contractor, Patrick A. Palmieri, David Forbes, and J. Don Richardson, "Exploring the Relationship between Underlying Dimensions of Posttraumatic Stress Disorder and Depression in a National, Trauma-Exposed Military Sample," *Journal of Affective Disorders* 133, no. 3 (October 2011): 477–80, http://www.ncbi.nlm.nih.gov/pubmed/21600663.

15 Ryan M. Engdahl, Jon D. Elhai, Don J. Richardson, and Christopher B. Frueh, "Comparing Posttraumatic Stress Disorder's Symptom Structure between Deployed and Nondeployed Veterans," *Psychological Assessment* 23, no. 1 (2011): 1–6, http://doi.apa.org/getdoi.CFm?doi=10.1037/a0020045.

16 Allan English, "Leadership and Operational Stress in the Canadian Forces," *Canadian Military Journal* 1, no. 3 (2000): 33–8.

17 Kelly M. J. Farley and Victor M. Catano, "The Battlefield as Workplace: Violence in Warfighting," in *Handbook of Workplace Violence*, 1–21 (London: Sage, 2006).

18 Deniz Fikretoglu, Alain Brunet, Stephane Guay, and David Pedlar, "Mental Health Treatment Seeking by Military Members with Posttraumatic Stress Disorder," *Canadian Journal of Psychiatry* 52, no. 2 (2007): 103–9.

19 Deniz Fikretoglu, Alain Brunet, Joaquin Poundja, Stéphane Guay, and David Pedlar, "Validation of the Deployment Risk and Resilience Inventory in French-Canadian Veterans: Findings on the Relation between Deployment Experiences and Postdeployment Health," *Canadian Journal of Psychiatry / Revue canadienne de psychiatrie* 51, no. 12 (October 2006): 755–63, http://www.ncbi.nlm.nih.gov/pubmed/17168250.

20 George A. Fraser, "The Use of a Synthetic Cannabinoid in the Management of Treatment-Resistant Nightmares in Posttraumatic Stress Disorder (PTSD)," *CNS Neuroscience & Therapeutics* 15, no. 1 (January 2009): 84–8, http://www.ncbi.nlm.nih.gov/pubmed/19228182.

21 Rhonda M. Gibson, "The Development of the Canadian Deployment Impact Scale for Assessing PTSD: A Psychometric Study" (PhD diss., University of Calgary, 1997).

22 Mark Humphries, "War's Long Shadow: Masculinity, Medicine, and the Gendered Politics of Trauma, 1914–1939," *Canadian Historical Review* 91, no. 3 (1 August 2010): 503–31, http://utpjournals.metapress.com/openurl.asp?genre=article &id=doi:10.3138/chr.91.3.503.

23 Rachel Kroch, "Living with Military-Related Posttraumatic Stress Disorder (PTSD): A Hermeneutic Phenomenological Study" (PhD diss., University of Calgary, 2009).

24 C. D. Lamerson and E. K. Kelloway, "Towards a Model of Peacekeeping Stress: Traumatic and Contextual Influences," *Canadian Psychology / Psychologie* canadienne

37, no. 4 (1996): 195–204, http://doi.apa.org/getdoi.cfm?doi=10.1037/0708-5591.37.4.195.

25 André Marin, Report to the Minister of National Defence by André Marin Ombudsman, Special Report: Systemic Treatment of CF Members with PTSD Complainant (Ottawa: Queen's Printer, 2001).

26 Mary McFadyen, A Long Road to Recovery: Battling Operational Stress Injuries, (Ottawa: Queen's Printer, 2008).

27 Richard J. McNally, "Troubles in Traumatology and Debunking Myths about Trauma and Memory," Canadian Journal of Psychiatry 50, no. 13 (November 2005): 817–22, http://www.ncbi.nlm.nih.gov/pubmed/17375869.

28 James A. Naifeh, Don J. Richardson, Kevin S. Del Ben, and Jon D. Elhai, "Heterogeneity in the Latent Structure of PTSD Symptoms among Canadian Veterans," Psychological Assessment 22, no. 3 (2010): 666–74, http://doi.apa.org/getdoi.cfm?doi=10.1037/a0019783.

29 Charles Nelson, Kate St Cyr, Bradley Corbett, Elisa Hurley, Shannon Gifford, Jon D. Elhai, and J. Donald Richardson, "Predictors of Posttraumatic Stress Disorder, Depression, and Suicidal Ideation among Canadian Forces Personnel in a National Canadian Military Health Survey," Journal of Psychiatric Research 45, no. 11 (November 2011): 1483–8, http://linkinghub.elsevier.com/retrieve/pii/S0022395611001300.

30 J. Pare, Post-traumatic Stress Disorder and the Mental Health of Military Personnel and Ceterans (Ottawa: Library of Parliament, 14 October 2011).

31 Greg Passey, "Mental Health, a Mounting Priority in the Canadian Forces," Canadian Psychiatry Aujourd'hui 5, no. 1 (2009): 445–6.

32 Luigi Pastò, Don McCreary, and Megan Thompson, Deployment Stressors, Coping, and Psychological Well-Being among Peacekeepers (Toronto: Defence Research and Development, n.d.).

33 Jordan Pekevski, "PTSD Symptom Cluster Associations with Alchohol Use and Physical Health Status in a Population of Veterans Exposed to Psychological Trauma" (PhD diss., University of South Dakota, 2011).

34 Emmanuel Popoola, "Intrinsic Spirituality and Posttraumatic Stress Disorder: A Focus on the Canadian Forces" (PhD diss., University of Phoenix, 2011).

35 Joaquin Poundja, Deniz Fikretoglu, and Alain Brunet, "The Co-occurrence of Posttraumatic Stress Disorder Symptoms and Pain: Is Depression a Mediator?," Journal of Traumatic Stress 19, no. 5 (2006): 747–51.

36 Joaquin Poundja, Deniz Fikretoglu, Stephane Guay, and Alain Brunet, "Validation of the French Version of the Brief Pain Inventory in Canadian Veterans Suffering from Traumatic Stress," Journal of Pain and Symptom Management 33, no. 6 (June 2007): 720–6, http://www.ncbi.nlm.nih.gov/pubmed/17531912.

37 Susan L. Ray, "Evolution of Posttraumatic Stress Disorder and Future Directions," Archives of Psychiatric Nursing 22, no. 4 (August 2008): 217–25, http://www.ncbi.nlm.nih.gov/pubmed/18640541.

38 Susan L. Ray, "The Experience of Contemporary Peacekeepers Healing from Trauma," Nursing Inquiry 16, no. 1 (March 2009): 53–63, http://www.ncbi.nlm.nih.gov/pubmed/19228304.

39 Susan L. Ray, "Contemporary Treatments for Psychological Trauma from the
    Perspective of Peacekeepers," *Canadian Journal of Nursing Research* 41, no. 2 (2009):
    114–28.
40 Susan L. Ray, "Embodiment and Embodied Engagement: Central Concerns for the
    Nursing Care of Contemporary Peacekeepers Suffering from Psychological Trauma,"
    Perspectives in Psychiatric Care 42, no. 2 (2006): 106–13.
41 Susan L. Ray, "Being in the World of Peacekeeping: Living the Unrepresentable," in
    Religion and Psychology, ed. Michael T. Evans and Emma D. Walker, 17–62 (New
    York: Nova Science Publishers, 2009).
42 Susan L. Ray, Julie Salverson, Sue Del-Mei, Dustin Garrett, Smita Misra, and Lauren
    Weinberg, "Dramatizing Research: The Experience of Contemporary Peacekeepers
    Healing from Trauma" (Paper presented at annual CIMVHR Forum, Kingston, 2011).
43 Susan L. Ray and Meredith Vanstone, "The Impact of PTSD on Veterans' Family
    Relationships: An Interpretative Phenomenological Inquiry," *International Journal of
    Nursing Studies* 46, no. 6 (June 2009): 838–47, http://linkinghub.elsevier.com/retrieve/
    pii/S0020748909000066.
44 Don Richardson, letter to the editor, *Canadian Journal of Psychiatry* 71, no. 8 (2010):
    1099–101.
45 J. Don Richardson, "Military-related PTSD in Canadian Veterans," *Canadian
    Psychiatry Aujourd'hui* 5, no. 1 (2009): 15–19.
46 J. Don Richardson, Kathy Darte, Stéphane Grenier, Allan English, and Joe Sharpe,
    "Operational Stress Injury Social Support: A Canadian Innovation in Professional
    Peer Support," *Canadian Military Journal* 9, no. 1 (2008): 57–64.
47 J. Don Richardson, Jon D. Elhai, and David J. Pedlar, "Association of PTSD and
    Depression with Medical and Specialist Care Utilization in Modern Peacekeeping
    Veterans in Canada with Health-Related Disabilities," *Journal of Clinical Psychiatry*
    67, no. 8 (2006): 1241–6.
48 J. Don Richardson, Jon D. Elhai, and Jitender Sarreen, "Predictors of Treatment
    Response in Canadian Combat and Peacekeeping Veterans with Military-Related
    Posttraumatic Stress Disorder," *Journal of Nervous and Mental Disease* 199, no. 9
    (September 2011): 639–45, http://www.ncbi.nlm.nih.gov/pubmed/21878776.
49 J. Don Richardson, Deniz Fikretoglu, Aihua Liu, and Diane McIntosh, "Aripiprazole
    Augmentation in the Treatment of Military-Related PTSD with Major Depression:
    A Retrospective Chart Review," *BMC Psychiatry* 11, no. 86 (January 2011),
    http://www.pubmedcentral.nih.gov/articlerender.fcgi?artid=3123270&tool=
    pmcentrez&rendertype=abstract.
50 J. Don Richardson, Mary Long, David E. Pedlar, and Jon D. Elhai, "Posttraumatic
    Stress Disorder and Health-Related Quality of Life among a Sample of Treatment
    and Pension-Seeking Deployed Canadian Forces Peacekeeping Veterans," *Canadian
    Journal of Psychiatry* 53, no. 9 (2008): 594–600.
51 J. Don Richardson, Diane McIntosh, Murray B. Stein, and Jitender Sareen, "Post-
    traumatic Stress Disorder: Guiding Management with Careful Assessment of
    Comorbid Mental and Physical Illness," *Mood and Anxiety Disorders Rounds* 1,
    no. 6 (2010): 1–6.

52 J. Don Richardson, Jordan Pekevski, and Jon D. Elhai, "Post-traumatic Stress Disorder and Health Problems among Medically Ill Canadian Peacekeeping Veterans," *Australian and New Zealand Journal of Psychiatry* 43 (2009): 366–72.

53 J. Don Richardson, James M. Thompson, Margaret Boswall, and Rakesh Jetly, , "Veteran Health Files: Horror Comes Home: Veterans with Posttraumatic Stress Disorder," *Canadian Family Physician* 56 (2010): 430–3.

54 Deniz Fikretoglu, Alain Brunet, Norbert Schmitz, Stephane Guay, and David Pedlar, "Posttraumatic Stress Disorder and Treatment Seeking in a Nationally Representative Canadian Military Sample," *Journal of Traumatic Stress* 19, no. 6 (2006): 847–58.

55 B. Rynor, "Veterans Stepping Forward for Treatment of Operational Stress Injuries," *Canadian Medical Association Journal* 182, no. 7 (22 March 2010): E281–2, http://www.cmaj.ca/cgi/doi/10.1503/cmaj.109-3213.

56 Jitender Sareen, Shay-Lee Belik, Tracie O. Afifi, Gordon Asmundson, Brian J. Cox, and Murray B. Stein, "Canadian Military Personnel's Population Attributable Fractions of Mental Disorders and Mental Health Service Use Associated with Combat and Peacekeeping Operations," *American Journal of Public Health* 98, no. 12 (December 2008): 2191–8, http://www.pubmedcentral.nih.gov/articlerender.fcgi?artid=2636534&tool=pmcentrez&rendertype=abstract.

57 Jitender Sareen, Brian J. Cox, Murray B. Stein, Tracie O. Afifi, Claire Fleet, and Gordon Asmundson, "Physical and Mental Comorbidity, Disability, and Suicidal Behavior Associated with Posttraumatic Stress Disorder in a Large Community Sample," *Psychosomatic Medicine* 69, no. 3 (April 2007): 242–8, http://www.ncbi.nlm.nih.gov/pubmed/17401056.

58 Jitender Sareen, Murray B. Stein, Siri Belik Thoresen, Shay-Lee Mark Zamorski, and Gordon Asmundson, "Is Peacekeeping Peaceful? A Systematic Review," *Canadian Journal of Psychiatry / Revue canadienne de psychiatrie* 55, no. 7 (July 2010): 464–72, http://www.ncbi.nlm.nih.gov/pubmed/20704774.

59 Deanne Simms, Susan O'Donnell, and Heather Molyneaux, The *Use of Virtual Reality in the Treatment of Posttraumatic Stress Disorder (PTSD)* (Fredricton: Queen's Printer, 2009).

60 Tom Spears, "Psychologic Scars Remain 50 Years after Dieppe Raid, Study of Canadian Veterans Finds," *Canadian Medical Association Journal / Journal de l'Association medicale canadienne* 153, no. 9 (1 November 1995): 1324–6, http://www.pubmedcentral.nih.gov/articlerender.fcgi?artid=1487483&tool=pmcentrez&rendertype=abstract.

61 Jennifer A. Stapleton, Gordon Asmundson, Meghan Woods, Steven Taylor, and Murray B. Stein, "Health Care Utilization by United Nations Peacekeeping Veterans and Depression Symptoms versus Those Without," *Military Medicine* 171 (June 2006): 562–7.

62 Statistics Canada, *Canadian Community Health Survey Cycle 1.2 Mental Health and Well-being: Canadian Forces Master File Documentation* (Ottawa, Queen's Printer, 2004).

63 Sherry H. Stewart, "Alcohol Abuse in Individuals Exposed to Trauma: A Critical Review," *Psychological Bulletin* 120, no. 1 (July 1996): 83–112, http://www.ncbi.nlm.nih.gov/pubmed/8711018.

64 Robert H. Stretch, "Effects of Service in Vietnam on Canadian Forces Military Personnel," *Armed Forces & Society* 16, no. 4 (1 July 1990): 571–85, http://afs.sagepub.com/content/16/4/571.

65 D Command Scientific Liaison, "Post-traumatic Stress Disorder and the Canadian Vietnam Veteran," *Journal of Traumatic Stress* 3, no. 2 (1990): 239–54.

66 Robert H. Stretch, "Psychohological Readjustment of Canadian Vietnam Veterans," *Journal of Consulting and Clinical Psychology* 59, no. 1 (1991): 188–9.

67 Kumar Vedantham, Alain Brunet, Richard Boyer, Daniel S. Weiss, Thomas J. Metzler, and Charles R. Marmar, "Posttraumatic Stress Disorder, Trauma Exposure, and the Current Health of Canadian Bus Drivers," *Canadian Journal of Psychiatry* 46 (2001): 149–55.

68 Erica Weir, "Veterans and Post-traumatic Stress Disorder," *Canadian Medical Association Journal* 163, no. 9 (2000): 1187.

69 Jeffrey S. Yarvis, Patrick S. Bordnick, Christina Spivey, and David Pedlar, "Subthreshold PTSD: A Comparison of Alcohol, Depression, and Health Problems in Canadian Peacekeepers with Different Levels of Traumatic Stress," *Stress, Trauma, and Crisis* 8 (April 2005): 195–213, http://www.tandfonline.com/doi/abs/10.1080/15434610590956949.

70 Jeffrey S. Yarvis and Laura Schiess, "Subthreshold Posttraumatic Stress Disorder (PTSD) as a Predictor of Depression, Alcohol Use, and Health Problems in Veterans," *Journal of Workplace Behavioral Health* 23, no. 4 (2008): 395–424.

71 Shannon Giddord, James Hutchinson, and Maggie Gibson, "Lifespan Considerations in the Psychological Treatment of Canadian Veterans with Post Traumatic Stress Disorder," in *Shaping the Future: Military and Veteran Health Research*, ed. Alice Aiken and Stéphanie Bélanger, 204–15 (Kingston: Canadian Defence Academy Press, 2011).

72 J. Don Richardson and Kate St Cyr, "Examining the Association between Psychiatric Ilness and Suicidal Ideation in Sample of Treatment-Seeking Canadian Peacekeeping and Combat Veterans with Posttraumatic Stress Disorder," *Canadian Journal of Psychiatry* 57, no. 8 (2012): 496–504.

73 Stéphane Grenier, Kath Darte, Alexandra Heber, and Don Richardson, "The Operational Stress Injury Social Support Program: A Peer Support Program in Collaboration between the Canadian Forces and Veterans Affairs Canada," in *Combat Stress Injury: Theory, Research, and Management*, ed. Charles R. Figley, William P. Nash, and Jonathan Shay, 261–94 (New York: Routledge, 2007).

74 Alexandra Heber, Stephane Grenier, Donald Richardson, and Kathy Darte, *Combining Clinical Treatment and Peer Support: A Unique Approach to Overcoming Stigma and Delivering Care* (Ottawa: Queen's Printer, 2006).

75 Rebecca A. Matteo, "The Economic Consequences of Post-traumatic Stress Disorder in Clients of Veterans Affairs Canada" (PhD diss., University of North Carolina at Chapel Hill, 2011).

76 Standing Committee on Veterans Affairs, *Support for Veterans and Other Victims of Posttraumatic Disorder* (Ottawa: Queen's Printer, 2007).

77 Jennifer A. Boisvert, Donald R. McCreary, Kristi D. Wright, and Gordon Asmundson, "Factorial Validity of the Center for Epidemiologic Studies–Depression

(CES-D) Scale in Military Peacekeepers," *Depression and Anxiety* 17, no. 1 (January 2003): 19–25, http://www.ncbi.nlm.nih.gov/pubmed/12577274.

78   Isabelle Savoie, Denise Morettin, Carolyn J. Green, and Arminée Kazanjian, "Systematic Review of the Role of Gender as a Health Determinant of Hospitalization for Depression," *International Journal of Technology Assessment in Health Care* 20, no. 2 (January 2004): 115–27, http://www.ncbi.nlm.nih.gov/pubmed/15209172.

79   Norman Shields, Michel White, and Michael Egan, "Dossiers sur la santé des anciens combattants: "Battlefield Blues" ambivalence face au traitement chez les vétérans souffrant de dépression," *Canadian Family Physician* 55 (2009): 799–802.

80   Shay-Lee Belik, Murray B. Stein, Gordon J. G. Asmundson, and Jitender Sareen, "Are Canadian Soldiers More Likely to Have Suicidal Ideation and Suicide Attempts Than Canadian Civilians?," *American Journal of Epidemiology* 172, no. 11 (October 2010): 1250–8.

81   Jitender Sareen and Shay-Lee Belik, "The Need for Outreach in Preventing Suicide among Young Veterans," *Public Library of Science Medicine* 6, no. 3 (3 March 2009): 0235–6, http://www.plosmedicine.org/article/info:doi/10.1371/journal.pmed.1000035.

82   A. Wong, M. Escobar, A. Lesage, M. Loyer, C. Vanier, and I. Sakinofsky, "Are un Peacekeepers at Risk for Suicide?," *Suicide & Life-Threatening Behavior* 31, no. 1 (January 2001): 103–12, http://www.ncbi.nlm.nih.gov/pubmed/11326764.

83   Mark Zamorski, *Report of the Canadian Forces Expert Panel on Suicide Prevention* (Ottawa: Queen's Printer, 2010).

84   Mark A. Zamorski, "Suicide Prevention in Military Organizations," *International Review of Psychiatry* 23 (April 2011): 173–80, http://www.ncbi.nlm.nih.gov/pubmed/21521087.

85   Statistics Canada, *Canadian Community Health Survey Cycle 1.2 Mental Health and Well-being: Canadian Forces Master File Documentation* (Ottawa: Queen's Printer, 2004).

86   Mark Zamorski, *Report on the Findings of the Enhanced Post-Deployment Screening of Those Returning from Op Archer / Task Force Afghanistan / Op Athena as of 11 Feb 2011* (Ottawa: Queen's Printer, 2011).

87   Tannis Y. Arbuckle and Urs Maag, "Individual Differences in Trajectory of Intellectual Development over 45 Years of Adulthood," *Psychology and Aging* 13, no. 4 (1998): 663–75.

88   D. P. Gold, D. Andres, J. Chaikelson, E. Schwartzman, and T. Arbuckle, "A Longitudinal Study of Competence in Elderly Veterans: The Role of Alcohol and Education," *Psychiatry* 54, no. 3 (August 1991): 238–50, http://www.ncbi.nlm.nih.gov/pubmed/1946825.

89   Dolores Pushkar Gold, David Andres, Jamshid Etezadi, Tannis Arbuckle, Alex Schwartzman, and June Chaikelson, "Structural Equation Model of Intellectual Change and Continuity and Predictors of Intelligence in Older Men," *Psychology and Aging* 10, no. 2 (June 1995): 294–303, http://www.ncbi.nlm.nih.gov/pubmed/7662188.

90   David William Molloy, Rosalie Russo, David Pedlar, and Michel Bédard, "Implementation of Advance Directives among Community-Dwelling Veterans," *Gerontologist* 40, no. 2 (April 2000): 213–17, http://www.ncbi.nlm.nih.gov/pubmed/10820924.

91 Jim Thompson, Michael Egan, Timothy Stultz, and Roland Chiasson, *Development of the Document: Dementia – A Resource for Health Professionals* (Charlottetown: Queen's Printer, 2009).

92 David J. Pedlar and David E. Biegel, "The Impact of Family Caregiver Attitudes on the Use of Community Services for Dementia Care," *Journal of Applied Gerontology* 18, no. 2 (1 June 1999): 201–21, http://jag.sagepub.com/cgi/doi/10.1177/073346489901800205.

93 Amber A. Mather, Murray B. Stein, and Jitender Sareen, "Social Anxiety Disorder and Social Fears in the Canadian Military: Prevalence, Comorbidity, Impairment, and Treatment-Seeking," *Journal of Psychiatric Research* 44, no. 14 (October 2010): 887–93, http://linkinghub.elsevier.com/retrieve/pii/S0022395610000543.

94 Vivian C. McAlister, "Composite Tissue Allotransplantation to Treat Veterans with Complex Amputation Injuries," in *Shaping the Future: Military and Veteran Health Research*, ed. Alice Aiken and Stéphanie Bélanger, 32–3 (Kingston: Canadian Defence Academy Press, 2011), 7.

95 Nathan Smith, review of *Veterans with a Vision: Canada's War Blinded in Peace and War, Canadian Historical Review* 92, no. 3 (2011): 565–6.

96 Stastistics Canada, *Canadian Forces Cancer and Mortality Study: Causes of Death* (Ottawa: Queen's Printer, 2011).

97 Statistics Canada, *The Canadian Persian Gulf Cohort Study: Detailed Report* (Ottawa: Queen's Printer, 2005).

98 Homer C. N. Tien, Sanjay Acharya, and Donald A. Redelmeier, "Preventing Deaths in the Canadian Military," *American Journal of Preventive Medicine* 38, no. 3 (March 2010): 331–9, http://www.ncbi.nlm.nih.gov/pubmed/20171536.

99 Janet Fast, Alison Yacyshyn, and Norah Keating, *Wounded Veterans, Wounded Families* (Edmonton: University of Alberta Press, 2008).

100 Jim Thompson and Mary Beth Maclean, *Evidence for Best Practices in the Managment of Disabilities: Executive Summary* (Charlottetown: Queen's Printer, 2009).

101 Paula C. Fletcher, Dawn M. Guthrie, Katherine Berg, and John P. Hirdes, "Risk Factors for Restriction in Activity Associated with Fear of Falling among Seniors within the Community," *Journal of Patient Safety* 6, no. 3 (September 2010): 187–91, http://www.ncbi.nlm.nih.gov/pubmed/21491793.

102 Dawn P. Gill, Dawn P. Guang Yong Zou, Gareth Jones, and Mark R. Speechley, "Comparison of Regression Models for the Analysis of Fall Risk Factors in Older Veterans," *Annals of Epidemiology* 19, no. 8 (August 2009): 523–30, http://www.ncbi.nlm.nih.gov/pubmed/19394862.

103 Dawn P. Gill, G. Y. Ou, Gareth R. Jones, and Mark Speechley, "Injurious Falls Are Associated with Lower Household but Higher Recreational Physical Activities in Community-Dwelling Older Male Veterans," *Gerontology* 54, no. 2 (January 2008): 106–15, http://www.ncbi.nlm.nih.gov/pubmed/18259094.

104 Mark Speechley, Shannon Belfry, Michael J. Borrie, Krista Bray Jenkyn, Richard Crilly, Dawn P. Gill, Sarena McLean, Paul Stolee, Anthony A. Vandervoort, and Gareth R. Jones, "Risk Factors for Falling among Community-Dwelling Veterans and Their Caregivers," *Canadian Journal on Aging / La revue canadienne du vieillissement* 24, no. 3 (31 March 2010): 261–74, http://www.journals.cambridge.org/abstract_S0714980800002890.

105 Lori E. Weeks, "An Examination of the Impact of Gender and Veteran Status on Falls among Implications for Targeting Falls among Community-Dwelling Seniors," *Community Health* 30, no. 2 (2007): 121–8.

106 Charles C. Engel, Kenneth C. Hyams, and Ken Scott, "Managing Future Gulf War Syndromes: International Lessons and New Models of Care," *Philosophical Transactions of the Royal Society of London. Series B, Biological Sciences* 361 (29 April 2006): 707–20, http://www.pubmedcentral.nih.gov/articlerender.fcgi?artid=1569617&tool=pmcentrez&rendertype=abstract.

107 G. A. Jamal, "Gulf War Syndrom: A Model for the Complexity of Biological and Environmental Interaction with Human Health," *Adverse Drug Reactions and Toxicological Reviews* 17, no. 1 (March 1998): 1–17, http://www.ncbi.nlm.nih.gov/pubmed/9638279.

108 Sharon Abel, *Risk Factors for the Development of Noise-Induced Hearing Loss in Canadian Forces Personnel* (Toronto: Queen's Printer, 2004).

109 Kenneth C. Hyams, James Riddle, David H. Trump, and John T. Graham, "Endemic Infectious Diseases and Biological Warfare during the Gulf War: A Decade of Analysis and Final Concerns," *American Journal of Tropical Medicine and Hygiene* 65, no. 5 (November 2001): 664–70, http://www.ncbi.nlm.nih.gov/pubmed/11716134.

110 Vilija R. Joyce, Paul G. Barnett, Ahmed M. Bayoumi, Susan C. Griffin, Tassos C. Kyriakides, Wei Yu, Vandana Sundaram, Mark Holodniy, Sheldon T. Brown, William Cameron, Mike Youle, Mark Sculpher, Aslam H. Anis, and Douglas K. Owens, "Health-Related Quality of Life in a Randomized Trial of Antiretroviral Therapy for Advanced HIV Disease," *Journal of Acquired Immune Deficiency Syndromes* 50, no. 1 (1 January 2009): 27–36, http://www.ncbi.nlm.nih.gov/pubmed/19295332.

111 Eileen M. Proctor, Judith L. Isaac-Renton, William B. Robertson, and William A. Black, "Strongyloidiasis in Canadian Far East War Veterans," *Canadian Medical Association Journal* 133 (1985): 876–78.

112 David Pichora, Randy Ellis, Tim Bryant, and John Rudan, "Advanced Real-Time 3D Imaging, Planning and Navigation in Orthopaedic Surgery," in *Shaping the Future: Military and Veteran Health Research*, ed. Alice Aiken and Stéphanie Bélanger, 37–51 (Kingston: Canadian Defence Academy Press, 2011).

113 Asaf Duraković, "Undiagnosed Illnesses and Radioactive Warfare," *Croatian Medical Journal* 44, no. 5 (October 2003): 520–32, http://www.ncbi.nlm.nih.gov/pubmed/14515407.

114 Hari Sharma, "Investigations of Environmental Impacts from the Deployment of Depleted Uranium Munitions," *Stop NATO!* (September 2003), http://www.stopnato.org.uk/du-watch/sharma/du-report.htm.

115 Jim Thompson, Helena Gauthier, Alain Poirier, Susan Baglole, and Stewart Macintosh Ma, *Nominal Rolls: Lessons Learned from Developing the "Mustard Gas List" Rehabilitation Directorate* (Charlottetown: Queen's Printer, 2010).

116 E. A. Ough, B. J. Lewis, W. S. Andrews, L. G. I. Bennett, R. G. V. Hancock, and K. Scott, "An Examination of Uranium Levels in Canadian Forces Personnel Who Served in the Gulf War and Kosovo," *Health Physics* 82, no. 4 (2002): 527–32.

117 Anne-Marie Boström, Deanna Van Soest, Betty Kolewaski, Doris L. Milke, and Carole A. Estabrooks, "Nutrition Status among Residents Living in a Veterans' Long-term Care Facility in Western Canada: A Pilot Study," *Journal of the American*

Medical Directors Association 12, no. 3 (March 2011): 217–25,
http://www.ncbi.nlm.nih.gov/pubmed/21333925.

118 Kathryn L. Hall, Caroline E. Denda, and Helen Yeung, "Dietary Vitamin D Intake among Elderly Residents in a Veterans' Centre," *Canadian Journal of Dietetic Practice and Research* 71, no. 1 (1 January 2010): 49–52.

119 Brendon Gurd and Jasmin K. Ma, "Potential Benefits of Interval Training for Active Military Personnel and Military Veterans," in *Shaping the Future: Military and Veteran Health Research*, ed. Alice Aiken and Stéphanie Bélanger, 52–67 (Kingston: Canadian Defence Academy Press, 2011).

120 M. A. Vaillandercourt and C. Bennett, "Editorial: Adherence to Lipid-Lowering Drug Therapy among Members of the Canadian Forces," *Military Medicine* 173, no. 7 (2008): 666–70.

121 Margaret C. Gibson, Gail Woodbury, Kim Hay, and Nancy Bol, "Pain Reports by Older Adults in Long-term Care: A Pilot Study of Changes over Time," *Pain Research & Management* 10, no. 3 (January 2005): 159–64, http://www.ncbi.nlm.nih.gov/pubmed/16175252.

122 Patricia L. Dobkin and Lucy J. Boothroyd, "Organizing Health Services for Patients with Chronic Pain: When There Is a Will There Is a Way," *Pain Medicine* 9, no. 7 (October 2008): 881–9, http://www.ncbi.nlm.nih.gov/pubmed/18950443.

123 James M. Thompson, Roland Chiasson, Patrick Loisel, Markus Besemann, and Tina Pranger, "Veteran Health Files: A Sailor's Pain – Veterans' Musculoskeletal Disorders, Chronic Pain, and Disability," *Canadian Family Physician* 55 (2009): 1085–8.

124 Markus Besemann, "Physical Rehabilitation Following Polytrauma: The Canadian Forces Physical Rehabilitation Program 2008–2011," *Canadian Journal of Surgery* 54, no. 6 (1 December 2011): S135–41, http://www.ncbi.nlm.nih.gov/pubmed/22099327.

125 P. Doyle, N. Maconochie, and M. Ryan, "Reproductive Health of Gulf War Veterans," *Philosophical Transactions of the Royal Society B: Biological Sciences* 361 (29 April 2006): 571–84, http://rstb.royalsocietypublishing.org/content/361/1468/571.

126 Mark A. Zamorski and Amanda M. Kelley, *Risky Driving Behaviour* (Ottawa: Queen's Printer, 2011).

127 Mary Tremblay, "Going Back to Civvy Street: A Historical Account of the Impact of the Everest and Jennings Wheelchair for Canadian World War II Veterans with Spinal Cord Injury," *Disability and Society* 11, no. 2 (2010): 37–41.

128 Charles Nelson et al., "Knowledge Gained from the Brief Traumatic Brain Injury Screen: Implications for Treating Canadian Military Personnel," *Military Medicine* 176, no. 2 (2011): 156–60.

129 James M. Thompson, *Persistent Symptoms Following Mild Traumatic Brain Injury (mTBI): A Resource for Clinicians and Staff* (Charlottetown: Queen's Printer, 2008).

130 Kerry Sudom, Mark Zamorski, and Bryan Garber, "Stigma and Barriers to Mental Health Care in Deployed Canadian Forces Personnel," *Military Medicine* 24, no. 4 (2012): 414–31.

131 Mark A. Zamorski, *Towards a Broader Conceptualization of Need, Stigma, and Barriers to Mental Health Care in Military Organizations: Recent Research Findings from the Canadian Forces* (Ottawa: Queen's Printer, 2003).

132 Sarah Louise Buydens, "The Lived Experience of Women Veterans of the Canadian Forces" (MA thesis, University of Victoria, 2002).

133 Kerry Sudom and J. A. Eyvindson, *Effects of Personnel Tempo on Military Members, Their Families, and the Organization: An Annotated Bibliography* (Ottawa: Queen's Printer, 2008).

134 David J. Pedlar and David E. Biegel, "The Impact of Family Caregiver Attitudes on the Use of Community Services for Dementia Care," *Journal of Applied Gerontology* 18, no. 2 (June 1999): 201–21.

135 Alysha D. Jones, "Intimate Partner Violence in Military Couples: A Review of the Literature," *Aggression and Violent Behavior* 17, no. 2 (March 2012): 147–57, http://linkinghub.elsevier.com/retrieve/pii/S1359178911001121.

136 Susan L. Ray, *A Downward Spiral: Homelessness among Canadian Forces and Allied Forces Veterans* (London: Human Resources and Skills Development Canada, 2011).

137 Susan L. Ray, "Social Covenant: Creating Sanctuary for Homeless Veterans," in *Veterans: Health Issues, Coping Strategies and Benefits,* ed. M. McCleod and C. S. Hewitt, 65–74 (Hauppauge, NY: Nova Science Publishers, 2012).

138 Susan L. Ray and Cheryl Forchuck, "The Experience of Homelessness among Canadian Forces and Allied Forces Veterans: Preliminary Findings," in *Shaping the Future: Military and Veteran Health Research,* ed. Alice Aiken and Stéphanie A. H. Bélanger, 269–84 (Kingston: Canadian Defence Academy Press, 2011).

139 Margaret Boswall, Suzanne O'Hanley, Nicole Caron-Boulet, and James M. Thompson, "Veteran Health Files: Forms for Father," *Canadian Family Physician* 56 (2010): 147–50.

140 James Struthers, "'They Suffered with Us and Should Be Compensated': Entitling Caregivers of Canada's Veterans," *Canadian Journal on Aging / La Revue canadienne du vieillissement* 26, no. 1 (2007): 117–32.

141 Standing Committee on Veterans Affairs, *A Timely Tune-up for the Living New Veterans Charter: Report of the Standing Committee on Veterans Affairs* (Ottawa: Queen's Printer, 2010).

142 Amy Buitenhuis and Alice B. Aiken, "A Comparison of Financial Programs Offered to 'Traditional' versus 'New' Veterans with Severe Disabilities: A New Class of Veteran?," in *Shaping the Future: Military and Veteran Health Research,* ed. Alice Aiken and Stéphanie Bélanger, 239–54 (Kingston: Canadian Defence Academy Press, 2011).

143 George Zimmerman and Wesley Weber, "Care for the Caregivers: A Program for Canadian Military Chaplains after Serving in NATO and United Nations Peacekeeping Missions in the 1990s," *Military Medicine* 165, no. 9 (2000): 687–90.

144 Jane A. Etherington, "From Combat to Classroom: Canadian Soldiers in Transiton" (MA thesis, Queen's University, 2012).

145 Canadian Medical Association, "BC Physicians Help Peacekeepers Fight Their Demons," *Canadian Medical Association Journal* 163, no. 9 (2000): 1183.

146 Jim Thompson, Jill Sweet, Alain Poirier, and Linda Van Til, *Suicide Ideation and Attempt Findings in the Survey on Transition to Civilian Life: Descriptive Analysis* (Charlottetown: Queen's Printer, 2011).

147 Jitender Sareen, "Emotional Costs of War and Peacekeeping High for Many Returning Soldiers," *Canadian Psychiatry Aujourd'hui* 5, no. 1 (2009): 446–7.

148 Jitender Sareen, Shay-Lee Belik, Murray B. Stein, and Gordon J. G. Asmundson, "Correlates of Perceived Need for Mental Health Care among Active Military

Personnel," *Psychiatric Services* 61, no. 1 (January 2010): 50–7, http://www.ncbi.nlm.nih.gov/pubmed/20044418.

149 Jitender Sareen, Brian J. Cox, Tracie O. Afifi, Murray B. Stein, Shay-Lee Belik, Graham Meadows, and Gordon J. G. Asmundson, "Combat and Peacekeeping Operations in Relation to Prevalence of Mental Disorders and Perceived Need for Mental Health Care," *Archives of General Psychiatry* 64, no. 7 (2007): 843–52.

150 M. C. Gibson, I. Gutmanis, H. Clarke, D. Wiltshire, A. Feron, and E. Gorman, "Staff Opinions about the Components of a Good Death in Long-term Care," *International Journal of Palliative Nursing* 14, no. 8 (2008): 374–81.

151 Auditor General, *Report of the Auditor General of Canada to the House of Commons: Chapter 4 – Military Health Care – National Defence* (Ottawa: Queen's Printer, 2007).

152 Minister of National Defence and Minister of Veterans Affairs Canada, *The Minister of National Defence and the Minister of Veterans Affairs Canada 2000 Annual Report to the Standing Committee on National Defence and Veterans Affairs on Quality of Life in the Canadian Forces* (Ottawa: Queen's Printer, 2000).

153 M. B. Maclean, L. Van Til, J. M. Thompson, D. Pedlar, A, Poirier, J. Adams, S. Hartigan, K. Sudom, *Life After Service Study: Data Collection Methodology for The Income Study and The Transition to Civilian Life Survey* (Government Report, Charlottetown, 2010).

154 Veteran Affairs Canada, *Literature Review: Care Trends for Seniors* (Government Report, Charlottetown, 1997).

155 Hollander Analytical Services, *Continuing Care Research Project Literature Review on the Cost-Effectiveness of Continuing Care Services* (Government Report, Victoria, 2006).

156 Margaret C. Gibson and Maryse Savoie, "Vet-Link: A New, National, Interdisciplinary Clinical-Research Network for Veterans Care," *Geriatrics Today* 6 (2003): 103–5.

157 Marcus J. Hollander, *Evaluation Framework for a Research Study on Continuing Care Services Provided by Veterans Affairs Canada (*Final Report, Charlottetown, 2004).

158 Mary Beth Maclean, James Thompson, and Alain Poirier, *Rehabilitation Needs of VAC Clients Post Eligibility for the SISIP Vocational Rehabilitation Program* (Government Report, Charlottetown, 2010).

159 Jo Ann Miller, Marcus Hollander, and Margaret MacAdams, *The Continuing Care Research Project for Veterans Affairs Canada and the Government of Ontario* (Government Report, Victoria, 2008).

160 Dave Pedlar, Wendy Lockhart, and Stewart Macintosh, "Canada's Veterans Independence Program: A Pioneer of 'Aging' at Home," *Health Papers* 10, no. 1 (2009): 79–83.

161 David Pedlar and John Walker, "The Overseas Service Veteran At Home Pilot: How Choice of Care May Affect Use of Nursing Home Beds and Waiting Lists," *Canadian Journal on Aging/ La revue canadienne du vieillissement* 23, no. 4 (31 March 2004): 367–9, http://www.journals.cambridge.org/abstract_S071498 0800003391.

162 John Sloan, Nicole Caron-Boulet, David Pedlar, James M. Thompson, "Veteran Health Files: Overgrown Lawn – Military Veteran No Longer Able to Maintain the Yard," *Canadian Family Physician* 55 (2009): 483–5.

163   Mark A Zamorski, *Evaluation of an Enhanced Post-deployment Health Screening Program for Canadian Forces Members Deployed on Operation APOLLO (Afghanistan/SW Asia) – Preliminary Findings and Action Plan* (Government Report, Ottawa, 2003).

164   Marlee Franz, "Results of a File Review of 350 Clients Who Have Participated in the Veterans Affairs Canada Rehabilitation Program, New Veterans Charter Evaluation," in *Shaping the Future: Military and Veteran Health Research*, ed. Alice Aiken and Stéphanie Bélanger, 323–41 (Canadian Defence Academy Press, 2011).

165   Gregory C. Gray and Han K. Kang, "Healthcare Utilization and Mortality Among Veterans of the Gulf War," *Philosophical Transactions of the Royal Society of London. Series B, Biological Sciences* 361 (29 April 2006): 553–69, http://www.pubmedcentral.nih.gov/articlerender.fcgi?artid=1569626&tool=pmcentrez&rendertype=abstract.

166   Gregory C. Gray, Gary D. Gackstetter, Han K. Kang, John T. Graham, Ken C. Scott, "After More Than 10 Years of Gulf War Veteran Medical Evaluations, What Have We Learned?," *American Journal of Preventive Medicine* 26, no. 5 (June 2004): 443–52, http://www.ncbi.nlm.nih.gov/pubmed/15165662.

167   James M. Thompson, Jill Sweet, and David Pedlar, *Preliminary Analysis of the CCHS 2.1 National Survey of the Health of Canadian Military Service Veterans* (Government Report, Charlottetown, 2012).

168   Timothy G. Black and Chiara Papile, "Making It on Civvy Street: An Online Survey of Canadian Veterans in Transition / Réussir sa transition vers la vie civile : Sondage en ligne des ex-membres des forces canadiennes en situation de transition," *Canadian Journal of Counselling and Psychotherapy* 44, no. 4 (2010): 383–401.

169   Ann-Renée Blais, Megan M. Thompson, Angela Febbraro, Donna Pickering, Don McCreary, *The Development of a Multidimensional Measure of Post-deployment Reintegration: Initial Psychometric Analyses & Descriptive Results – Final Report to Director General Health Services Quality of Life* (Government Report, Toronto, 2003).

170   Ann-Renée Blais, Megan M. Thompson, and Donald R. McCreary, *Post-deployment Reintegration Measure: Psychometric Replication and Preliminary Validation Results* (Government Report, Toronto, 2006).

171   Bryan G. Garber and Mark A. Zamorski, "Evaluation of a Third-location Decompression Program for Canadian Forces Members Returning from Afghanistan," *Military Medicine* 177, no. 4 (April 2012): 397–403, http://www.ncbi.nlm.nih.gov/pubmed/22594129.

172   Deanne Marie Gervais, "Intergenerational Life Review Group With Canadian World War II Veterans and Canadian Peacekeepers" (MA thesis, University of British Columbia, 2001).

173   Jamie G. H. Hacker Hughes, Mark Earnshaw, Neil Greenberg, Rod Eldridge, Nicola T. Fear, Claire French, Martin P. Deahl, and Simon Wessely, "The Use of Psychological Decompression in Military Operational Environments," *Military Medicine* 173, no. 6 (June 2008): 534–8, http://www.ncbi.nlm.nih.gov/pubmed/18595415.

174   M. B. Maclean, A. Poirier, and J. Sweet, *Veterans Independence Program Need – Indicators from the Survey on Transition to Civilian Life* (Government Report, Charlottetown, 2011).

175 Mary Beth Maclean, Alain Poirier, and Jim Thompson, *Contact with Veterans Not in Receipt of VAC Benefits – Data from the Survey on Transition to Civilian Life* (Government Report, Charlottetown, 2011).

176 M. B. Maclean, J. Sweet, and A. Poirier, *Effectiveness of Transition Screening – Evidence from the Survey on Transition to Civilian Life* (Government Report, Charlottetown, 2011).

177 Mary Beth Maclean, Jill Sweet, and Alain Poirier, *Income Adequacy: Comparing Pre- and Post- Military Incomes of Medical and Non-Medical Releases* (Government Report, Charlottetown, 2011).

178 M. B. Maclean, J. Sweet, and A. Poirier, *Effectiveness of Career Transition Services* (Government Report, Charlottetown, 2011).

179 Mary Beth Maclean, Jill Sweet, and Alain Poirier, *Predictors of Persistent Low Income* (Government Report, Charlottetown, 2012).

180 Mary Beth Maclean, Linda Van Til, Jim Thompson, David Pedlar, Alain Poirier, Jonathan Adams, Shannon Hartigan, Kerry Sudom, Catherine Campbell, *Life After Service Study: Data Collection Methodology for The Income Study and The Transition to Civilian Life Survey* (Government Report, Charlottetown, 2012).

181 Victor W. Marshal, Rebecca Matteo, and David Pedlar, *Post-military Experiences of Veterans Affairs Canada Clients: The Need for Military Release Readiness* (Government Report, Chapel Hill, NC, USA, 2005).

182 Victor W. Marshall, Rebecca Matteo, and David Pedlar, *Work-related Experience and Financial Security of Veterans Affairs Canada Clients: Contrasting Medical and Non-medical Discharge* (Government Report, Chapel Hill. NC, USA 2005).

183 André Marin, *From Tents to Sheets: An Analysis of the CF Experience with Third Location Decompression After Deployment* (Government Report, Ottawa, 2004).

184 Helmets to Hardhats Canada, *Helmets to Hardhats Canada Buisness Plan* (Report, Ottawa, 2012), http://www.buildingtrades.ca/.

185 Tina Pranger, Kelly Murphy, and James M. Thompson, "Veteran Health Files: Shaken World – Coping with Transition to Civilian Life," *Canadian Family Physician* 55, no. 1 (2009): 159–61.

186 S. L. Ray and K. Heaslip, "Canadian Military Transitioning to Civilian Life: A Discussion Paper," *Journal of Psychiatric and Mental Health Nursing* 18, no. 3 (10 April 2011): 198–204, http://doi.wiley.com/10.1111/j.1365-2850.2010.01652.x.

187 Michel Rossignol, *Afghanistan: Military Personnel and Operational Stress Injuries* (Government Report, Ottawa, 2007).

188 Michael Neil Sorsdahl, "Re-entry and Transition Factors for Returning Canadian Forces Military Members From Overseas Deployments" (PhD dissertation, University of British Columbia, 2010).

189 Michael Neil Sorsdahl, "Interpersonal Trust in the Canadian Forces Transition Program for Peacekeepers and Veterans" (MA thesis, University of Victoria, 2005).

190 Wendy Sullivan-Kwantes, Angela R. Febbraro, and Ann-Renee Blais, *Air Force Post-deployment Reintegration: A Qualitative Study* (Government Report, Toronto, 2005).

191 Jim Thompson, Marc Corbière, Linda Van Til, Tina Pranger, Norman Shields, May Wong, Chantal Basque, *BECES-V: Modification of the BECES Tool (Barriers to Employment and Coping Efficacy Scales) for Veterans with Mental Health Problems Reintegrating in the Workplace* (Government Report, Charlottetown, 2011).

192 Jim Thompson, Mary Beth MacLean, Linda Van Til, Jill Sweet, Alain Poirier, and David Pedlar, *Survey on Transition to Civilian Life: Report on Regular Force Veterans* (Charlottetown: Queen's Printer, 2011).

193 Jim Thompson and Alain Poirier, *Descriptive Cross Tables from the Survey on Transition to Civilian Life* (Charlottetown: Queen's Printer, 2012).

194 Jim Thompson and Alain Poirier, *Survey on Transition to Civilian Life: Veterans Not Receiving Benefits from VAC* (Charlottetown: Queen's Printer, 2011).

195 Marvin J. Westwood, Timothy G. Black, and Holly McLean, "A Re-entry Program for Peacekeeping Soldiers: Promoting Personal and Career Transition," *Canadian Journal of Counselling* 36, no. 3 (2002): 221–32.

196 Marvin J. Westwood, Holly McLean, Douglas Cave, William Borgen, and Paul Slakov, "Coming Home: A Group-Based Approach for Assisting Military Veterans in Transition," *Journal for Specialists in Group Work* 35, no. 1 (21 January 2010): 44–68, http://www.tandfonline.com/doi/abs/10.1080/01933920903466059.

197 Mark A. Zamorski, Kim Guest, Suzanne Bailey, and Bryan G. Garber, *Beyond Battlemind: Evaluation of a New Mental Health Training Program for Canadian Forces Personnel Participating in Third-Location Decompression* (Ottawa: Queen's Printer, 2012).

198 Heather M. Foran, Bryan G. Garber, Mark A. Zamorski, Mariane Wray, Kathleen Mulligan, Neil Greenberg, Carl Andrew Castro, and Amy B. Adler, *Post-Deployment Military Mental Health Training: Cross-National Evaluations* (Ottawa: Queen's Printer, 2011).

199 Rakesh Jetly, "Psychiatric Lessons Learned in Kandahar," *Canadian Journal of Surgery / Journal canadien de chirurgie* 54, no. 6 (December 2011): 142–4, http://www.pubmedcentral.nih.gov/articlerender.fcgi?artid=3322650&tool=pmcentrez&rendertype=abstract

200 Kathryn Basham, "Weaving a Tapestry of Resilience and Challenges, Commentary: Clinical Assessment of Canadian Military Couples," *Clinical Social Work Journal* 37, no. 4 (5 November 2009): 340–5, http://www.springerlink.com/index/10.1007/s10615-008-0176-y.

201 Megan M. Thompson, Monique A. M. Gignac, *A Model of Psychological Adaptation in Peace Support Operations: An Overview* (Ottawa: Queen's Printer, 2001).

202 Jon D. Elhai, J. Don Richardson, and David J. Pedlar, "Predictors of General Medical and Psychological Treatment Use among a National Sample of Peacekeeping Veterans with Health Problems," *Journal of Anxiety Disorders* 21, no. 4 (January 2007): 580–9, http://www.ncbi.nlm.nih.gov/pubmed/16965892.

203 David K. Conn, Ian Ferguson, K. Mandelman, and Carol Ward, "Psychotropic Drug Utilization in Long-term-Care Facilities for the Elderly in Ontario, Canada," *International Psychogeriatrics* 11, no. 3 (September 1999): 223–33, http://www.ncbi.nlm.nih.gov/pubmed/10547123.

204 Chelsea Clark, "Not Attributable to Service: First World War Veterans' 'Second Battle' with the Canadian Pension System" (MA thesis, University of Calgary, 2009).

205 Gerontological Advisory Council, *Keeping the Promise: The Future of Health Benefits for Canada's War Veterans* (Charlottetown: Queen's Printer, 2006).

206 Victor W. Marshall and Rebecca A. Matteo, *Canadian Forces Clients of Veterans Affairs Canada: "Risk Factors" for Post-Release Socioeconomic Well-Being* (Government Report, Chapel Hill, NC, 2004).

207 Peter Neary, "'Without the Stigma of Pauperism': Canadian Veterans in the 1930s," *British Journal of Canadian Studies* 22, no. 1 (1936): 32–61.

208 Canadian Forces Advisory Council, *Honouring Canada's Commitment: "Opportunity with Security" for Canadian Forces Veterans and Their Families in the 21st Century* (Ottawa: Queen's Printer, 2004).

209 Ellen M. Gee and Margeny A. Boyce, "Veterans and Veterans Legislation in Canada: An Historical Overview," *Canadian Journal on Aging* 7, no. 3 (1988): 204–17.

210 Paul C. Hébert, Ken Flegel, Matthew B. Stanbrook, and Noni MacDonald, "Editorial: No Privacy of Health Information in Canada's Armed Forces," *Canadian Medical Association Journal* 183, no. 3 (2011): E167–8.

211 Mary Tremblay, "The Right to the Best Medical Care: Dr W. P. Warner and the Canadian Department of Veterans Affairs, 1945–55," *Canadian Bulletin of Medical History* 15 (1998): 3–25.

212 Allan English, "Not Written in Stone: Social Covenants and Resourcing Military and Veterans Health Care in Canada," in *Shaping the Future: Military and Veteran Health Research*, ed. Alice Aiken and Stéphanie Bélanger, 230–8 (Kingston: Canadian Defence Academy Press, 2011).

12

Exploring the Relationships between Untreated Adverse Childhood Events and Substance Abuse, and Their Impact on PTSD Relapse Rates among Canadian Military Veterans

JOHN WHELAN

Abstract

Chart data for 108 CF veterans were reviewed in an exploratory study of the relationships between adverse childhood events (ACE), substance use disorders (SUD), and post traumatic stress disorder (PTSD) relapse rates. Data were compared for two veteran groups: one group treated previously for PTSD ($n = 57$) and a second group of untreated veterans undergoing initial PTSD assessment ($n = 51$). Interview data, and responses to the Detailed Assessment of PTSD Scale (DAPS) and the Personality Assessment Inventory (PAI) were submitted to formal statistical analysis. The results indicated that a history of developmental abuse, cluster B personality traits, and adolescent and military substance abuse were associated with PTSD relapse among veterans treated previously within exposure-based, cognitive-behavioural therapy (CBT-PE). The implications of veteran accounts of unreported physical and sexual abuse, and ongoing use of substances during prior treatment (i.e., CBT-PE) are discussed. The findings support recommendations that clinicians conduct developmentally-focused assessments for personnel presenting with military-related trauma. Results also provide support for a formal study aimed at validating screening protocols to identify clients at risk for relapse after treatment, and to tailor treatment regimes with particular assessment profiles. The chapter ends with a discussion of a conceptual model to guide future research.

Introduction

The impetus for this project came from clinical interviews with clients referred through Veterans Affairs Canada for reassessment and treatment of post traumatic stress disorder (PTSD). These veterans had completed exposure-based treatment previously, but during reassessments they continued to meet criteria for PTSD and disclosed developmental and substance abuse histories that were widely discrepant from the accounts described in baseline assessments conducted when they were still serving. This study investigates the impact of these undisclosed, potentially traumatizing events (PTEs) and substance use disorders (SUDs) on reported post-treatment declines. Specifically, the study explores the extent to which adverse childhood events (ACE) and SUDs were represented among these relapsing veterans, compared to veterans who were seeking assessment and treatment for a first time. Readers should note that the term relapse is used here to refer to spontaneous return of fear responses noted in the literature for anxiety disorders, including PTSD, following successful exposure treatment.[1]

Relevant Literature

Review of Front Line Treatments for PTSD

Cognitive-behavioural therapies (CBT) and exposure therapies, in particular, have been studied extensively and are deemed to be the preferred psychological treatment for PTSD.[2] Treatment standards for PTSD also recommend pharmacotherapy (e.g., sertraline, paroxetine) as part of interventions.[3] Despite the proven efficacy of psychotherapy and psychotropic interventions, a worrisome concern for clinicians, following the identified needs of earlier detection and easier access to treatment, is the persistence of trauma symptoms in approximately 50% of cases in some populations.[4] Early treatment termination by clients and symptom persistence because of co-morbid conditions (e.g., substance abuse, personality disorders, developmental trauma) contribute to observed post-treatment declines.[5] In fact, over 90% of those with PTSD are estimated to exhibit other Axis I disorders, including major depression, anxiety disorders, suicidality, and Axis II concerns (e.g., borderline and antisocial personality disorders).[6] Despite its proven effectiveness for discrete event trauma, recent studies have raised concerns over the comparative effectiveness of CBT-based interventions in managing multiple traumas and chronic addiction.[7] In the treatment of chronic interpersonal abuse, questions have also been raised over the adequacy of the construct of PTSD as a discrete-event disorder.[8] An alternative view that has gained attention holds that many of the co-morbid issues seen among PTSD clients (e.g. substance abuse and cluster B traits, such as affective instability, identity problems, negative relationships, and self-harm) are reflective of a broader constellation of reactions to trauma, namely complex PTSD.[9] This literature appears to present challenges to the PTSD construct and emphasizes the importance of adopting additional treatment approaches to psychological trauma that are sensitive to the full scope of life experiences.

Relationships between ACE and Adult-Onset PTSD

Childhood trauma has been identified as a stable predictor of adult-onset psychological distress, including depression, sexual disturbances, PTSD, substance use disorders, high PTSD symptom severity, and poor treatment outcomes.[10] A history of two or more traumatic events involving assaultive violence in childhood has been associated with a nearly five-fold greater risk that a traumatic event in adulthood will develop into PTSD.[11] Results from a 2012 large cross-sectional survey of the U.S. population noted a dose–response relationship between frequency of childhood physical assaults and subsequent psychiatric disorders (i.e., attention deficit hyperactivity disorder, PTSD, and bipolar disorder).[12] In terms of military PTSD, while studies have linked increased rates with direct combat experience (e.g., firefights), recent studies of U.S. combat soldiers from Iraq and Afghanistan found that ACE (e.g., childhood physical and sexual abuse, living with a mentally ill caregiver, witnessing domestic violence) played a critical role in the development of post-deployment depression and PTSD.[13] A somewhat provocative study of veterans from the Lebanon war assessed at baseline and again at follow-up (1983 and 2002 respectively) concluded that stressful experiences during childhood played a more significant role in the development of future PTSD than events during combat.[14] In sum, the findings from the literature emphasize the importance of understanding lifelong experiences in conceptualizing and treating PTSD, even in cases of military trauma.

Relationships among PTSD, SUD, and ACE

Among treatment-seeking substance-abuse clients, trauma histories are common and are linked with more severe substance use and higher psychiatric distress.[15] Estimates of PTSD rates among SUD clients vary from a high of 40% to 90%, with lower-end estimates of between 20% and 30%.[16] A Polish study reported that more than 80% of patients undergoing treatment for alcohol dependence reported at least one PTE and that approximately 60% of them reported multiple PTEs.[17] Other studies have reported illicit drug use estimates among military veterans of between 25% and 56%.[18] In a study of pathological gamblers, approximately 89% of them met criteria for a PTSD diagnosis.[19] Various theories have been advanced over the past eighty or more years to explain addictive behaviours, each one coming and going out of favour over time.[20] Over the past fifteen years, promising advances in understanding substance overuse and behavioural preoccupations (e.g., food, gambling, sex) have come from the field of trauma research.[21] This research has found generally that PTSD predates the onset of SUDs,[22] highlighting the function of various psychoactive substances and other behaviours in helping distressed people "self-medicate" overwhelming emotional and physiological states.[23] Several clinical studies suggest that a history of sexual abuse is common among individuals who are obese or who exhibit disordered eating.[24] Clients diagnosed with PTSD frequently report that they use alcohol, heroin, marijuana, benzodiazepines, and other depressant medications to help them sleep, reduce irritability and hyper-vigilance, and control excessive startle response, and that they often use prescription analgesics to reduce intrusive memories.[25] Consistent with this self-medication hypothesis, individuals with both SUD and PTSD problems often report a "drinking-to-cope motive" triggered by trauma memories.[26] These findings represent a body of evidence emphasizing complex interrelationships between ACEs and adult trauma reactions, and the role of self-medication motives for clients entering substance abuse and/or trauma-focused treatment.[27]

Purpose of Study

The literature outlines complex relationships between ACE, SUD, and adult PTSD, and the difficulties in treating these issues successfully when they are co-morbid. Much of the available research has focused on civilian populations, whereas the available military research tends to focus on diagnosing and treating combat exposure as a central feature of PTSD. This study is the first to investigate the effects of ACE and SUD among Canadian military veterans who have undergone PTSD treatment for operationally related trauma and have relapsed. Consistent with the literature, it is hypothesized that relapsed veterans will report higher levels of childhood sexual and physical abuse, and higher rates of SUD compared to the broader population of PTSD veterans.

Methods

A retrospective chart review was conducted for approximately 225 veterans referred for assessment and treatment at a private clinic in the Atlantic region during the period 2008–11. The clinic employs four psychologists who work primarily with serving and retired members of the military and RCMP. All clients were assessed by one of the psychologists and reviewed by the senior psychologist prior to release of final reports to Veterans Affairs Canada. PTSD diagnoses were based on the results of clinical interviews and equivalent findings from the Clinician-Administered PTSD Scale (CAPS)[28] and the Detailed Assessment of PTSD Scale (DAPS). Given the normative data and attention to associated features provided by the DAPS, only results from this measure were included in the study.

Ethical Considerations

The research proposal was reviewed with Veterans Affairs Canada and with the provincial regulatory body for psychologists. Given that client confidentiality was assured, that no other risks to participants had been identified, and with the potential of contributing to the understanding of military PTSD, permission was granted by both organizations to proceed with the study.

Inclusion/Exclusion Criteria

Participant charts were included for review if the assessment diagnosis met the criteria for operationally-related PTSD, and if the resulting profiles for completed DAPS and PAI were psychometrically valid. Participant charts were excluded from analysis if they met criteria for another OSI (e.g., major depressive disorder or panic disorder) but did not meet criteria for a PTSD diagnosis, and if they were an RCMP veteran.

Measures

Clinical Interviews

Participants were asked about their life situation since leaving the military; developmental, family, and military experiences; history of substance use; and clarification of responses to the standardized measures. Other information included age, marital and family status, military rank, service element, and deployment history.

Personality Assessment Inventory (PAI)

The PAI[29] is a multi-scale test of psychological functioning comprising twenty-two non-overlapping scales (e.g., depression, anxiety, aggression) in adults; the 2008 update[30] includes interpretive scoring software. The PAI contains validity scales (to measure possible faking, exaggeration, or defensiveness), clinical scales corresponding to psychiatric diagnostic categories, treatment risk factors (e.g., suicidal ideation), and interpersonal functioning. Respondents are asked to rate their responses on a four-point scale. The scale is written at a grade four level and takes approximately forty-five minutes to complete. Response profiles are compared to two normative groups: equivalent demographic groups and a normative psychiatric group. The test manual provides extensive psychometric data; Cronbach's alpha ratings for the clinical and treatment scale ranges are .82 to .93. Test-retest reliability over a two-week period ranged from .67 to .90. The test manual provides tables outlining good discriminant and convergent studies with a number of other psychological measures.

Detailed Assessment of Post Traumatic Stress (DAPS)

The DAPS[31] is a 105-item inventory providing detailed information on various criterion A events (e.g., natural disasters, war, rape, physical assault, child abuse), psychological reactions (cognitive, emotional, and dissociative), post traumatic stress symptoms (re-experiencing, avoidance, hyper-arousal), and level of post traumatic impairment. Respondents are asked to rate their answers on a five-point graduated scale. It is appropriate for clients aged eighteen to ninety-one years and takes twenty to thirty minutes to complete. The event focus of the DAPS allows for tentative DSM–IV diagnoses of post traumatic stress disorder (PTSD) and acute stress disorder (ASD). Two validity scales evaluate under- and over-report of symptoms, and three supplementary scales evaluate event-related dissociation, substance abuse, and suicidality. Standardization studies of the DAPS involved a normative group of adults reporting at least one DSM–IV-type trauma; clinical and non-clinical validity subjects; and a university student group. Cronbach's alpha ratings for the clinical scales were estimated at .88 to .92 (Cronbach's alpha). Diagnoses of PTSD have good sensitivity (.88) and specificity (.86) when compared to the Clinician-Administered PTSD Scale (CAPS).

Results

Description of Participants

Charts were selected for 108 former members of the CF assessed at a private clinic in the Atlantic region. Participants were separated into two groups: veterans treated previously for PTSD ($n = 57$; 90% male; 10% female; average age: 44 years; service element: 44% Army; 37% Navy; 14% Air Force; 5% combined service) and untreated veterans ($n = 51$; 92% male; 8% female; average age: 50 years; service element: 47% Army; 49% Navy; 2% Air Force; 2% combined service). T tests of between-group differences for the demographic variables were non-significant at $\alpha = .01$.[32]

Analysis Design

Given the exploratory nature of this study, the initial question was whether a set of variables measuring PTSD symptoms/behaviours could predict degree of relapse. The population of all veterans with PTSD was represented by the fifty-one clients who had not received treatment; the fifty-seven patients who relapsed after treatment represented the population of patients expected to relapse after treatment. Hence, the relapsed population (TRT = 1) were considered to be a subset of the broader PTSD population (TRT = 0). This relationship placed limits on the questions that could be answered from the data. For example, it was not possible to estimate the probability that a patient would relapse after treatment. The question that could be answered was whether there was a difference in the set of predictors between the population of all PTSD veterans and the subpopulation that will relapse.

Table 12.1 | Probability estimates for categorical predictors

	$\hat{P}_{0,TRT=0}$	$\hat{P}_{0,TRT=1}$	z-statistic	p-value
Adolescent substance abuse	0.8235	0.3509	5.7127	0.0000
Military substance abuse	0.6667	0.1754	5.9158	0.0000
Childhood sexual abuse	0.8431	0.5965	2.9875	0.0014
Childhood physical abuse	0.6667	0.5263	1.5020	0.0665

Results of Data Analysis

Data were analyzed through MATLAB.[33] Visual comparison of the PAI and DAPS sub-scale distributions for the two groups revealed considerable overlap for most variables, with the exception of the variable BOR (i.e., comprising PAI subscales measuring the cluster B traits: affective instability, identity problems, negative relationships, self-harm). The analysis of between-group mean difference ($\mu_{TRT=0}$ = 34.6, $\mu_{TRT=1}$ = 41.5) was significant (t = 3.11, df = 106, p = .002). As shown in table 12.1, categorical predictors separated the two groups. In each case, the null hypothesis, probability that the variable was zero and the same for both populations, was rejected. As shown, all variables indicated significant differences between the two populations (α set at .10 for exploratory results).

Investigating Relationships between the Categorical Predictors for Treatment Group and BOR Scores

Frequency distributions for ASUD and MSUD by TRT group showed that a greater proportion of the TRT = 1 group reported a history of substance abuse (86%) compared with TRT = 0 (34%). The distribution for CSA and CPA by TRT group showed that a greater proportion of TRT = 1 group reported a history of sexual and physical abuse (68%), compared to the TRT = 0 group (41%). Inspection of the distribution of CSA and CPA rates for average BOR scores showed that for the TRT = 0 group, a history involving both types of abuse corresponded to the highest average BOR score of 40; in comparison for TRT = 1, both types of abuse corresponded to a much higher average BOR score of 52.

Formal Analysis of the Data

Analysis of the categorical predictors by TRT group was not possible, as many of the combinations contained fewer than two data points. Partitioning of the variable "Score" based on a summation of responses (i.e., 0 or 1 on ASUD, MSUD, CSA, and CPA with possible score totals of 0 to 4) into level 1 (score < 3) and level

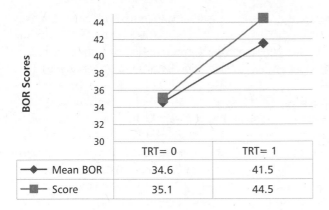

	TRT= 0	TRT= 1
◆— Mean BOR	34.6	41.5
■— Score	35.1	44.5

Figure 12.1 | Results of ANOVA for score and BOR by TRT group. Significant differences between TRT = 0 and TRT = 1 are shown for mean BOR and Score predictors.

2 (score > 3) by TRT was carried out. This procedure showed that 53% of the TRT = 1 group had Score totals less than three, compared with 82% in the TRT = 0 group. By comparison, 47% of TRT = 1 group had Score > 3, compared to 18% for the TRT = 0 group. As shown in figure 12.1, ANOVA results were significant for the predictors, Score (F = 4.31, p < .04) and BOR (F = 8.74, p < .004). The TRT = 0 and TRT = 1 groups had significantly different mean values for BOR (34.6 versus 41.5, p = 0.04). The predictor Score showed a significant effect on mean BOR values, p = 0.004, with a mean of 35.1 when Score < 3 and 44.5 when Score > 3. The interaction was non-significant.

Discussion

The purpose of this study was to investigate ACE and SUD rates among relapsed veterans and untreated veterans diagnosed with PTSD. Consistent with the hypothesis, the results indicated that relapsed veterans had a significantly higher incidence of childhood sexual and physical abuse, and higher adolescent and military substance-abuse rates. While not hypothesized, higher cluster B personality traits were also found among the relapsed veteran group. Among the untreated group, with the stated assumption that they were representative of the broader population of veterans with PTSD, rates of 34% for SUD and 41% for developmental abuse were found. These rates are noteworthy and are consistent with the literature, emphasizing the importance of including screening measures specific to SUD and ACE issues for all assessments of military-related trauma. Of greater concern was the finding that 86% of relapsed veterans reported SUDs and that 68% of these clients reported histories of sexual and physical abuse. This finding raises considerable concern, especially in light of the elevated scores on the PAI borderline personality scale (e.g., affective instability, identity problems, negative relationships, and risks of self-harm) for members of this group. An important question is whether clients with these complex presentations are appropriate for trauma exposure therapy as a first-line intervention because there is possibility of symptom exacerbation.[34]

The finding of wide discrepancies in ACE and SUD reports between reassessment results and the baseline assessments, which was the impetus for this study, now takes on tremendous significance in light of the results. The differences can be explained, in part, by client reports that they were not asked if ACE or SUD occurred during their early development. For those who acknowledged being asked, they either denied these events or downplayed the frequency/severity because of several concerns: information would be placed in their medical files, information could bias the treatment focus of caregivers, and their reports of military OSIs would not be taken seriously. In some cases, veterans stated they discussed developmental abuse and substance abuse with their clinicians, but this information was not consistently reported in the baseline assessments. While possibly driven by career concerns by clients or by concerns about remaining focused on operational issues by clinicians, the absence of this information in the record has serious implications for treatment planning. It can also have direct effects for subsequent health-care providers who may need to rely on these records where veterans are referred for "PTSD treatment only" in the community following release from the CF. There is the risk that subsequent clinicians may re-engage these veterans in similar CBT-PE therapy for PTSD and recreate similar treatment outcomes, while other interventions (e.g., integrated harm-reduction focused PTSD-SUD treatment or developmentally focused trauma group therapy) are not considered because of incomplete information in the record.

These findings suggest a need to reconsider the range of accepted PTSD treatment options in managing military PTSD. For instance, treated veterans often reported an inability to maintain an alcohol abstinence requirement before and during their trauma-focused work, sometimes creating conflicts with their health teams. Alternatively, recent studies challenge the generally accepted wisdom of this treatment expectation and suggest instead that trauma-focused CBT can help clients with PTSD-SUD without an abstinence requirement and without escalating symptoms of either problem.[35] According to these studies, these clients may even differentially benefit from a trauma-focused model over ones that do not focus on PTSD symptoms. A well-controlled, randomized study reported equivalent outcomes for clients engaging in CBT therapy without an abstinence requirement, compared with clients undergoing standard addiction treatment followed by trauma therapy.[36] Even so, the findings from the present study suggest that trauma interventions likely need to be conducted within a developmental perspective. Potential program formats include the ninety-day, multi-modal residential program for developmental trauma and military PTSD as outlined by Busittil and an integrated PTSD-SUD program developed by Ford and Russo.[37] Likewise, a group-based program offered to clients of Veterans Affairs Canada using a developmental trauma approach showed positive results over a nine-month period for trauma symptoms, general mental health, and quality of life outcomes.[38]

Limitations and Future Research

This study provides information on the relationships among ACE, SUD, and PTSD relapse among military veterans. It also reinforces the importance of conducting developmentally focused assessments for military personnel who report operational stress injuries. The study advances our understanding of the complexities facing trauma clinicians and clients and suggests alternative treatment options for military clients with particular assessment profiles.

There are important limitations to the findings. First, the results are not generalizable to the broader population of military personnel who develop PTSD. Indeed, there may have been a selection bias in that particular military veterans may have been referred to this centre, given its focus on treating co-morbid PTSD-SUD. Second, in the absence of a true control group for those who had been treated previously, it was not possible to compare these results with a veteran group with developmental abuse histories who did not relapse. Inclusion of a control group would allow for identification of other factors that may have influenced treatment outcomes for the treated veterans (e.g., chain of command support for the member's medical status at the unit level). Finally, the emphasis in this study on alcohol and illicit substances is likely overly restrictive in terms of the potential range of self-medicating behaviours among traumatized clients.

For future research, a conceptual model is outlined in figure 12.2. While a broad theoretical discussion of the framework is beyond the purpose and scope of this paper, the proposed model is outlined here as a basis for further discussion. Consistent with the literature described earlier, there are direct relationships between developmental abuse and specific behavioural reactions (ADHD, early substance abuse, aggression).[39] This literature posits that developmental abuse can also contribute significantly to rates of adult-onset PTSD following subsequent traumas.[40] One hypothesized (and testable) outcome of veterans' efforts to distance themselves from negative developmental memories and stressful social/familial environments might include seeking out environments that provide structure, separation from earlier experiences, and the prospect of a more hopeful identity. Entering military service may provide an opportunity to cultivate an entirely different view of self and the world. Military culture has been described as institutionalized masculinity, which prizes values such as self-reliance, emotional inexpression and self-control, and risk-taking.[41] It is possible that these values and the clearly defined pathway to masculine identity may be particularly attractive to people who have experienced powerlessness and lack of purpose earlier in life. The proposed model of PTSD relapse suggests the possibility that an OSI can result in a breach of this acquired military masculine identity, leaving the person disoriented

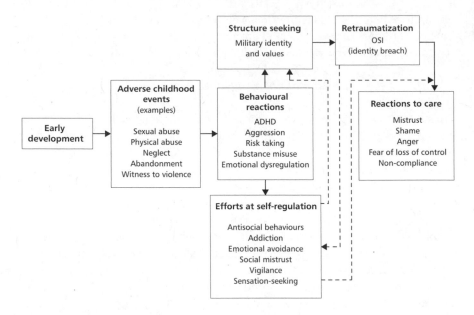

Figure 12.2 | Proposed conceptual model of the relationships between adverse childhood events and PTSD relapse among military veterans

and unprotected from the effects of developmental experiences. Indeed, many of the study participants described being stigmatized and robbed of their honour when diagnosed with PTSD. A recent cogent review of the history of psychological trauma among U.S. soldiers argued that stigma of PTSD is likely to continue within military cultures until a different masculinity is adopted within the broader social context.[42] An important research question could focus on whether reactions to traumatic exposures and the reluctance to seek/accept help represent military members' adherence to acquired masculine values or whether the sequelae of prior developmental abuse present formidable challenges to the requirement during treatment to process intense emotional reactions. To summarize, a better understanding of the determinants of client behaviours that challenge the course of treatment, including mistrust of care-providers, lack of engagement, and emotional avoidance may help explain the noted problems of non-compliance and early termination among PTSD clients.

Conclusion

The results of this study offer support for additional formal inquiry aimed at developing measures to identify specific profiles for veterans with PTSD and to match these veterans with appropriate interventions. An exploration of the complex relationships between early life development and military service may provide a better understanding of the etiology and trajectories of trauma reactions among military personnel. Alternative treatments could help address the problems of early treatment termination and treatment relapse among clients. The hope of such endeavours would be to provide a larger proportion of traumatized military personnel the possibility of recovery and retention within their military careers.

Notes

1   J. T. Bonnow and W. C. Follette, "A Functional Analytic Conceptualization of Retraumatization: Implications for Clinical Assessment," in *Retraumatization: Assessment, Treatment, and Prevention*, ed. M. P. Duckworth and V. M. Follette, 129–62 (New York: Routledge, 2012).

2   B. A. Sharpless and J. P. Barber, "A Clinician's Guide to PTSD Treatments for Returning Veterans," *Professional Psychology Research Practice* 42, no. 1 (2011): 8–15; N. J. Kitchiner, N. P. Roberts, D. Wilcox, and J. I. Bisson, "Systematic Review and Meta-Analysis of Psychosocial Interventions for Veterans of Military," *European Journal of Psychotraumatology* 3 (2012): http://www.eurojnlofpsychotraumatol.net/index.php/ejpt/article/view/19267.

3   L. N. Ravindran and M. B. Stein, "Pharmacotherapy of PTSD: Premises, Principles, and Priorities," *Brain Research* 13 (2009): 24–39; D. Kozarić-Kovačić, "Psychopharmacotherapy of Posttraumatic Stress Disorder," *Croatian Medical Journal* 49 (2008): 459–75.

4   K. Nilamadhab, "Cognitive Behavioral Therapy for the Treatment of Post-Traumatic Stress Disorder: A Review," *Neuropsychiatric Disease and Treatment* 7 (2011): 167–81; D. G. Baker, C. M. Nievergelt, and V. B. Risbrough, "Posttraumatic Stress Disorder: Emerging Concepts of Pharmacotherapy," *Expert Opinion on Emerging Drugs* 14, no. 2 (2009): 251–72.

5   M. A. Schottenbauer, C. R. Glass, D. B. Arnkoff, and S. H. Gray, "Contributions of Psychodynamic Approaches to Treatment of PTSD and Trauma: A Review of the Empirical Treatment and Psychopathology Literature," *Psychiatry* 71, no. 1 (2008): 13–34; P. J. Brown, R. L. Stout, and T. Mueller, "Substance Use Disorder and Posttraumatic Stress Disorder Comorbidity: Addiction and Psychiatric Treatment Rates," *Psychology of Addictive Behaviors* 13, no. 2 (1999): 115–22; M. Tull, M. Jakupcak, M. McFadden, and L. Roemer, "The Role of Negative Affect Intensity and the Fear of Emotions in Posttraumatic Stress Symptom Severity among Victims of Childhood Interpersonal Violence," *Journal of Nervous and Mental Disease* 195, no. 7 (2007): 580–7; A. R. Rademaker, E. Vermetten, and R. J. Kleber, "Multimodal Exposure-Based Group Treatment for Peacekeepers with PTSD: A Preliminary Evaluation," *Military Psychology* 21 (2009): 482–96.

6   D. Richardson, D. McIntosh, J. Sareen, and M. B. Stein, "Post-Traumatic Stress Disorder: Guiding Management with Careful Assessment of Comorbid Mental and Physical Illness," in *Shaping the Future: Military and Veteran Health Research*, ed. A. B. Aiken and S. A. H. Belanger, 216–29 (Kingston: Canadian Defence Academy, 2011); J. S. Cacciola, J. M. Koppenhavera, A. I. Altermana, and J. R. McKay,

"Posttraumatic Stress Disorder and Other Psychopathology in Substance Abusing Patients," *Drug and Alcohol Dependence* 101, nos 1–2 (2009): 27–33.

7 J. D. Ford, J. Hawke, S. Alessi, D. Ledgerwood, and N. Petry, "Psychological Trauma and PTSD Symptoms as Predictors of Substance Dependence Treatment Outcomes," *Behaviour Research and Therapy* 45 (2007): 2417–31; B. E. Wampold, Z. E. Imel, K. M. Laska, S. Benish, S. D. Miller, C. Fluckiger, A. C. Del Re, T. P. Baardseth, and S. Budge, "Determining What Works in the Treatment of PTSD," *Clinical Psychology Review* 30 (2010): 923–33; S. B. Norman, S. R. Tate, K. G. Anderson, and S. A. Brown, "Do Trauma History and PTSD Symptoms Influence Addiction Relapse Context?," *Drug and Alcohol Dependence* 6 (2007): 89–96.

8 P. K. Connor, D. J. Higgins, "The 'HEALTH' Model – Part 1: Treatment Program Guidelines for complex PTSD," *Sexual and Relationship Therapy* 23 (2008): 293–303; A. M. Fritch, M. Mishkind, M. A. Reger, and G. A. Gahm, "The Impact of Childhood Abuse and Combat-Related Trauma on Post Deployment Adjustment," *Journal of Traumatic Stress* 23 (2010): 248–54; J. M. Currier, J. M. Holland, and D. Allen, "Attachment and Mental Health Symptoms among U.S. Afghanistan and Iraq Veterans Seeking Health Care Services," *Journal of Traumatic Stress* 25 (2012): 633–40; J. Fox and B. Pease, "Military Deployment, Masculinity and Trauma: Reviewing the Connections," *Journal of Men's Studies* 20, no. 1 (2012): 16–31.

9 T. Luxenberg, J. Spinazzola, and B. van der Kolk, "Complex Trauma and Disorders of Extreme Stress (DESNOS) Diagnosis, Part 1: Assessment," *Directions in Psychiatry* 21 (2001): 373–92; J. L. Herman, "Complex PTSD: A Syndrome in Survivors of Prolonged and Repeated Trauma," *Journal of Trauma Stress* 5 (1992): 377–91; C. Spitzer, C. Chevalier, M. Gillner, H. J. Freyberger, and S. Barnow, "Complex Posttraumatic Stress Disorder and Child Maltreatment in Forensic Inpatients," *Journal of Forensic Psychiatry & Psychology* 17, no. 2 (2006): 204–16.

10 B. F. Fuemmeler, F. J. McClernon, and J. C. Beckham, "Adverse Childhood Events Are Associated with Obesity and Disordered Eating: Results from a U.S. Population-Based Survey of Young Adults," *Journal of Traumatic Stress* 22 (2009): 329–33; K. H. Walter, K. J. Horsey, P. A. Palmieri, and S. E. Hobfoll, "The Role of Protective Self-Cognitions in the Relationship between Childhood Trauma and Later Resource Loss," *Journal of Traumatic Stress* 23 (2010): 264–73; J. A. Schumacher, S. F. Coffey, and P. R. Stasiewicz, "Symptom Severity: Alcohol Craving, and Age of Trauma Onset in Childhood and Adolescent Trauma Survivors with Comorbid Alcohol Dependence and Posttraumatic Stress Disorder," *American Journal on Addictions* 15 (2006): 422–5.

11 N. Breslau, H. D. Chilcoat, R. C. Kessler, and G. C. Davis, "Previous Exposure to Trauma and PTSD Effects of Subsequent Trauma: Results from the Detroit Area Survey of Trauma," *American Journal of Psychiatry* 156 (1999): 902–7.

12 L. Sugaya, D. S. Hasin, M. Olfson, K. H. Lin, and B. F. Grant, "Child Physical Abuse and Adult Mental Health: A National Study," *Journal of Traumatic Stress* 25 (2012): 384–92.

13 O. A. Cabrera, C. W. Hoge, P. D. Bliese, C. A. Castro, and S. C. Messer, "Childhood Adversity and Combat as Predictors of Depression and Post-Traumatic Stress in Deployed Troops," *American Journal of Preventative Medicine* 33 (2007): 77–82; E. E. Van Voorhees, E. A. Dedert, P. S. Calhoun, M. Brancu, J. Runnals, J. C. Beckham,

and VA Mid-Atlantic MIRECC Workgroup, "Childhood Trauma Exposure in Iraq and Afghanistan War Era Veterans: Implications for Posttraumatic Stress Disorder Symptoms and Adult Functional Social Support," *Child Abuse & Neglect* 36, no. 5 (2012): 423–32.

14 Z. Solomon, S. Zur-Noah, D. Horesh, G. Zerach, and G. Keinan, "The Contribution of Stressful Life Events throughout the Life Cycle to Combat-Induced Psychopathology," *Journal of Traumatic Stress* 21, no. 3 (2008): 318–25.

15 W. Langeland, N. Draijer, and D. N. van den Brink, "Trauma and Dissociation in Treatment-Seeking Alcoholics: Towards a Resolution of Inconsistent Findings," *Comprehensive Psychiatry* 43 (2002): 195–203; G. L. de Bernardo, M. Newcomb, A. Toth, G. Richey, and R. Mendoza, "Comorbid Psychiatric and Alcohol Abuse/ Dependency Disorders: Psychosocial Stress, Abuse, and Personal History Factors of Those in Treatment," *Journal of Addictive Disorders* 21 (2002): 43–59; S. E. Back, S. C. Soone, T. Killeen, B. S. Dansky, and K. T. Brady, "Comparative Profiles of Women with PTSD and Comorbid Cocaine or Alcohol Dependence," *American Journal of Drug and Alcohol Abuse* 29 (2003): 169–89.

16 P. C. Ouimette, R. H. Moos, and P. J. Brown, "Substance Use Disorder – Posttraumatic Stress Disorder Comorbidity: A Survey of Treatments and Proposed Practice Guidelines," in *Trauma and Substance Abuse: Causes, Consequences, and Treatment of Comorbid Disorders*, ed. P. C. Ouimette and P. J. Brown, 91–110 (Washington, DC: American Psychological Association (2003); S. B. Norman, S. R. Tate, K. G. Anderson, and S. A. Brown, "Do Trauma History and PTSD Symptoms Influence Addiction Relapse Context?," *Drug and Alcohol Dependence* 90, no. 1 (2007): 89–96.

17 M. Draganand, M. Lis-Turlejska, "Lifetime Exposure to Potentially Traumatic Events in a Sample of Alcohol-Dependent Patients in Poland," *Journal of Traumatic Stress* 20 (2007): 1041–51.

18 J. I. Ruzek, "Concurrent Posttraumatic Stress Disorder and Substance Use Disorder among Veterans: Evidence and Treatment Issues," in Ouimette and Brown, *Trauma and Substance Abuse*, 191–207.

19 D. M. Ledgerwood and N. M. Petry, "Posttraumatic Stress Disorder Symptoms in Treatment-Seeking Pathological Gamblers," *Journal of Traumatic Stress* 19, no. 3 (2006): 411–16.

20 J. J. Whelan, "A Study of Treatment Outcomes for Canadian Forces Members Who Have Received an Intervention for Alcohol Abuse" (PhD diss., University of New Brunswick, 2001).

21 J. J. Whelan, "Treatment of Comorbid PTSD and SUD: A Review of the Literature" (presentation to Treatment Standards Committee, Department of National Defence, Ottawa, 2003).

22 H. D. Chilcoat and C. Menard, "Epidemiological Investigations: Comorbidity of Posttraumatic Stress Disorder and Substance Use Disorder," in Ouimette and Brown, *Trauma and Substance Abuse*, 9–28; C. Zlotnick, D. M. Johnson, R. L. Stout, W. H. Zywiak, J. E. Johnson, and R. J. Schneider, "Childhood Abuse and Intake Severity in Alcohol Disorder Patients," *Journal of Traumatic Stress* 19, no. 6 (2006): 949–59; C. Raghavan and S. Kingston, "Child Sexual Abuse and Posttraumatic Stress Disorder:

The Role of Age at First Use of Substances and Lifetime Traumatic Events," *Journal of Traumatic Stress* 19, no. 2 (2006): 269–78.

23 S. H. Stewart and P. J. Conrod, "Psychosocial Models of Functional Associations be-tween Posttraumatic Stress Disorder and Substance Use Disorder," in Ouimette and Brown, *Trauma and Substance Abuse*, 29–55.

24 B. F. Fuemmeler, F. J. McClernon, and J. C. Beckham, "Adverse Childhood Events Are Associated with Obesity and Disordered Eating: Results from a U.S. Population-Based Survey of Young Adults," *Journal of Traumatic Stress* 22, no. 4 (2009): 329–33.

25 R. K. Inaba, "Alcohol Expectancies among Substance Abusing Vietnam Veterans with Posttraumatic Stress Disorder" (PhD diss., California School of Professional Psychology, 1997); P. C. Ouimette, K. Humphreys, R. H. Moos, J. W. Finney, R. Cronkite, and B. Federman, "Self-Help Group Participation among Substance Use Disorder Patients with Posttraumatic Stress Disorder," *Journal of Substance Abuse Treatment* 20 (2001): 25–32; Stewart and Conrod, "Psychosocial Models of Functional Associations."

26 T. O'Hare, C. Shen, and M. Sherrer, "High-Risk Behaviors and Drinking-to-Cope as Mediators of Lifetime Abuse and PTSD Symptoms in Clients with Severe Mental Illness," *Journal of Traumatic Stress* 23 (2010): 255–63; S. Kingston and C. Raghavan, "The Relationship of Sexual Abuse, Early Initiation of Substance Use, and Adolescent Trauma to PTSD," *Journal of Traumatic Stress* 22 (2009): 65–8.

27 D. A. Hien, A. N. Campbell, L. M. Ruglass, M.-C. Hu, and T. Killeen, "The Role of Alcohol Misuse in PTSD Outcomes for Women in Community Treatment: A Secondary Analysis of NIDA's Women and Trauma Study," *Drug and Alcohol Dependence* 111 (2010): 114–19.

28 D. Blake, F. Weathers, L. Nagy, D. Kaloupek, D. Charney, and T. Keane, *Clinician-Administered PTSD Scale for DSM-IV* (West Haven: National Center for Posttraumatic Stress Disorder Behavioral Science Division – Boston Neurosciences Division, 1998); D. Blake, F. Weathers, L. Nagy, D. Kaloupek, G. Klauminzer, D. Charney, T. Keane, and T. C. Buckley, *Instruction Manual: Clinician-Administered PTSD Scale (CAPS)* (West Haven: National Center for Posttraumatic Stress Disorder Behavioral Science Division – Boston Neurosciences Division, 2000).

29 L. C. Morey, *Personality Assessment Inventory Professional Manual* (Lutz, FL: Psychological Assessment Resources, 1991).

30 L.C. Morey, *PAI Software Portfolio*, version 3 (Lutz, FL: Psychological Assessment Resources, 2008).

31 J. Briere, *DAPS: Detailed Assessment of Posttraumatic Stress Professional Manual* (Odessa, FL: Psychological Assessment Resources, 2001).

32 R. G. Pagano, *Understanding Statistics in the Behavioral Sciences*, 3rd ed. (New York: West Publishing, 1997).

33 Mathworks Inc., *MATLAB: The Language of Technical Computing* (Natick, MA: Mathworks, 1994–2012).

34 L. A. Frye and C. R. Spates, "Prolonged Exposure, Mindfulness, and Emotion Regulation for the Treatment of PTSD," *Clinical Case Studies* 11, no. 3 (2012): 184–200; E. B. Foa, L. A. Zoellner, N. C. Feeny, E. A. Hembree, and J. Alvarez-Conrad, "Does Imaginal Exposure Exacerbate PTSD Symptoms?," *Journal of Consulting and Clinical Psychology* 70, no. 4 (2002): 1022–8; J. T. Levitt and M. Cloitre, "A Clinician's Guide

to STAIR/MPE: Treatment for PTSD Related to Childhood Abuse," *Cognitive and Behavioral Practice* 12 (2005): 40–52.

35 S. B. Norman, S. R. Tate, K. G. Anderson, and S. A. Brown, "Do Trauma History and PTSD Symptoms Influence Addiction Relapse Context?," *Drug and Alcohol Dependence* 90 (2007): 89–96.

36 K. Mills, M. Teesson, S. E. Back, K. T. Brady, A. L. Baker, S. Hopwood, C. Sannibale, E. L. Barrett, S. Merz, J. Rosenfeld, and P. L. Ewer, "Integrated Exposure-Based Therapy for Co-occurring Posttraumatic Stress Disorder and Substance Dependence," *Journal of the American Medical Association* 308, no. 7 (2012): 690–9.

37 W. Busuttil, "The Development of a 90-Day Residential Program for the Treatment of Complex Posttraumatic Stress Disorder," *Journal of Aggression, Maltreatment, & Trauma* 12 (2006): 29–55; J. D. Ford and E. Russo, "Trauma-Focused, Present-Centered, Emotional Self-Regulation Approach to Integrated Treatment for Posttraumatic Stress and Addiction: Trauma Adaptive Recovery Group Education and Therapy (TARGET)," *American Journal of Psychotherapy* 60, no. 4 (2006): 335–55.

38 J. J. Whelan, "Outcome Evaluation of the Trauma Relapse Prevention Group (TRPG) Program for Canadian Military Veterans Diagnosed with Chronic PTSD" (report submitted to Veterans Affairs Canada, Charlottetown, 2010); Whelan, "Trauma Relapse Prevention Group (TRPG) Leader's Guide" (unpublished, 2009).

39 D. Weinstein, D. Staffelbach, and M. Biaggio, "Attention-Deficit Hyperactivity Disorder and Posttraumatic Stress Disorder: Differential Diagnosis in Childhood Sexual Abuse," *Clinical Psychology Review* 20, no. 3 (2000): 359–78; S. A. Husain, M. A. Allwood, and D. J. Bell, "The Relationship between PTSD Symptoms and Attention Problems in Children Exposed to the Bosnian War," *Journal of Emotional and Behavioral Disorders* 16, no. 1 (2008): 52–62.

40 L. Irish, S. A. Ostrowski, W. Fallon, E. Spoonster, M. van Dulmen, E. M. Sledjeski, and D. L. Delahanty, "Trauma History Characteristics and Subsequent PTSD Symptoms in Motor Vehicle Accident Victims," *Journal of Traumatic Stress* 21 (2008): 377–84; E. Triffleman, C. R. Marmar, K. L. Delucchi, and H. Ronfeldt, "Childhood Trauma and Posttraumatic Stress Disorder in Substance Abuse Inpatients," *Journal of Nervous and Mental Disease* 183, no. 3 (1995): 172–6.

41 J. A. Morrison, "Masculinity Moderates the Relationship between Symptoms of PTSD and Cardiac-Related Health Behaviors in Male Veterans," *Psychology of Men & Masculinity* 13, no. 2 (2012): 158–65; H. A. Garcia, E. P. Finley, and W. Lorber, "A Preliminary Study of the Association between Traditional Masculine Behavioral Norms and PTSD symptoms in Iraq and Afghanistan Veterans," *Psychology of Men & Masculinity* 12, no. 1 (2011): 55–63; S. M. Burns and J. R. Mahalik, "Suicide and Dominant Masculinity Norms among Current and Former United States Military Servicemen," *Professional Psychology: Research and Practice* 42, no. 5 (2011): 347–53.

42 C. Jarvis, "If He Comes Home Nervous: U.S. World War II Neuropsychiatric Casualties and Postwar Masculinities," *Journal of Men's Studies* 17, no. 2 (2009): 97–115.

13

Evidence-Based Treatments for Military-Related PTSD: A Review of Advances in Psychotherapy

MAYA ROTH, KATE ST CYR, AND
ALEXANDRA MCINTYRE-SMITH

Abstract

The objective of the current review is to (1) review the published literature of evidence-based psychotherapeutic modalities with an emphasis on the use of these treatments for military-related PTSD, (2) provide a brief overview of treatment considerations when working with military-related PTSD, and (3) describe recent advances in the treatment of military-related PTSD, in particular, the concept of moral injury, and the impact of these advances on the efficiency and effectiveness of psychotherapy for military-related PTSD.

Methods: Literature reviews were conducted to identify evidence for prolonged exposure (PE) therapy, cognitive-processing therapy (CPT), and eye movement desensitization and reprocessing therapy (EMDR). Additional reviews were conducted to determine the evidence base for the inclusion of interventions targeting moral injury in the treatment protocol.

Findings and conclusions: Previous research indicates that PE and CPT are highly effective in treating individuals with PTSD, including combat-related PTSD, and should be considered by clinicians seeking to treat active military personnel and military veterans who meet diagnostic criteria for PTSD. The literature base for EMDR was less conclusive but may be beneficial to individuals when trauma-focused therapy is contraindicated. Finally, early research suggests that the inclusion of the concept of moral injury in treatment sessions may benefit military members and veterans with PTSD.

Introduction

Military-Related Post Traumatic Stress Disorder

Research suggests that participation in peacekeeping missions and exposure to combat are associated with increased risk of developing psychiatric conditions,

such as post traumatic stress disorder (PTSD),[1] and that lifetime prevalence estimates of PTSD among military personnel and veterans range from 9% to 30%.[2] As
such, PTSD continues to be a significant concern for the Canadian Forces (CF).
Previous research indicates that there is a self-perceived need for mental health
service utilization following deployment on combat or peacekeeping missions
among CF personnel, and that a considerable proportion of military personnel
who acknowledge a need for treatment will seek it.[3]

Treatment for military-related PTSD may consist of pharmaco-therapy, psychotherapy, or a combination of the two. PTSD can be treated with an array of psychotropic medications, each with varying degrees of success in symptom reduction.
Likewise, a number of unique psychotherapies, each with distinctive components,
may be used in the treatment of military-related PTSD; and, similarly, evidence for
some of these modalities is more promising than that of others. The most promising psychotherapies, often referred to as evidence-based treatments, are typically
trauma-focused and may follow a manualized protocol, which ensures the clinician adheres to the treatment procedure. Examples of trauma-focused treatments
for which the evidence base is strong include prolonged exposure (PE) therapy
and cognitive processing therapy (CPT);[4] these modalities will be discussed at
greater length in the following section.

Despite well-documented success, the results of a 2004 survey suggests that
evidence-based psychotherapies tend to be used relatively infrequently by mental
health practitioners within the United States Veterans Health Administration.[5] It
is uncertain at this point whether mental health care providers to Canadian military members and veterans are similar to their U.S. counterparts in the provision
of evidence-based psychotherapy. As such, the objectives of the current research
are (1) to provide a review of the literature relating to the use of evidence-based
psychotherapies for military-related PTSD, (2) to offer a brief overview of important treatment considerations when working with military personnel with PTSD,
and (3) to describe some advances in the treatment of military-related PTSD
and their potential impact on the delivery of evidence-based psychotherapy for
military-related PTSD.

Methods

Literature reviews were conducted in the months of October and November 2012
using PsycInfo and the following search terms: *military and veterans with post
traumatic stress disorder, PTSD, military-related PTSD, trauma,* and *psychological
trauma* as well as *evidence-based psychotherapy, evidence-based treatment,* and
evidence-based therapy. Abstracts of identified published manuscripts were reviewed for relevance to our study, and reference lists of highly pertinent publications were also reviewed for additional publications of interest. From there, the
authors focused on three psychotherapies for which a number of peer-reviewed
manuscripts were available: prolonged exposure therapy, cognitive processing

therapy, and eye movement desensitization and reprocessing. However, while the authors of this chapter attempted to include all appropriate manuscripts, regardless of the nature of the findings, we acknowledge that the information included in the following sections may not be exhaustive, particularly because the literature reviews were limited to academic journal articles published in English.

Results

Evidence-Based Psychotherapies

Trauma-focused cognitive-behavioural interventions have been shown to effectively reduce symptoms of PTSD in an array of populations, including military veterans.[6] While these strategies vary in their content and delivery mechanisms, all aim to combine anxiety management and elements of cognitive restructuring with psycho-education to alleviate symptoms of PTSD.[7]

Prolonged Exposure

Prolonged exposure (PE) belongs to the family of exposure therapy (ET). These modalities involve guiding the patient through a traumatic experience repetitively until exposure to the traumatic memory or stimuli no longer evokes a fear response.[8] PE is characterized by two essential components: imaginal exposure (i.e., repeated retelling of the traumatic event) and in vivo exposure (i.e., repeated encounters with situations, people, places, or objects that evoke the emotional, cognitive, and behavioural fear structure related to the traumatic event).[9] PE further builds upon these components by uniting elements of imaginal and in vivo exposure with psycho-education, breathing retraining, and post-imaginal exposure processing, which includes cognitive restructuring, in a manualized protocol,[10] with the goal to confront and emotionally process the trauma. This goal is rooted in the overall treatment rationale that cognitive and situational avoidance, as well as negative beliefs about self and the world, maintain PTSD. Foa and colleagues (2007) assert that imaginal and in vivo exposure directly target avoidance and dysfunctional beliefs, and that they promote emotional engagement with the traumatic event so that it can be processed and PTSD can be ameliorated.[11] Delivery of the PE protocol occurs over eight to twelve standardized, audiotaped ninety-minute sessions,[12] and objectives for each session are provided in the manual. Weekly homework of listening to the audiotaped session, reviewing handouts or readings, in vivo exposure exercises, and breathing exercises are also a key part of the treatment protocol.[13]

A small number of controlled studies have demonstrated the effectiveness of PE for military-related PTSD. Schnurr and colleagues (2007) demonstrated that despite increased dropout rates, participants who received a course of PE were more likely to lose their PTSD diagnosis and achieve total remission than participants in a present-centred therapy comparison group.[14] Another study by Rauch and colleagues (2009) was limited by its small sample size ($N = 10$) and lack of controlled design; however, significant treatment gains resulted, and 50 per cent of the sample no longer met criteria for PTSD following treatment with the manualized PE treatment protocol.[15] Tuerk and colleagues (2011) determined that PE had the potential to be effective at treating military-related PTSD when implemented in Veterans Affairs Medical Centers when used in controlled clinical studies.[16] A study detailing the dissemination strategy of PE among the U.S. Veterans Health Administration found that the use of PE had positive effects on patient outcomes.[17]

Other studies have evaluated the effectiveness of PE delivered by telehealth services. Two of these studies (by Gros[18] and Tuerk[19]) compared the use of PE delivered by telehealth to PE delivered in person. Both studies found that significant treatment gains were attained, regardless of delivery method; however, the Tuerk study found that individuals in the telehealth group were less likely to complete treatment, while the Gros study reported slightly larger decreases in PTSD and depressive symptom severity among individuals receiving PE in person.

Despite the relatively small number of controlled studies that have examined the utility of PE for military-related PTSD, the evidence of its effectiveness was sufficient for a number of national and international organizations to have identified PE as a first-line psychotherapeutic treatment for individuals with military-related PTSD, including the U.S. Veterans Health Administration and the International Society for Traumatic Stress Studies (ISTSS).[20] PE is the only psychotherapy recommended by the Institute of Medicine (IOM) as an effective treatment of combat-related PTSD.[21]

Cognitive Processing Therapy

Cognitive processing therapy (CPT) is a manualized treatment protocol for PTSD based on a social cognitive theory of PTSD (the primary focus is on the way in which traumatized individuals construe and cope with a traumatic event). The theory suggests that PTSD develops when the natural recovery process is disrupted or stalled and hypothesizes that cognitive stuck points (trauma-related thoughts and beliefs) interfere with recovery. Resick and colleagues (2006) suggest that trauma sufferers are vulnerable to develop stuck points because the nature and aftereffects of traumatic events are often inherently incongruent with previously held beliefs about self, others, and the world, and that these stuck points are maintained as a result of how individuals attempt to integrate the memory of the traumatic event with pre-existing beliefs.[22]

Similarly to PE, CPT is a highly structured intervention that focuses on largely cognitive interventions to identify, challenge, and modify stuck points. It is delivered to patients over twelve hour-long sessions and incorporates some degree of cognitive and emotional exposure to the traumatic event through (1) a written account exercise, (2) examination of the impact that the traumatic event has had on their post-trauma functioning, (3) an impact statement, and (4) differentiation between emotions that occurred during the trauma (natural emotions) and those that are based on interpretations of the traumatic event (manufactured emotions).[23] Finally, five cognitive themes (safety, trust, power-control, esteem, and intimacy) are discussed in treatment. Treatment of military-related PTSD with CPT, like PE, involves the use of weekly assignments, which are typically started in sessions and completed as homework.[24]

While the literature base for the efficacy of CPT for military-related PTSD is relatively small, results have been positive. In a waitlist-control study by Monson and colleagues (2006), the authors found that participants in the CPT group experienced significant reductions in their PTSD symptom severity, compared to the waitlist-control group, and that 40% of participants in the CPT group no longer met diagnostic criteria for PTSD at the post-treatment assessment.[25] Another study demonstrated that Operation Enduring Freedom and Operation Iraqi Freedom veterans reported less severe symptoms of PTSD following a course of CPT (Chard et al., 2010). Interestingly, high post-treatment symptom severity was positively associated with number of sessions attended, suggesting that providing CPT for a substantially greater number of sessions than the twelve prescribed in the treatment protocol may not be beneficial.[26]

Other studies have demonstrated the effectiveness of modified CPT for military-related PTSD. Alvarez and colleagues (2011) compared the effectiveness of group CPT to other trauma-focused group treatment as usual (TAU) in a residential program for PTSD. At discharge from the program, participants in the CPT group had greater symptom improvement and were more likely to be classified as "recovered" or "improved" than the TAU group.[27] Similarly, Morland and colleagues (2011) examined the feasibility of providing group CPT by videoconferencing. They found that participants in both the videoconferencing and in-person groups had clinically meaningful reductions in PTSD symptomatology post-treatment, and that there were no significant differences in treatment outcomes between groups.[28]

On the basis of the available evidence, CPT has been identified as an appropriate first-line psychotherapeutic treatment for military-related PTSD by the U.S. Veterans Health Administration.[29]

Eye Movement Desensitization and Reprocessing Therapy

Like PE, eye movement desensitization and reprocessing (EMDR) belongs to the family of exposure therapies. It combines the use of eye movements with imaginal exposure to help patients cognitively process traumatic experiences.[30] During a typical EMDR session, patients are asked to recall a scene from the traumatic event and, while visually tracking the therapist's finger, which is moving back and forth approximately eighteen inches away from the patient's face, focus on bodily sensations of distress. This is repeated, starting with the worst scene from the traumatic event, over a number of sessions, until the memory no longer produces high levels of emotional and cognitive distress. Sessions usually conclude with a debriefing.[31]

EMDR has been, to some extent, less widely accepted as an evidence-based treatment modality for PTSD, despite recommendations that it be used as a first-line psychotherapeutic treatment for PTSD by the American Psychiatric Association, the U.K. National Institute for Health and Clinical Excellence, the Australian National Health and Medical Research Council, ISTSS, and the U.S. Veterans Administration / Department of Defense; and a second-line treatment modality by the IOM.[32] It has been suggested that some of the hesitation to endorse EMDR as an evidence-based treatment may be attributed to premature claims of EMDR as a proven treatment for PTSD,[33] and/or because, at its core, EMDR is a variant of exposure therapy; the eye movements unique to its protocol are not vital to achieving treatment outcomes.[34] Recent research has aimed to dispel some of these concerns and to provide an empirical base of evidence upon which more accurate claims can be made; however, recent studies examining the utility of EMDR for PTSD in civilian samples have reported mixed results,[35] and results of military-specific studies demonstrate mixed results as well. A recent meta-analysis by Albright and Thyer reviewed six controlled studies and three quasi-experimental studies to better understand whether there is a strong evidence base for EMDR as an empirically supported treatment for military-related PTSD.[36] They found that four of the studies included in the analysis[37] reported no significant improvement in PTSD symptomatology, while the remaining five studies[38] showed some degree of improvement. It is worth noting, however, that all of the studies included in the meta-analysis exhibited important limitations, including small sample size, lack of adherence to treatment protocols, and the lack of generalizability to veterans of the recent conflicts in Iraq and Afghanistan. More recent studies (i.e., Russell, 2006;[39] Russell et al., 2007;[40] Silver et al., 2008[41]) have reported more promising results but were also subject to many of the limitations noted above.

The relative lack of a strong evidence base for EMDR in comparison to the support for PE and CPT may therefore be a combination of scientific resistance and paucity of large, representative studies. There is evidence to suggest that EMDR may be a suitable treatment option for certain military personnel and veterans, particularly for individuals for whom PE or CPT is not a viable option.

Treatment Considerations for Military-Related PTSD

Challenges of Implementing Evidence-Based Psychotherapy

A number of treatment considerations unique to military personnel and veterans may be important to consider when implementing evidence-based treatments for PTSD. First, some research indicates that the successful delivery of exposure therapies with military veterans may be challenging.[42] Engagement in trauma-focused therapies may be unproductive or even detrimental for individuals who are experiencing significant guilt related to their traumatic experiences.[43] Because other research findings suggest that up to 30% of military veterans with symptoms of PTSD may experience symptoms of survivor guilt following their traumatic experiences, there may be significant barriers to achieving an optimal outcome with interventions like PE, CPT, and EMDR.[44] While PE, through post-imaginal exposure processing, and CPT, through cognitive restructuring of stuck points, may address survivor guilt and guilt/shame about their role within the traumatic event, a focus on guilt and the moral/ethical ramifications of the traumatic event are not central to these interventions. Furthermore, it has been suggested that heavy alcohol use, which is common in approximately 20%–25% of military veterans,[45] may slow or hinder treatment gains that would otherwise be made in PE. The Center for the Treatment and Study of Anxiety is examining the efficacy of combined PE and treatment for alcohol use disorders in a largely civilian population, which may, upon completion, prove to be informative for clinicians treating military-related PTSD. Finally, it is worthwhile noting that the provision of trauma-focused treatment in "real-life" situations may vary from the controlled studies upon which trauma-focused therapies have gained widespread acceptance. These studies aim to ensure adherence to the rigid protocols that often accompany trauma-focused therapies, which may pose a challenge for the practising clinician, and at times report elevated treatment dropout rates when compared to less intensive treatments.[46] However, it is essential to note that many of these concerns can be addressed by maintaining flexibility in the administration of a trauma-focused therapy, even when using a manualized protocol. Clinicians providing trauma-focused therapy to military personnel and veterans can make slight modifications to the protocol (i.e., repeating the material of a particular session; completing the content of the protocol in slightly fewer or slightly more sessions than typically prescribed) in order to meet the unique needs of each patient.[47] Minor deviations such as these may reduce the risk of premature dropout.

Incorporation of Military Culture and Moral Injury

It is also vital for clinicians providing evidence-based trauma-focused therapies to military personnel and veterans to remember to incorporate military culture into the treatment protocol. This may occur through the use of military-specific terminology, clinician knowledge of relevant military values and roles, and clinician understanding of cultural differences across military branches.[48] Addressing the concept of moral injury has also been recently identified as a potentially useful component in the treatment of military-related PTSD. Potentially morally injurious incidents, such as instigating, failing to prevent, or witnessing events that contradict one's moral beliefs, are not uncommon wartime experiences, and the consequences may have a profound effect on emotional, psychological, spiritual, and social well-being.[49] These experiences may damage one's views of self and the world, and may result in changes in ethical attitudes or behaviour, changes in or loss of spirituality, increased feelings of guilt, shame, anger, or isolation, decreased trust in others and in society as a whole, and poor self-care or increased self-harm.[50] Both CPT and PE can be used to address the issue of moral injury within their respective protocols; however, certain cases may warrant further discussion of moral injury than the CPT and PE protocols permit. Nonetheless, these trauma-focused protocols may help identify military personnel and veterans experiencing significant symptoms of moral injury and may provide a starting point for intensive moral injury work, such as the novel adaptive disclosure intervention, a combat-specific, trauma-focused psychotherapy that specifically aims to address moral injury and traumatic loss.[51]

Conclusions

While the treatment of military-related PTSD is a complex and challenging field, research demonstrates that, with the right treatment for the right patient, PTSD can successfully be treated. Evidenced-based, trauma-focused therapies that address the concept of moral injury and allow the clinician to incorporate military culture are considered the gold standard in the psychotherapeutic treatment of military-related PTSD.

Notes

1   Charles W. Hoge, Carl A. Castro, Stephen C. Messer, Dennis McGurk, Dave I. Cotting, and Robert L. Koffman, "Combat Duty in Iraq and Afghanistan, Mental Health Problems, and Barriers to Care," *New England Journal of Medicine*, 351, no. 1 (2004): 13–22; Charles S. Milliken, Jennifer L. Auchterlonie, and Charles W. Hoge, "Longitudinal Assessment of Mental Health Problems among Active and Reserve Component Soldiers Returning from the Iraq War," *Journal of the American Medical Association* 298, no. 18 (2007): 2141–8; Jitender Sareen, Brian J. Cox, Murray B. Stein, Tracie O. Afifi, Claire Fleet, and Gordon J. Asmundson, "Physical and Mental Comorbidity, Disability, and Suicidal Behavior Associated with Posttraumatic Stress Disorder in a Large Community Sample," *Psychosomatic Medicine* 69, no. 3 (2007): 242–8.
2   Charles W. Hoge, Artin Terhakopian, Carl A. Castro, Stephen C. Messer, and Charles C. Engel, "Association of Posttraumatic Stress Disorder with Somatic Symptoms, Health Care Visits, and Absenteeism among Iraq War Veterans," *American Journal of Psychiatry* 164, no. 1 (2007): 150–3; Coady B. Lapierre, Andria F. Schwegler, and Bill J. LaBauve, "Posttraumatic Stress and Depression Symptoms in Soldiers Returning from Combat Operations in Iraq and Afghanistan," *Journal of Traumatic Stress* 20, no. 6 (2007): 933–43; Karen H. Seal, Daniel Bertenthal, Christian R. Miner, Saunak Sen, and Charles Marmar, "Bringing the War Back Home: Mental Health Disorders

among 103,788 US Veterans Returning from Iraq and Afghanistan Seen at VA Facilities," *Archives of Internal Medicine* 167, no. 5 (2007): 476–82; Josefin Sundin, Nicola T. Fear, Amy Iversen, Roberto J. Rona, and Simon Wessely, "PTSD after Deployment to Iraq: Conflicting Rates, Conflicting Claims," *Psychological Medicine* 40, no. 3 (2010): 367–82.

3 Deniz Fikretoglu, Alain Brunet, Stephane Guay, and David Pedlar, "Mental Health Treatment Seeking by Military Members with Posttraumatic Stress Disorder: Findings on Rates, Characteristics, and Predictors from a Nationally Representative Canadian Military Sample," *Canadian Journal of Psychiatry* 52, no. 2 (2007): 103–10; Jitender Sareen, Brian J. Cox, Tracie O. Afifi, Murray B. Stein, Shay-Lee Belik, Graham Meadows, and Gordon J. G. Asmundson, "Combat and Peacekeeping Operations in Relation to Prevalence of Mental Disorders and Perceived Need for Mental Health Care: Findings from a Large Representative Sample of Military Personnel," *Archives of Psychiatry* 64, no. 7 (2007): 843–52.

4 Barbara O. Rothbaum, Elizabeth A. Meadows, Patricia Resick, and David W. Foy, "Cognitive-Behavioral Therapy," in *Effective Treatments for Posttraumatic Stress Disorder: Practice Guidelines from the International Society for Traumatic Stress Studies,* ed. Edna B. Foa, Matthew Friedman, and Terrence M. Keane, 60–83 (New York: Guilford, 2000); Isaac Marks, Karina Lovell, Homa Noshirvani, Maria Livanou, and Sian Thrasher, "Treatment of Posttraumatic Stress Disorder by Exposure and/or Cognitive Restructuring: A Controlled Study," *Archives of General Psychiatry* 55, no. 4 (1998): 317–25.

5 Craig S. Rosen, Helen C. Chow, John F. Finney, Mark A. Greenbaum, Rudolf H. Moos, Javaid I. Sheikh, and Jerome A. Yesavage, "VA Practice Patterns and Practice Guidelines for Treating Posttraumatic Stress Disorder," *Journal of Traumatic Stress* 17, no. 3 (2004): 213–22.

6 Elizabeth A. Hembree, Edna B. Foa, Nicole M. Dorfan, Gordon P. Street, Jeanne Kowalski, and Xin Tu, "Do Patients Drop Out Prematurely from Exposure Therapy for PTSD?," *Journal of Traumatic Stress* 16, no. 6 (2003): 555–62; Patricia A. Resick, Pallavi Nishith, Terri L. Weaver, Millie C. Astin, and Catherine A. Feuer, "A Comparison of Cognitive-Processing Therapy with Prolonged Exposure and a Waiting Condition for the Treatment of Chronic Posttraumatic Stress Disorder in Female Rape Victims," *Journal of Consulting and Clinical Psychology* 70, no. 4 (2002): 867–79; Sheila A. Rauch, Erin Defever, Todd Favorite, Anne Duroe, Cecily Garrity, Brian Martis, and Israel Liberzon, "Prolonged Exposure for PTSD in a Veterans Health Administration PTSD Clinic," *Journal of Traumatic Stress* 22, no. 1 (2009): 60–4; Peter W. Tuerk, Matthew Yoder, Anouk Grubaugh, Hugh Myrick, Mark Hamner, and Ron Acierno, "Prolonged Exposure Therapy for Combat Related Posttraumatic Stress Disorder: An Examination of Treatment Effectiveness for Veterans of the Wars in Afghanistan and Iraq," *Journal of Anxiety Disorders* 25, no. 3 (2011): 397–403.

7 Management of Post-Traumatic Stress Working Group, *VA/DoD Clinical Practice Guideline for Management of Post-Traumatic Stress* (Washington, DC: Department of Veterans Affairs/Department of Defence, 2010).

8 Paula P. Schnurr, Matthew J. Friedman, David W. Foy, M. Tracie Shea, Frank Y. Hsieh, Philip W. Lavori, Shirley M. Glynn, Melissa Wattenberg, and Nancy C.

Bernardy, "Randomized Trial of Trauma-Focused Group Therapy for Posttraumatic Stress Disorder," *Archives of General Psychiatry* 60, no. 5 (2003): 481–9.

9   Edna B. Foa, Diana E. Hearst, Constance V. Dancu, Elizabeth A. Hembree, and Lisa H. Jaycox, "Prolonged Exposure (PE) Manual" (Philadelphia: Medical College of Pennsylvania, Eastern Pennsylvania Psychiatric Institute, 1994).

10   Edna B. Foa, Barbara O. Rothbaum, and Jami M. Furr, "Augmenting Exposure Therapy with Other CBT Procedures," *Psychiatric Annals* 33, no. 1 (2003): 47–53.

11   Edna B. Foa, Elizabeth Hembree, and Barbara O. Rothbaum, *Prolonged Exposure Therapy for PTSD: Emotional Processing of Traumatic Experiences, Therapist Guide* (New York: Oxford University Press, 2007).

12   Edna B. Foa, and B. O. Rothbaum, *Treating the Trauma of Rape: A Cognitive-Behavioral Therapy for PTSD* (New York: Guilford, 1998).

13   Edna B. Foa, Elizabeth A. Hembree, Shawn P. Cahill, Sheila A. M. Rauch, David S. Riggs, Norah C. Feeny, and Elna Yadin, "Randomized Trial of Prolonged Exposure for Posttraumatic Stress Disorder with and without Cognitive Restructuring: Outcome at Academic and Community Clinics," *Journal of Consulting and Clinical Psychology* 73, no. 5 (2005): 953–64; Patricia A. Resick, Pallavi Nishith, Terri L. Weaver, Millie C. Astin, and Catherine A. Feuer, "A Comparison of Cognitive-Processing Therapy with Prolonged Exposure and a Waiting Condition for the Treatment of Chronic Posttraumatic Stress Disorder in Female Rape Victims," *Journal of Consulting and Clinical Psychology* 70, no. 4 (2002): 867–79.

14   Paula P. Schnurr, Matthew J. Friedman, Charles C. Engel, Edna B. Foa, M. Tracie Shea, Bruce K. Chow, Patricia A. Resick, Veronica Thurston, Susan M. Orsillo, Rodney Haug, Carole Turner, and Nancy Bernardy, "Cognitive Behavioral Therapy for Posttraumatic Stress Disorder in Women: A Randomized Controlled Trial," *Journal of the American Medical Association* 297, no. 8 (2007): 820–30.

15   Sheila A. M. Rauch, Erin Defever, Todd Favorite, Anne Duroe, Cecily Garrity, Brian Martis, and Israel Liberzon, "Prolonged Exposure for PTSD in a Veterans Health Administration Clinic," *Journal of Traumatic Stress* 22, no. 1 (2009): 60–4.

16   Peter W. Tuerk, Matthew Yoder, Anouk Grubaugh, Hugh Myrick, Mark Hamner, and Ron Acierno, "Prolonged Exposure Therapy for Combat Related Posttraumatic Stress Disorder: An Examination of Treatment Effectiveness for Veterans of the Wars in Afghanistan and Iraq," *Journal of Anxiety Disorders* 25, no. 3 (2011): 397–403.

17   Bradley E. Karlin, Josef I. Ruzek, Kathleen M. Chard, Afsoon Eftekhari, Candice M. Monson, Elizabeth A. Hembree, Patricia A. Resick, and Edna B. Foa, "Dissemination of Evidence-Based Psychological Treatments for Posttraumatic Stress Disorder in the Veterans Health Administration," *Journal of Traumatic Stress* 23, no. 6 (2010): 663–73.

18   Daniel F. Gros, Matthew Yoder, Peter W. Tuerk, Brian E. Lozano, and Ron Acierno, "Exposure Therapy for PTSD Delivered to Veterans via Telehealth: Predictors of Treatment Completion and Comparison to Treatment Delivered in Person," *Behavioural Therapy* 42, no. 2 (2011): 276–83.

19   Peter W. Tuerk, Matthew Yoder, Kenneth J. Ruggiero, Daniel F. Gros, and Ron Acierno, "A Pilot Study of Prolonged Exposure Therapy for Posttraumatic Stress Disorder Delivered via Telehealth Technology," *Journal of Traumatic Stress* 23, no. 1 (2010): 116–23.

20 Karlin et al., "Dissemination of Evidence-Based Psychological Treatments"; David
     Forbes, Mark Creamer, Jonathan I. Bisson, Judith A. Cohen, Bruce E. Crow, Edna
     B. Foa, Matthew J. Friedman, Terrence M. Keane, Harold S. Kudler, and Robert J.
     Ursano, "A Guide to Guidelines for the Treatment of PTSD and Related Conditions,"
     Journal of Traumatic Stress 23, no. 5 (2010): 537–52.

21 Institute of Medicine, *Treatment of Posttraumatic Stress Disorder: An Assessment of
     the Evidence* (Washington, DC: National Academies, 2008).

22 Patricia A. Resick, Candice M. Monson, and Kathleen M. Chard, *Cognitive Processing
     Therapy Treatment Manual: Veteran/Military Version* (Boston, MA: Veterans
     Administration, 2006).

23 Ibid.

24 Ibid.

25 Candice M. Monson, Paula P. Schnurr, Patricia A. Resick, Matthew J. Friedman,
     Yinong Young-Xu, and Susan P. Stevens, "Cognitive Processing Therapy for Veterans
     with Military-Related Posttraumatic Stress Disorder," *Journal of Consulting and
     Clinical Psychology* 74, no. 5 (2006): 898–907.

26 Kathleen M. Chard, Jeremiah A. Schumm, Gina P. Owens, and Sara M. Cottingham,
     "A Comparison of OEF and OIF veterans and Vietnam Veterans Receiving Cognitive
     Processing Therapy," *Journal of Traumatic Stress* 23, no. 1 (2010): 25–32.

27 Jennifer Alvarez, Caitlin McLean, Alex H. S. Harris, Craig S. Rosen, Josef I. Ruzek,
     and Rachel Kimerling, "The Comparative Effectiveness of Cognitive Processing
     Therapy for Male Veterans Treated in a VHA Posttraumatic Stress Disorder
     Residential Rehabilitation Program," *Journal of Consulting and Clinical Psychology* 79,
     no. 5 (2011): 590–9.

28 Leslie A. Morland, Anna K. Hynes, Margaret-Anne Mackintosh, Patricia A. Resick,
     and Kathleen M. Chard, "Group Cognitive Processing Therapy Delivered to Veterans
     via Telehealth: A Pilot Cohort," *Journal of Traumatic Stress* 24, no. 4 (2011): 465–9.

29 Karlin et al., "Dissemination of Evidence-Based Psychological Treatments."

30 Francine Shapiro, *Eye Movement Desensitization and Reprocessing: Level II Manual*
     (Pacific Grove, CA: EMDR, 1993).

31 John G. Carlson, Claude M. Chemtob, Kristin Rusnak, Nancy L. Hedlund, and Miles
     Y. Muraoka, "Eye Movement Desensitization and Reprocessing (EMDR) Treatment
     for Combat-Related Posttraumatic Stress Disorder," *Journal of Traumatic Stress* 11, no.
     1 (1998): 3–24; Lee Hyer and Jeffrey M. Brandsma, "EMDR Minus Eye Movements
     Equals Good Psychotherapy," *Journal of Traumatic Stress* 10, no. 3 (1997): 515–22.

32 Forbes et al., "A Guide to Guidelines."

33 James D. Herbert, Scott O. Lilienfeld, Jeffrey M. Lohr, Robert W. Montgomery,
     William T. O'Donohue, Gerald M. Rosen, and David F. Tolin, "Science and
     Pseudoscience in the Development of Eye Movement Desensitization and
     Reprocessing: Implications for Clinical Psychology," *Clinical Psychology Review* 20,
     no. 8 (2000): 945–71.

34 Lisa M. Najavits, "Psychosocial Treatments for Posttraumatic Stress Disorder," in *A
     Guide to Treatments That Work*, ed. Peter E. Nathan and Jack M. Gorman, 513–30
     (New York: Oxford University Press, 2007); David L. Albright and Bruce Thyer,
     "Does EMDR Reduce Post-Traumatic Stress Disorder Symptomatology in Combat

Veterans?," *Behavioral Interventions* 25, no. 1 (2010): 1–19; Hyer and Brandsma, "EMDR Minus Eye Movements Equals Good Psychotherapy."

35 Grant J. Devilly and Susan H. Spence, "The Relative Efficacy and Treatment Distress of EMDR and a Cognitive Behavioral Protocol in the Amelioration of Post Traumatic Stress Disorder," *Journal of Anxiety Disorders* 13, nos 1–2 (1999): 131–57; Gail Ironson, Blanche V. Freund, Jennifer L. Strauss, and Jessie Williams, "Comparison for Two Treatments for Posttraumatic Stress: A Community-Based Study of EMDR and Prolonged Exposure," *Journal of Clinical Psychology* 58, no. 1 (2002): 113–28; Steven Taylor, Dana S. Thordarson, Louise Maxfield, Ingrid C. Federoff, Karina Lovell, and John Ogrodniczuk, "Comparative Efficacy, Speed, and Adverse Effects of Three PTSD Treatments: Exposure Therapy, EMDR, and Relaxation Training," *Journal of Consulting and Clinical Psychology* 71, no. 2 (2003): 330–8; Barbara O. Rothbaum, Millie C. Astin, and Fred Marsteller, "Prolonged Exposure versus Eye Movement Desensitization and Reprocessing (EMDR) for PTSD Rape Victims," *Journal of Traumatic Stress* 18, no. 6 (2005): 607–16; Claude M. Chemtob, David F. Tolin, Bessel A. van der Kolk, and Roger K. Pitman, "Eye Movement Desensitization and Reprocessing," in Foa, Keane, and Friedman, *Effective Treatments for PTSD*, 333–5.

36 Albright and Thyer, "Does EMDR Reduce Post-Traumatic Stress Disorder Symptomatology."

37 Patrick A. Boudewyns, Steven A. Stwertka, Lee A. Hyer, James W. Albrecht, and Edwin V. Sperr, "Eye Movement Desensitization and Reprocessing: A Pilot Study," *Behavioural Therapist* 16, no. 2 (1993): 30–3; James A. Jensen, "An Investigation of Eye Movement Desensitization and Reprocessing (EMD/R) as a Treatment for Posttraumatic Stress Disorder (PTSD) Symptoms of Vietnam Combat Veterans," *Behavioural Therapy* 25, no. 2 (1994): 311–25; Grant J. Devilly, Susan H. Spence, and Ronald M. Rapee, "Statistical and Reliable Change with Eye Movement Desensitization and Reprocessing: Treating Trauma with a Veteran Population," *Behavioural Therapy* 29, no. 3 (1998): 435–55; Michael L. Macklin, Linda J. Metzger, Natasha B. Lasko, Nancy J. Berry, Scott P. Orr, and Roger K. Pitman, "Five-Year Follow-up Study of Eye Movement Desensitization and Reprocessing Therapy for Combat Related Posttraumatic Stress Disorder," *Comprehensive Psychiatry* 41, no. 1 (2000): 24–7.

38 Steven M. Silver, Alvin Brooks, and Jeanne Obenchain, "Treatment of Vietnam War Veterans with PTSD: A Comparison of Eye Movement Desensitization and Reprocessing, Biofeedback, and Relaxation Training," *Journal of Traumatic Stress* 8, no. 2 (1995): 337–42; Patrick A. Boudewyns and Lee A. Hyer, "Eye Movement Desensitization and Reprocessing (EMDR) as Treatment for Post-Traumatic Stress Disorder (PTSD)," *Clinical Psychology Psychotherapy* 3, no. 3 (1996): 185–95; Roger K. Pitman, Scott P. Orr, Bruce Altman, Ronald E. Longpre, Roger E. Poire, and Michael L. Macklin, "Emotional Processing during Eye-Movement Desensitization and Reprocessing Therapy of Vietnam Veterans with Chronic Post-Traumatic Stress Disorder," *Comprehensive Psychiatry* 37, no. 6 (1996): 419–29; John G. Carlson, Claude M. Chemtob, Kristin Rusnak, Nancy L. Hedlund, and Miles Y. Muraoka, "Eye Movement Desensitization and Reprocessing for Combat-Related Posttraumatic Stress Disorder," *Journal of Traumatic Stress* 11, no. 1 (1998): 3–24; Susan Rogers, Steven Silver, James Goss, Jeanne Obenchain, Amy Willis, and Robert L. Whitney,

"A Single Session, Controlled Group Study of Flooding and Eye Movement Desensitization and Reprocessing in Treating Posttraumatic Stress Disorder among Vietnam War Veterans: Preliminary Data," *Journal of Anxiety Disorders* 13, nos 1–2 (1999): 119–30.

39 Mark C. Russell, "Treating Combat-Related Stress Disorders: A Multiple Case Study Utilizing Eye Movement Desensitization and Reprocessing (EMDR) with Battlefield Casualties from the Iraqi War," *Military Psychology* 18, no. 1 (2006): 1–18.

40 Mark C. Russell, Steven M. Silver, Susan Rogers, and Jolee N. Darnell, "Responding to a Identified Need: A Joint Department of Defense / Department of Veterans Affairs Training Program in Eye Movement Desensitization and Reprocessing (EMDR) for Clinicians Providing Trauma Services," *International Journal of Stress Management* 14, no. 1 (2007): 61–71.

41 Steven M. Silver, Susan Rogers, and Mark C. Russell, "Eye Movement Desensitization and Reprocessing (EMDR) in the Treatment of War Veterans," *Journal of Clinical Psychology* 64, no. 8 (2008): 947–57.

42 Shirley M. Glynn, Spencer Eth, Eugenia T. Randolph, David W. Foy, Marleen Urbaltis, Laurie Boxer, George G. Paz, Gregory B. Leong, Gregory Firman, Jonathan D. Salk, Jeffrey W. Katzman, and Judith Crowthers, "A Test of Behavioral Family Therapy to Augment Exposure for Combat-Related Posttraumatic Stress Disorder," *Journal of Consulting and Clinical Psychology* 67, no. 2 (1999): 243–51; David W. Foy, Bruce Kagan, Charles McDermott, Gregory Leskin, R. Carl Sipprelle, and George Paz, "Practical Parameters in the Use of Flooding for Treating Chronic PTSD," *Clinical Psychology and Psychotherapy* 3, no. 3 (1996): 169–75.

43 Edna B. Foa and Richard J. McNally, "Mechanics of Change in Exposure Therapy," in *Current Controversies in the Anxiety Disorders*, ed. Ronald M. Rapee, 329–43 (New York: Guilford, 1996); Agnes van Minnen, Arnoud Arntz, and Ger P. J. Keijsers, "Prolonged Exposure in Patients with Chronic PTSD: Predictors of Treatment Outcome and Dropout," *Behaviour Research Therapy* 40, no. 4 (2002): 439–57.

44 Zahava Solomon and Mario Mikulincer, "Trajectories of PTSD: A 20-Year Longitudinal Study," *American Journal of Psychiatry* 163, no. 4 (2006): 659–66.

45 Amy C. Iversen, Lauren van Staden, Jamie H. Hughes, Tess Browne, Lisa Hull, John Hall, Neil Greenberg, Roberto J. Rona, Matthew Hotopf, Simon Wessely, and Nicola T. Fear, "The Prevalence of Common Mental Disorders and PTSD in the UK Military: Using Data from a Clinical Interview-Based Study," *BMC Psychiatry* 9 (2009): 68, doi:10.1186/1471-244X-9-68; Hoge et al., "Combat Duty in Iraq and Afghanistan"; Milliken, Auchterlonie, and Hoge, "Longitudinal Assessment of Mental Health Problems."

46 Roger K. Pitman, Bruce Altman, Evan Greenwald, Ronald E. Longpre, Michael L. Macklin, Roger E. Poire, and Gail S. Steketee, "Psychiatric Complication during Flooding Therapy for Posttraumatic Stress Disorder," *Journal of Clinical Psychiatry* 52, no. 1 (1991): 17–20; Roger K. Pitman, Scott P. Orr, Bruce Altman, Ronald E. Longpre, Roger E. Poire, and Michael L. Macklin, "Emotional Processing and Outcome of Imaginal Flooding Therapy in Vietnam Veterans with Chronic Posttraumatic Stress Disorder," *Comprehensive Psychiatry* 37, no. 6 (1996): 409–18; N. Tarrier, Hazel Pilgrim, Claire Sommerfield, Brian Faragher, Martina Reynolds, Elizabeth Graham, and Christine Barrowclough, "A Randomized Trial of Cognitive Therapy

and Imaginal Exposure in the Treatment of Chronic Posttraumatic Stress Disorder," *Journal of Consulting and Clinical Psychology* 67, no. 1 (1999): 13–18; Edward S. Kubany and Frederick P. Manke, "Cognitive Therapy for Trauma-Related Guilt: Conceptual Bases and Treatment Outlines," *Cognitive and Behavioral Practice* 2, no. 1 (1995): 27–61.

47 Lisa H. Jaycox and Edna B. Foa, "Obstacles in Implementing Exposure Therapy for PTSD: Case Discussions and Practical Solutions," *Clinical Psychology and Psychotherapy* 3, no. 3 (1996): 176–84; Barbara O. Rothbaum and Ann C. Schwartz, "Exposure Therapy for Posttraumatic Stress Disorder," *American Journal of Psychotherapy* 56, no. 1 (2002): 59–75.

48 Michael R. DeVries, H. Kent Hughes, Harvey Watson, and Bret A. Moore, "Understanding the Military Culture," in *Handbook of Counseling Military Couples*, ed. Bret A. Moore, 7–18 (New York: Taylor and Francis Group, 2012).

49 Brett T. Litz, Nathan Stein, Eileen Delaney, Leslie Lebowitz, William P. Nash, Caroline Silva, and Shira Maguen, "Moral Injury and Moral Repair in War Veterans: A Preliminary Model and Intervention Strategy," *Clinical Psychology Review* 29, no. 8 (2009): 695–706.

50 Kent D. Drescher and David W. Foy, "When They Come Home: Posttraumatic Stress, Moral Injury, and Spiritual Consequences for Veterans," *Reflective Practice: Formation and Supervision in Ministry* 28 (2012): 85–102.

51 Matt J. Gray, Yonit Schorr, William Nash, Leslie Lebowitz, Amy Amidon, Amy Lansing, Melissa Maglione, Ariel J. Lang, and Brett Litz, "Adaptive Disclosure: An Open Trial of a Novel Exposure-Based Intervention for Service Members with Combat-Related Psychological Stress Injuries," *Behavioural Therapy* 43, no. 2 (2011): 407–15.

14

Service Use in an Outpatient Clinic for Current and Veteran Military and RCMP Members

JENNIFER C. LAFORCE, DEBBIE L. WHITNEY,
AND KRISTEN N. KLASSEN

Abstract

Military, Veteran, and RCMP clients engage in a variety of outpatient mental health treatments through the Winnipeg OSI Clinic. Similar to most outpatient settings, service use is mutually regulated by clinicians and clients. Files of 393 discharged clients were reviewed in order to determine typical service use and the factors that predict the number of sessions received. Clinical symptom severity did not differentiate the type of services in which clients engaged. Retired, veteran, older clients were overrepresented in the group that received a formal assessment but no therapy, whereas current Canadian Forces members were much more likely to engage in therapy than use assessment services only. In predicting volume of service use, it appears important to attend to diagnostic complexity as knowing clients' diagnoses, and in particular co-morbidities, provided significantly more information than just being aware of the intensity of their reported symptoms or demographic variables.

Introduction

The intense and sustained demands of both military and police service are associated with the development of mental health conditions such as post traumatic stress disorder (PTSD), depression, substance abuse, and other anxiety disorders.[1] Within the Canadian Forces (CF), a survey conducted in 2001 found the prevalence of mental health disorders in the past year to be 15%, with depression at 6.9% and PTSD at 2.3%.[2] The survey also found that the experiences of combat exposure and/or witnessing atrocities had the strongest association with mental health disorders. Since then, approximately 30,000 Canadian soldiers have been deployed in support of the war in Afghanistan, and a current estimate is that 30% of soldiers deployed in a combat zone will experience mental health difficulties sometime within their lifetime and 10% will experience a severe form of PTSD within their lifetime.[3] Estimates of PTSD prevalence among police officers vary widely, with a Canadian study of police officers finding 32% of their trauma-exposed volunteer sample screening positive for PTSD.[4]

There are now effective, evidence-based psychotherapies for a wide variety of mental health disorders, including PTSD.[5] However, for groups with rigorous performance standards like the military and police, there is concern that psychological barriers to care (e.g., stigma, negative attitudes about treatment, and lack of concern about sub-threshold conditions) may discourage treatment seeking.[6]

In the Canadian context, there have been substantial efforts to reduce stigma and provide access to appropriate specialist care. The term *operational stress injury* (OSI) has been widely adopted within the CF and Veterans Affairs Canada (VAC) as a more inclusive term to refer to a broad range of persistent psychological difficulties that may result from service.[7] VAC has also established a network of OSI clinics across the country, which provide assessment and treatment of OSIs. Services are available to current and veteran members of the CF and the Royal Canadian Mounted Police (RCMP) and affected family members.

These OSI clinics are structured to provide interdisciplinary and evidence-based care, with access to psychiatric medication consultation and management, a range of psychotherapy services, clinical support services, and family services.[8] Within the OSI clinics, service length is not determined by administrative limits; rather, service type and length are jointly regulated by clinician and client choice as a result of individualized case planning. Evidence-based psychotherapy and pharmacotherapy are used flexibly, and clients often receive concurrent or sequential services from multiple professionals. Treatment may be changed if gains are not being made, and clients may receive more than one form of treatment before they are discharged. When there are co-morbid conditions, aspects of a variety of therapies may be combined to address needs. When clients recover earlier than anticipated, therapy may be ended before an entire treatment protocol has been completed.

Previous research showed that treatment-as-usual (a combination of evidence-based psychotherapy and pharmaco-therapy) within an OSI clinic produced positive results one year later for Canadian veterans with service-related PTSD, as symptoms of PTSD, depression, and anxiety were all significantly reduced following treatment.[9] Intriguingly, those seen for longer durations (six months or more) were reported to have made the greater gains;[10] however, there is not clear agreement that those people with longer durations of therapy always do better.[11] Although it is encouraging to know that these individualized treatments produce results, it also would be helpful to know more about how clients use the services available to them.

The goal of this research was two-fold: to describe current service use patterns of outpatient clients of the Winnipeg OSI Clinic and to explore client variables that differentiated service use both in *type* and *volume* of service. Service use was examined with reference to whether or not clients engaged in formal assessment services and/or received psychotherapy. Next to intake, these were the highest volume service categories. It was assumed that most clients would proceed from intake to formal assessment to psychotherapy, given the program design. No hypotheses were made about the demographic variables that would predict the type of service used; however, we expected that individual differences would be more apparent in examining the volume of service use. Specifically, we expected those with more severe symptoms at intake would use more services and that diagnostic complexity (i.e., the presence of multiple diagnoses) would be more predictive of session volume than symptom severity alone.

Methods

Clinical Research Database

Clinic use patterns were identified by examining data from the Clinical Research Database at the Winnipeg OSI clinic. Since 2009, clients of the Winnipeg OSI clinic have been asked for consent to use routinely collected demographic and clinical data for research. Between 2009 and 2012, 242 clients have been approached for consent by research staff, and over 96% have consented to allow the data to be used. A retrospective chart review was conducted on files from 2004 to 2009, which added data from an additional 329 clients for a total of 571 clients. This total included some instances where the same individual is represented multiple times (i.e., if he or she accessed services at multiple times). The resulting Clinical Research Database contains demographic variables – variables related to clinical symptoms and diagnoses – and indications of type and volume of service use. The database and associated research projects have been approved by the University of Manitoba Health Research Ethics Board.

Inclusion Criteria

A single client may be represented in the database multiple times if referred more than once. In order to ensure that an individual client was represented only once in this research, we selected the data corresponding to a client's first referral where (a) at least one service session was received and (b) the file had been closed by 30 September 2012. This study focused on clients who were current or veteran members of the CF or RCMP; family members were not included in these analyses. Because we wanted to represent the full range of clients who access service, there were no exclusion criteria related to clinical symptoms nor severity.

Services

The clinical services received were coded as follows:

Intake

All intake sessions were clinical interviews that followed a semi-structured format and covered informed consent for OSI clinic services, presenting concerns, illness and interpersonal history, and clarified expectations for services.

Assessment

Assessment sessions were diagnostic interviews conducted by either a registered psychologist or psychiatrist. Assessments often were used to clarify diagnosis, recommend and plan treatment, and/or meet administrative requests such as determining eligibility for VAC disability awards. The standard psychiatric assessment was one session, whereas the standard psychological assessment was three sessions.

Psychotherapy

Psychotherapy sessions were conducted by either a registered psychologist or registered social worker. Most were individual therapy sessions, but couples and family sessions also were included. Psychotherapy approaches covered a broad range of evidenced-based treatments including prolonged exposure, cognitive processing therapy, eye movement desensitization and reprocessing, behavioural activation, cognitive-behaviour therapies (for depression, generalized anxiety disorder, obsessive compulsive disorder, panic disorder, and pain), acceptance and commitment therapy, aspects of dialectical behaviour therapy, seeking safety, mindfulness-based stress reduction, cognitive-behavioural conjoint therapy for PTSD, and emotion focused couple therapy. Psychotherapies were provided primarily as individual treatment, with couple-based treatment and group treatments also available.

Treatment decisions, including which empirically based treatment would be used and length of treatment, were determined on an individual basis collaboratively between the therapist and client. The OSI clinic interdisciplinary team of clinicians met weekly to discuss and provide consultation on treatment decisions.

Psychiatric Treatment

Treatment sessions conducted by a psychiatrist were coded as psychiatric treatment and often included but were not limited to medication-based therapy.

Supportive Counselling

Supportive counselling sessions were provided by a registered psychiatric nurse, most often supporting clients who were on a waitlist for other clinic services.

Measures

PTSD Checklist–Military Version

The PTSD Checklist–Military Version (PCL–M)[12] is a seventeen-item self-report questionnaire that assesses PTSD symptom severity. Respondents are asked to indicate how much the problem described in the statement has bothered them over the last month on a scale from 1 (Not at all) to 5 (Extremely). Each of the seventeen statements corresponds to one of the seventeen *Diagnostic and Statistical Manual,* version IV (*DSM–IV*) diagnostic criteria for PTSD. The military version orients the respondent at the beginning of the questionnaire by stating veterans sometimes have these problems in response to military experiences. The first eight items also reference "a stressful military experience." A total score is calculated by summing the items with higher scores indicating greater severity (range = 17–85). A score of fifty is often used within military populations to differentiate the clinical from the non-clinical range.[13] The PCL is the second-most prevalent self-report instrument used by traumatic stress professionals.[14] It has excellent internal consistency across different veteran populations, sexual assault survivors, and motor vehicle accident survivors (Cronbach's αs ranging from .94 to .97). Test-retest reliability over two to three days for Vietnam veterans was excellent (Pearson r = .96).[15]

Beck Depression Inventory–II

The Beck Depression Inventory–II (BDI–II)[16] is a twenty-one-item self-report questionnaire that is used to assess the severity of symptoms of depression. Each item includes a four-point scale (range 0–3) with statements starting with the absence of a symptom and then presenting ascending levels of severity. Respondents chose a statement which best described how they have been feeling over the previous two weeks. Items are summed to provide a total score (range = 0–63). It has excellent internal consistency (Cronbach's αs ranging from .92 to .93), test-retest reliability over one week (Pearson r = .93), and shows appropriate convergent and discriminate validity with other measures.[17]

Beck Anxiety Inventory

The Beck Anxiety Inventory (BAI)[18] is a twenty-one-item questionnaire that measures severity of anxiety symptoms that are minimally shared with depression. Respondents are asked to indicate how bothered they were by each of twenty-one symptoms over the last week on a scale with four options ranging from Not at all (scored 0) to Severely I could barely stand it (scored 3). Items are summed to provide a total score (range = 0–63). The BAI has excellent internal consistency (Cronbach's αs ranging from .85 to .93), adequate test-retest reliability (Pearson r

= .75),[19] and has good discriminant validity, correlating better with other anxiety than depression measures.[20]

Diagnosis

In recording diagnosis, preference was given for diagnoses made by OSI clinic psychologists or psychiatrists as part of a comprehensive diagnostic assessment that often included both unstructured and semi-structured clinical interviews (e.g., the use of the Clinician-Administered PTSD Scale [CAPS]).[21] Where the clinical file contained multiple diagnostic reports, the diagnosis of the professional with the most experience with the client was selected. When diagnostic reports from the OSI clinic were not present, diagnoses were recorded from outside professional reports. Diagnoses were categorized as (1) PTSD, (2) depression (for either major depressive disorder or dysthymia), (3) other anxiety (for generalized anxiety disorder, panic disorder, social phobia, or specific phobia), (4) substance related (for any substance-related condition other than a disorder in sustained full remission), (5) pain (for pain disorder associated with psychological factors or associated with both psychological factors and a general medical condition), (6) other (for other Axis I disorders including bipolar, eating disorders, nightmare disorder, primary insomnia, intermittent explosive disorder, and pathological gambling), and (7) Axis II (for any personality disorder or specific traits listed on Axis II of the DSM–IV multi-axial diagnosis); the presence of either deferred diagnosis or no diagnosis on Axis II also was noted.

Discharge Reason

At discharge, the primary clinician recorded the reason for discharge as (1) goals met, indicating that the initial referral request was satisfied, (2) services declined, indicating further services were offered but the client declined them, (3) client discontinued, indicating that in the midst of a service the client discontinued contact unexpectedly, (4) referred out, indicating the client was referred to other services outside of the osi clinic, (5) inactive / no contact, indicating the file was closed following an unexpected three-month period when there was no contact from the client or the client scheduled and failed to show for three consecutive appointments, or (6) deceased, if the client had died.

Results

Descriptions of Clients

There were 363 clients identified as meeting the inclusion criteria. The majority (61.7%) were serving members of the CF. Just over a third of clients were referred by VAC, including 120 CF veterans, 3 RCMP veterans, and 1 veteran of service in a

Table 14.1 | Client demographics, work service variables, and clinical symptoms at start of service

	n (%)	M (SD)
DEMOGRAPHIC		
Age in years		41.86 (14.27)
Male (*n* = 363)	330 (90.9)	
Marital status (*n* = 363)		
Married / common-law	246 (67.8)	
Divorced/separated/widowed	53 (14.6)	
Never married	64 (17.6)	
Children (*n* = 360)		
No. of children		1.60 (1.50)
Have children	255 (70.8)	
Education (*n* = 355)		
< Grade 12	62 (17.5)	
Grade 12	175 (49.3)	
> Grade 12	118 (33.2)	
Employment (*n* = 360)		
Full time	264 (73.3)	
Not working	58 (16.1)	
Retired	38 (10.6)	
DUTY-RELATED		
Referral source (*n* = 363)		
VAC	124 (34.2)	
CF	224 (61.7)	
RCMP	15 (4.1)	
Years in CF/RCMP service (*n* = 355)		14.70 (8.41)
No. of overseas deployments (*n* = 343)		2.03 (1.60)
No. of RCMP postings (*n* = 16)	5.39 (3.48)	
CLINICAL SYMPTOMS		
BDI–II (*n* = 275)		26.56 (11.49)
BAI (*n* = 278)		21.85 (12.52)
PCL–M (*n* = 303)		55.35 (13.92)
Re-experiencing		3.12 (0.99)
Avoidance/numbing		3.14 (0.91)
Hyperarousal		3.53 (0.91)

Table 14.2 | Client diagnoses (*n* = 346)

	n *(%)*
Axis I	
PTSD	207 (59.8)
Depression-related	168 (48.6)
Other anxiety	63 (18.2)
Substance related	55 (15.9)
Pain	50 (14.5)
Adjustment disorder	33 (9.5)
Axis II	
Disorder or specific traits listed	56 (16.2)
Deferred	73 (21.1)
No diagnosis on Axis II	217 (62.7)
Axis I co-morbidity	
No diagnosis	26 (7.5)
1 diagnosis	126 (36.4)
2 diagnoses	121 (35.0)
3 or more diagnoses	73 (20.1)

foreign country's military. Only a minority of clients were serving RCMP members (4.1%). The majority of clients were male (90.9%). Most had at least a high school education (82.5%). Average age was 41.86 (*SD* = 14.27) years, with an average of 14.70 (*SD* = 8.41) years of service. Current or former CF clients had an average of 2.03 overseas deployments, and current or former RCMP clients reported an average of 5.39 postings. Just over two-thirds of the sample was married or living with common-law partners, and 70.8% reported having children, with a median of two children. The majority of clients were working (68.9% full-time, 2.5% part-time, 1.4% students), although 10.6% were not working at all as the result of disability, a leave of absence, or unspecified reasons. Table 14.1 provides further details.

Clients reported significant clinical symptoms at intake. Mean scores for PCL–M, BDI–II, and BAI, are reported in table 14.1. These scores fall within accepted clinical ranges for PTSD, depression, and anxiety symptoms, respectively.

Diagnostic co-morbidity was common, as over half the sample had two or more diagnoses, with PTSD and depression being the most common diagnoses. See table 14.2 for further information on diagnoses.

Services Received by Clients

The three primary services were intake, assessment, and psychotherapy, as these were the services accessed by the greatest number of clients (95% of clients had an

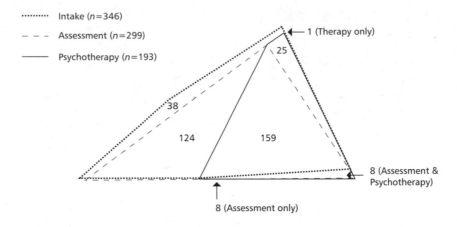

Figure 14.1 | Proportional representation of number of clients using intake, assessment, and psychotherapy services

intake, 82% had an assessment, and 53% had psychotherapy). Figure 14.1 depicts the proportion of the 363 clients who used intake, assessment, and psychotherapy services. The progression for the modal client was intake to assessment to treatment. Most clients went on to other services after intake (n = 331, 91%), with only 32 clients (9%) being discharged after intake. There were 132 (36%) clients who received assessments but did not go on to psychotherapy. Of the 193 clients who participated in psychotherapy, 167 also had assessments, but 26 received psychotherapy without participating in a formal assessment in the OSI clinic.

Not represented in figure 14.1 are psychiatric treatment services and supportive counselling services. There were 74 clients who received psychiatric treatment (i.e., 20% of all clients), 70 of whom participated in a formal assessment and 51 of whom also received psychotherapy, and 37 clients received supportive counselling (i.e., 10% of all clients), 31 of whom participated in a formal assessment and 25 of whom also received psychotherapy.

Client Differences in Service Use Patterns

In order to determine if any of the demographic, duty-related, or clinical variables presented earlier differentiated clients who only received intake (intake only; n = 32) from those who received assessments but no further service (assessment only; n = 132) and/or those who received therapy (psychotherapy; n = 193), a series of one-way analyses of variance (ANOVAs) for continuous variables and chi-squares for categorical variables were run.

Mean age differed across service use groups (i.e., intake only, assessment only, psychotherapy), $F(2, 354)$ = 8.20, p < .001. Subsequent pair-wise comparisons (with the Bonferroni correction) revealed that the group that received assessment only was significantly older (M = 45.70, SD = 17.16) than the psychotherapy group (M = 39.26, SD = 11.81), although neither group was significantly different from the intake only group (M = 42.10, SD = 12.35). There were significant associations between service use and referral source ($\chi^2(9)$ = 17.85, p < .01) and between service use and employment status ($\chi^2(4)$ = 15.01, p < .01). These contingency tables are presented in table 14.3. In order to better understand these associations, the standardized residuals for the observations were examined, with residuals falling outside of ± 1.96, reflecting observations that were significantly different from what was expected, p < .05. An examination of the standardized residuals revealed that both VAC-referred clients and retired clients were more likely to be in the assessment only group and less likely to be in the psychotherapy group than expected. The opposite pattern was observed for CF-referred clients, who were more likely to be in the psychotherapy group and less likely to be in the assessment only group than expected. No variable appeared to differentiate the intake only group from other service use groups.

None of the questionnaires administered at intake (PCL–M, BDI–II, BAI) showed significant differences across service use, Fs ranged from 0.94 to 0.003, ps > .39. However, the number of diagnoses differentiated service use, $F(2, 337)$ = 6.44, p < .01. Subsequent pair-wise comparisons (with the Bonferroni correction) revealed that the psychotherapy group had significantly more diagnoses than the assessment only group (psychotherapy M = 1.88, SD = 0.94; assessment only M = 1.51, SD = 0.95). The intake only group (M = 1.53, SD = 1.01) did not differ significantly from either of the other two groups.

The association between service use and discharge reason was significant ($\chi^2(8)$ = 80.11, p < .001), indicating that people were discharged from the clinic for different reasons, depending on their service use group. Only one client was discharged because of death and was removed from this analysis. An examination of the standardized residuals (presented in table 14.3) revealed that intake only clients were more likely to be discharged because services were declined or they were referred out and less likely to be discharged with goals met than expected. In contrast, fewer therapy clients were discharged because services were declined than expected. Repeated analysis with the categories "Client Discontinued" with "Inactive / No contact" combined did not alter this pattern of results.

Volume of Service Use

Distribution of Session Volume

The distribution of total number of sessions that clients participated in across all services is presented in figure 14.2. Although the mean number of sessions was 15.45 (SD = 23.91), the median was 5 (range: 1–171), with a third of clients having 3

Table 14.3. Cross-tabulation of referral source, employment status, and discharge reason by service use

	Intake only	Assessment only	Psychotherapy
REFERRAL SOURCE			
DND			
Count (expected count)	16 (19.7)	67 (81.3)	137 (118.9)
Standardized residual	-0.8	-1.6	1.7
VAC			
Count (expected count)	15 (11.0)	60 (45.5)	48 (66.5)
Standardized residual	1.2	2.2	-2.3
RCMP			
Count (expected count)	1 (1.3)	5 (5.2)	8 (7.6)
Standardized residual	-0.2	-0.1	0.2
EMPLOYMENT STATUS			
Employed			
Count (expected count)	22 (22.9)	92 (97.7)	148 (141.4)
Standardized residual	-0.2	-0.6	0.6
Not working			
Count (expected count)	8 (4.7)	16 (20.1)	30 (29.1)
Standardized residual	1.5	-0.9	0.2
Retired			
Count (expected count)	1 (3.3)	24 (14.2)	13 (20.5)
Standardized residual	-1.3	2.6	-1.7
DISCHARGE REASON			
Declined			
Count (expected count)	11 (1.9)	6 (7.8)	4 (11.3)
Standardized residual	6.6	-0.6	-2.2
Goals met			
Count (expected count)	8 (19.2)	90 (79.3)	116 (115.4)
Standardized residual	-2.6	1.2	0.1
Client discontinued			
Count (expected count)	1 (3.1)	13 (13.0)	21 (18.9)
Standardized residual	-1.2	–	0.5
Referred out			
Count (expected count)	9 (2.6)	7 (10.8)	13 (15.6)
Standardized residual	4.0	-1.1	-0.7
Inactive / no contact			
Count (expected count)	3 (5.1)	16 (21.1)	38 (30.7)
Standardized residual	-0.9	-1.1	1.3

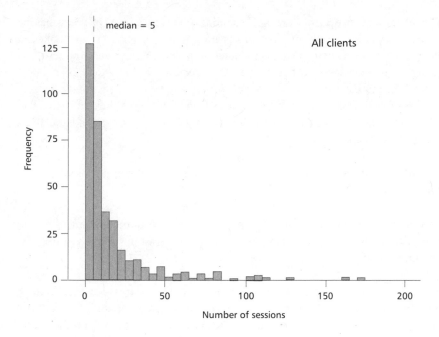

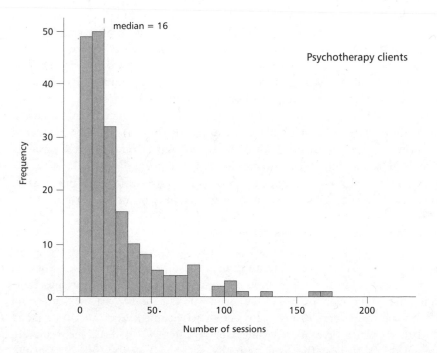

Figure 14.2 | Total number of sessions across all services for all clients and psychotherapy clients

or fewer sessions, two-thirds having 13 sessions or fewer, and 85% of clients having 30 or fewer sessions. Total number of sessions across all services was looked at for the subset of 193 clients who participated in psychotherapy, with the resulting histogram also displayed in figure 14.2. As expected, psychotherapy clients participated in more sessions with a mean of 26.37 (SD = 28.56) sessions across all services and a median number of 16 sessions (range: 2–171). A third of clients had 10 or fewer sessions, two-thirds had 24 sessions or fewer, and 85% of clients had 48 or fewer sessions.

Predicting Session Volume from Duty-Related Variables, Demographics, and Clinical Symptoms

Given that session volume is not normally distributed, with both strong skew and kurtosis (as depicted in figure 14.2), the natural log of session volume was used for subsequent analyses.

In order to determine what variables best predicted the total number of sessions across all services, the natural log of session volume was regressed onto three blocks of variables. This first block included duty-related variables (i.e., referral source (coded as VAC or CF), years of service at time of referral, and number of deployments). The second block included demographic variables (i.e., age at intake, children (coded yes or no), married (coded yes or no), working (coded yes or no), retired (coded yes or no)) and the final block included clinical symptoms at intake (i.e., BDI–II, BAI, and PCL–M scores). Given the exploratory nature of this research, variables were entered within each block using a forward stepwise method.

In the first block of service related variables, none of the identified variables were associated strongly enough with session volume to be entered in the model. In the second block of demographic variables, only age was entered in the analysis, and in the final step, of all the clinical measures, only the PCL–M score was entered in the model. See table 14.4 for more details. Although significant, these variables accounted for very little of the variance in session frequency (i.e., final R^2 = .04[22]).

When this analysis was repeated for the log of therapy sessions, not one variable showed a strong enough association to be entered into the model.

Predicting Session Volume from Diagnosis

In order to determine the relationship between diagnoses and session volume, the natural log of session volume was regressed onto dichotomous variables indicating the presence or absence of the diagnostic categories of PTSD, depression, other anxiety, substance related, pain, Axis II, adjustment, and other (as defined in Method), which were entered using a forward stepwise method. The results are presented in table 14.5. The resulting model accounted for 9% of the variance in total number of sessions and included PTSD, depression, and pain.

Table 14.4 | Multiple regression to predict log (total number of sessions) given work-service variables, demographic variables, and initial clinical symptoms

Step	B	SE B	β
Step 1			
No variables entered in this step			
Step 2			
Constant	2.69	0.27	
Age	-0.02	0.01	-0.16*
Step 3			
Constant	2.01	0.42	
Age	-0.02	0.01	-0.15*
PCL–M	0.01	0.01	0.13*

Note: $R^2 = .03$ for step 2, $\Delta R^2 = .02$ for step 3 ($p < .02$)

* $p < .05$

Table 14.5 | Multiple regression to predict log (total number of sessions) given presence of diagnostic categories

Step	B	SE B	β
Step 1			
Constant	1.66	0.10	
PTSD	0.56	0.13	0.22***
Step 2			
Constant	1.49	0.12	
PTSD	0.54	0.13	0.22***
Depression	0.37	0.13	0.15**
Step 3			
Constant	1.42	0.12	
PTSD	0.55	0.13	0.22***
Depression	0.36	0.13	0.15**
Pain	0.48	0.18	0.14**

Note: $R^2 = .05$ for step 1, $\Delta R^2 = .02$ for step 2 ($p < .01$), $\Delta R^2 = .02$ for step 3 ($p < .01$)

* $p < .05$; ** $p < .01$; *** $p < .001$

Table 14.6 | Multiple regression to predict log (total number of sessions) given presence of diagnostic categories

Step	B	SE B	β
Step 1			
Constant	2.26	0.37	
Age	-0.02	0.01	-0.21***
PCL–M	0.01	0.01	0.14*
Step 2			
Constant	2.02	0.37	
Age	-0.01	0.01	-0.16**
PCL–M	0.00	0.01	0.05
PTSD	0.49	0.15	0.20**
Depression	0.27	0.14	0.11
Pain	0.40	0.19	0.12*
Step 3			
Constant	1.83	0.37	
Age	-0.14	0.01	
PCL–M	0.01	0.01	
PTSD	0.79	0.22	
Depression	0.72	0.23	
Pain	-0.08	0.40	
PTSD x Depression	-0.79	0.29	
PTSD x Pain	-0.71	0.54	
Depression x Pain	0.28	0.56	
PTSD x Depression x Pain	-0.26	0.74	

Note: $R^2 = .07$ for step 1, $\Delta R^2 = .06$ for step 2 ($p < .001$), $\Delta R^2 = .04$ for step 3 ($p < .05$)

* $p < .05$; ** $p < .01$; *** $p < .001$

Predicting Session Volume Including Diagnostic Complexity in the Model

In order to test the hypothesis that diagnostic complexity would be particularly important in predicting session volume, the natural log of session volume was regressed onto three blocks of variables. The first block forced the entry of age at intake and initial PCL score as determined by the first regression. The next block forced the entry of PTSD, depression, and pain as determined in the second regression. The third block represented co-morbidity and contained all interaction variables among the diagnoses of PTSD, depression, and pain. The results are in table 14.6. The first block of variables accounted for 7% of the variance of session volume. In step 2, the addition of the diagnoses variables (i.e., PTSD, depression, and pain) significantly improved the model, which then accounted for 13% of the variance of session volume. However, at this step, clients' self-reported PTSD symptom intensity was no longer a significant predictor. Adding information about co-morbidity further significantly improved the model, now accounting for 16%[23] of the total variance.

Discussion

Although the modal client received both formal assessment and then therapy after intake, there were subgroups of clients with other service use patterns. Case planning for the modal client would be relevant for just over half of clients seen at the OSI clinic. The remainder of clients used clinic services in different configurations, and it is important to understand what might make their needs different.

Clinical symptom severity did not differentiate the type of services in which clients engaged. That is, initial levels of depression, anxiety, or PTSD symptoms did not differentiate those clients who discharged following only intake services from those who received a formal assessment but no psychotherapy from those who received psychotherapy as part of their service. However, when examining the demographic variables, retired, veteran, older clients were overrepresented in the group that received a formal assessment but no therapy, whereas CF personnel were much more likely to engage in therapy than use assessment services only. It is tempting to assume that this difference is explained by cohort-related differences in the acceptability of psychotherapy; however, other research has shown that both active members and veterans demonstrate similar reluctance to use mental health services and report similar barriers to care.[24] Likewise no difference was found in treatment drop-out rates between older and younger veterans.[25] Barriers to care often are conceptualized in three categories: stigma, organizational barriers, and negative attitudes toward treatment.[26] It is possible that the CF clients encountered fewer organizational barriers to care (e.g., might more easily take time away from work than veterans; can access treatment by telehealth from their workplace).

In predicting volume of service use, it appears important to attend to diagnostic complexity. Knowing clients' diagnoses and, in particular, co-morbidities provided significantly more information than just being aware of the intensity of their reported symptoms. In this research, the information available at the start of services regarding duty-related factors, demographics, and self-reported symptom severity provided little useful information to anticipate how much service an individual would use. Even using more liberal techniques to select variables for the regression equations, the resulting model contained only age and self-reported PTSD symptom severity and accounted for only 4% of the variance in volume of service used. Knowing whether or not an individual was diagnosed with PTSD, depression-related conditions, and/or pain-related conditions significantly improved the model, with the resulting model accounting for 13% of session volume. Knowing about co-morbidity (represented as interactions among diagnoses in the model) significantly improved the model further, with the final model accounting for 16% of the variance. This finding aligns with results from inpatient studies where clients with multiple diagnoses are typically committed to hospital more often and for greater lengths of time.[27]

Limiting the analysis to psychotherapy clients resulted in higher session volumes (median = 13 sessions) than including all possible clients (median = 5 sessions). This result is not surprising, given that psychotherapy tends to be a higher session volume activity than assessment, support, or psychiatric services. Although a minority of clients receive an extraordinary number of sessions (15% had 48 or more sessions), the majority of clients experienced a volume of service consistent with standardized treatment protocols (often around 8–12 sessions).[28] This volume of sessions also is similar to what was described by Watkins and colleagues in their report on mental health services for American veterans, which identified an average of twelve psychotherapy sessions across all mental health conditions.[29]

Session volume was not normally distributed as one would expect with data bounded on the left side (i.e., impossible to have < 1 session) but not the right side (i.e., theoretically unlimited number of sessions possible). We decided to retain outliers and used the natural log transformation of the number of sessions for the analyses, as this reflected the clinical reality that, although most clients receive typical amounts of service, a minority of clients receive vastly more. Research that arbitrarily excludes atypical clients fails to fully represent the actual context in which care is provided.

The great variability in session volume is not surprising, given the heterogeneity of this population, both in reasons for accessing services and in presenting needs. Although the majority of clients are referred for primary treatment of OSIs, a substantial number of clients access the OSI clinic to complement professional services they receive in the community (e.g., referred solely for a psychiatric consult or to determine eligibility for a different service or benefit). Likewise, some clients present with more complex situations, including unstable social support networks, which complicate recovery. Clients also likely improve at different rates and opt to leave therapy once they have achieved what they perceive to be a *good enough level*.[30] That is, those clients who get better more quickly may be more likely to leave early, whereas clients who improve more slowly (as would be expected with increasing co-morbidity) may be more likely to benefit from more sessions. Although our first-line treatments benefit most clients, they do not benefit all.[31] Clients with complex needs, who are failed by shorter-term treatments, do respond to more involved, comprehensive protocols such as dialectical behaviour therapy.[32]

Limitations

This research is limited by its focus on an existing clinical sample (all clients of one specific clinic) with its inherent lack of control. In particular, the assessing clinician was not independent from the treating clinician in most cases. Not all program options were available to all clients (e.g., over the 8-year period covered by this research, different therapy groups were offered at some times but not others). Some individuals attended services outside of the clinic, and that service use is not represented within these data. Although the structure of the program emphasizes providing evidence-based treatments, we do not know from these data exactly what treatments were used or how closely those protocols were followed.

Given that this research included only discharged clients, it provides a more complete representation of earlier clients and more recent clients who used services briefly, rather than those who accessed services within the year and are still receiving services. The nature of this research was exploratory, and the number of analyses used in the earlier sets of analyses to understand how client characteristics related to service use created a higher likelihood of Type I errors. Our measure of reasons for discharge was also entirely clinician-based; we do not know if the client's reasons for discharge varied across the service use groups.

This research also did not look at the outcomes of service delivery (either in client satisfaction or symptom improvement). Accordingly, no inferences can be made about the effectiveness of the services described. With lower-volume users, we cannot differentiate successful short-term service delivery (e.g., provided psychoeducation in a way that best matched an individual's current stage of change) from working with clients who terminated prematurely but could have benefitted from greater service involvement at that time. Likewise, with higher-volume users, we cannot differentiate clients with exceptionally complex needs who required correspondingly exceptional session volumes from those who were provided with more service than they really needed.

Future Research

The next steps for this project will be to expand the analysis to identify and understand how service use relates to symptom change over time, by expanding these analyses to look at reported levels of clinical symptoms at discharge. Ideally, we would like to be able to predict the best service constellations to offer which clients, taking care to neither underservice nor over-service clients in order to maximize resource use and most efficiently use the time clients invest in receiving services.

As complex and uncontrolled as these data can be, we believe it is important to use analytic techniques to better understand heterogeneous groups such as outpatient clients and heterogeneous settings such as outpatient clinics with a range of services and flexible service delivery models. This is the context within which many individuals receive treatment. Without normative data, clinicians may naturally focus on complex or more complicated cases, which can skew awareness of how services are being delivered. Accordingly it is important to balance clinical appreciation of key issues within the context of objective data. This information helps us understand actual service use better, assists in planning for future de-mands, and provides a foundation from which to consider program changes and improvements.

Notes

1 N. S. Bell, P. R. Hunt, T. C. Harford, and A. Kay, "Deployment to a Combat Zone and Other Risk Factors for Mental Health–Related Disability Discharge from the U.S. Army: 1994–2007," *Journal of Traumatic Stress* 24 (2011): 34–43; B. A. Chopko and R. C. Schwartz, "Correlates of Career Traumatization and Symptomatology among Active-Duty Police Officers," *Criminal Justice Studies* 25 (2012): 83–95.

2 J. Sareen, B. J. Cox, T. O. Afifi, M. B. Stein, S. Belik, G. Meadows, and G. J. G. Asmundson, "Combat and Peacekeeping Operations in Relation to Prevalence of Mental Disorders and Perceived Need for Mental Health Care: Findings from a Large Representative Sample of Military Personnel," *Archives of General Psychiatry* 64 (2007): 843–52.

3 J. Pare, *Post-Traumatic Stress Disorder and the Mental Health of Military Personnel and Veterans* (Ottawa: Library of Parliament, 2011).

4 G. J. G. Asmundson and J. A. Stapleton, "Associations between Dimensions of Anxiety Sensitivity and PTSD Symptom Clusters in Active-Duty Police Officers," *Cognitive Behaviour Therapy* 37 (2008): 66–75.

5 R. Bradley, J. Greene, E. Russ, L. Dutra, and W. Westen, "A Multidimensional Meta-Analysis of Psychotherapy for PTSD," *American Journal of Psychiatry* 162 (2005): 214–27; M. M. Steenkamp and B. T. Litz, "Psychotherapy for Military-Related Posttraumatic Stress Disorder: Review of the Evidence," *Clinical Psychology Review* 33 (2013): 45–53.

6 Steenkamp and Litz, "Psychotherapy for Military-Related Posttraumatic Stress Disorder"; M. A. Zamorski, "Towards a Broader Conceptualization of Need, Stigma and Barriers to Mental Health Care in Military Organizations: Recent Research Findings from the Canadian Forces," *RTO Human Factors and Medicine Panel (HFM) Symposium, Bergen, Norway, April 2011*, http://www.rto.nato.int/abstracts.aspx.

7 Operational Stress Injury Social Support, "What Are Operational Stress Injuries?," 2006, http://www.osiss.ca/engraph/what_e.asp?sidecat=1&txt=2; Veterans Affairs Canada, "What Is an Operational Stress Injury?," http://www.veterans.gc.ca/eng/mental-health/support/factssha.

8 National Centre for Operational Stress Injuries Network Development and Coordination Sector, *Guidelines for Operational Stress Injury Clinics* (Ste Anne, QC: National Centre for Operational Stress Injuries Network Development and Coordination Sector, 2011).

9 J. D. Richardson, J. D. Elhai, and J. Sareen, "Predictors of Treatment Response in Canadian Combat and Peacekeeping Veterans with Military-Related Posttraumatic Stress Disorder," *Journal of Nervous and Mental Disease* 199 (2011): 639–45.

10 Ibid.

11 K. I. Howard, S. M. Kopta, M. S. Krause, and D. E. Orlinsky, "The Dose–Effect Relationship in Psychotherapy," *American Psychologist* 41 (1986): 159–64; see S. A.

Baldwin, A. Berkeljon, D. C. Atkins, J. A. Olsen, and S. L. Nielsen, "Rates of Change in Naturalistic Psychotherapy: Contrasting Dose–Effect and Good-Enough Level Models of Change," *Journal of Consulting and Clinical Psychology* 77 (2009): 203–11; M. Barkham, J. Connell, W. B. Stiles, J. N. Miles, F. Margison, C. Evans, and J. Mellor-Clark, "Dose–Effect Relations and Responsive Regulation of Treatment Duration: The Good Enough Level," *Journal of Consulting and Clinical Psychology* 74 (2006): 160–7; W. B. Stiles, M. Barkham, J. Connell, and J. Mellor-Clark, "Responsive Regulation of Treatment Duration in Routine Practice in United Kingdom Primary Care Settings: Replication in a Larger Sample," *Journal of Consulting and Clinical Psychology* 76 (2008): 298–305.

12 P. D. Bliese, K. M. Wright, A. B. Adler, O. Cabrera, C. A. Castro, and C. Hoge, "Validating the Primary Care Posttraumatic Stress Disorder Screen and the Posttraumatic Stress Disorder Checklist with Soldiers Returning from Combat," *Journal of Consulting and Clinical Psychology* 76 (2008): 272–81; F. W. Weathers, J. A. Huska, and T. M. Keane *PCL–M for DSM–IV* (Boston, MA: National Center for PTSD-Behavioral Science Division, 1991).

13 S. M. Orsillo, "Measures for Acute Stress Disorder and Posttraumatic Stress Disorder," in *Practitioner's Guide to Empirically Based Measures of Anxiety*, ed. M. M. Antony, S. M. Orsillo, and L. Roemer, 255–308 (New York: Kluwer Academic / Plenum Publishers, 2001).

14 J. D. Elhai, M. J. Gray, T. B. Kashdaon, and C. L. Franklin, "Which Instruments Are Most Commonly Used to Assess Traumatic Event Exposure and Posttraumatic Effects?: A Survey of Traumatic Stress Professionals," *Journal of Traumatic Stress* 18 (2005): 541–5.

15 Orsillo, "Measures for Acute Stress Disorder and Posttraumatic Stress Disorder."

16 A. Beck, R. Steer, and G. Brown, *Manual for Beck Depression Inventory – II* (San Antonio, TX: Psychological Corporation, 1996).

17 Ibid.

18 A. Beck and R. Steer, *Manual for the Beck Anxiety Inventory* (San Antonio, TX: Psychological Corporation, 1993).

19 Ibid.

20 L. Roemer, "Measures of Anxiety and Related Constructs," in Antony, Orsillo, and Roemer, *Practitioner's Guide to Empirically Based Measures of Anxiety*, 49–83.

21 D. Blake, F. Weathers, L. N. Nagy, D. Kaloupek, G. Klauminzer, D. Charney, T. Keane, and T. C. Buckley. *Clinician-Administered PTSD Scale (CAPS): Instruction Manual* (West Haven, CT: National Center for Posttraumatic Stress Disorder, 2000).

22 The difference between the total $R^2 = .04$ and the values presented stepwise in table 14.4 (i.e., $R^2 = .03 + .02$) is due to rounding error.

23 The difference between the total $R^2 = .17$ and the values presented stepwise in table 14.6 (i.e., $R^2 = .07 + .06 + .04$) is due to rounding error.

24 D. Fikretoglu, A. Brunet, S. Guay, and D. Pedlar, "Mental Health Treatment Seeking by Military Members with Posttraumatic Stress Disorder: Findings on Rates, Characteristics and Predictors from a Nationally Representative Canadian Military Sample," *Canadian Journal of Psychiatry* 52 (2007): 103–9; C. W. Hoge, "Interventions for War-Related Posttraumatic Stress Disorder: Meeting Veterans Where They Are," *JAMA* 306 (2011): 549–51.

25 K. M. Chard, J. A. Schumm, G. P. Owens, and S. M. Cottingham, "A Comparison of OEF and OIF Veterans and Vietnam Veterans Receiving Cognitive Processing Therapy," *Journal of Traumatic Stress* 23 (2010): 25–32.

26 P. Y. Kim, T. W. Britt, R. P. Klocko, L. A. Riviere, and A. B. Adler, "Stigma, Negative Attitudes about Treatment and Utilization of Mental Health Care among Soldiers," *Military Psychology* 23 (2011): 65–81.

27 E. M. Magallón-Neri, G. Canalda, J. E. De la Fuente, M. Forns, R. García, E. González, and J. Castro-Fornieles, "The Influence of Personality Disorders on the Use of Mental Health Services in Adolescents with Psychiatric Disorders," *Comprehensive Psychiatry* 53 (2012): 509–15.

28 American Psychiatric Association, "Practice Guideline for the Treatment of Patients with Major Depressive Disorder (Revision)," *American Journal of Psychiatry* 151 (2000): 1–36.

29 Baldwin et al., "Rates of Change in Naturalistic Psychotherapy"; Barkham et al., "Dose–Effect Relations and Responsive Regulation of Treatment Duration"; Stiles et al., "Dose–Effect Relations and Responsive Regulation of Treatment Duration."

30 Ibid.

31 Bradley et al., "Multidimensional Meta-Analysis of Psychotherapy for PTSD."

32 C. J. Robins and A. L. Chapman, "Dialectical Behavior Therapy: Current Status, Recent Developments, and Future Directions," *Journal of Personality Disorders* 18 (2004): 73–89; C. R. Koons, C. J. Robins, J. L. Tweed, T. R. Lynch, A. M. Gonzalez, J. Q. Morse, G. K. Bishop, M. I. Butterfield, and L. A. Bastian, "Efficacy of Dialectical Behavior Therapy in Women Veterans with Borderline Personality Disorder," *Behavior Therapy* 32 (2001): 371–90.

15

Integration of Chiropractic Services into the United States Veterans Health Administration

STEVEN R. PASSMORE AND ANTHONY J. LISI

Abstract

This chapter is a narrative review of the integration of chiropractic care into the Veterans Health Administration in the United States. The provision of chiropractic services at existing and additional Veterans Health Administration sites continues to expand. This chapter illustrates the process through which chiropractic care was integrated into the Veterans Health Administration in the United States, how it has evolved, and describes its clinical context for the benefit of veterans.

The Initial Onsite Veterans Health Administration Chiropractic Integration

Every honourably discharged veteran of military service in the United States is entitled to chiropractic care through the Veterans Health Administration (VHA). The Veterans Health Administration is the largest network of health-care facilities in the United States, employs more than 15,000 physicians, and has an operational size similar to the province of Ontario.[1] Services at Veterans Health Administration facilities include the spectrum of specialties from medicine, surgery, pharmacy, physical therapy, dentistry, optometry, podiatry, and most recently chiropractic care. The integration of the chiropractic profession occurred in response to patient demand and government legislation.

In the United States, the federal Public Law 107-135 was passed in 2001, with section 204 pertaining to the program for the "provision of chiropractic care and services to veterans."[2] To proceed with the integration, a committee of external experts was formed as defined in part g of section 204.[3] The Chiropractic Advisory Committee consisted of eleven members (2 female), who were appointed by the secretary of veterans affairs.[4] Characteristics of the clinical, academic, and military backgrounds of the appointed committee members were diverse. There were five chiropractors, two medical doctors, one osteopath, one physician's assistant, and one clinical manager of rehabilitation at a VHA site.[5] Two of the clinicians also held PHDs.[6] Several committee members were military veterans; branches represented were the Navy (5), Navy Reserve (1), Marine Corps (1), and the National Guard (1).[7] Academic affiliations by committee members were held at chiropractic (3) and other academic institutions (4).[8] Multiple committee members also held positions at national or international chiropractic (4) or medical (2) professional service organizations.[9]

The role of the Chiropractic Advisory Committee was to assist and advise the secretary of veterans affairs on the development and implementation of the chiropractic health program in the Department of Veterans Affairs. Specifically, the committee provided advice on the protocols governing "referral to chiropractors," "direct access to chiropractic care," the "scope of practice of chiropractic practitioners." Additional missions of the committee were to create a "definition of services to be provided" and attend to "other matters" deemed "appropriate" by the secretary. The committee was instructed to meet up to three times annually and was scheduled to dissolve on 31 December 2004.[10]

Prior to dissolving in 2004, the Chiropractic Advisory Committee submitted thirty-eight recommendations for the development and implementation of the chiropractic health program.[11] The recommendations were categorized under six headings: Qualifications for Employment; Scope of Practice; Services to Be Provided (Privileges); Access to Chiropractic Care; Referrals to and from Doctors of Chiropractic; and Integration of Chiropractic Care into the VHA.[12] The complete list of recommendation topics as stratified by headings can be found in table 15.1.

The CHA is divided into twenty-one geographically distinct regions defined as Veterans Integrated Service Networks (VISNs).[13] Section 204 part c states that the "Secretary will designate at least one site for such program in each geographic service area" of the VHA.[14] Each VISN consists of medical centres (hospitals), and community-based outpatient clinics (CBOCs). In line with the federal mandate, in 2004–05 an initial group of twenty-six sites were identified, and the first onsite chiropractors were appointed as either employees or contractors. Responsibility for hiring or contracting was turned over to each of the facilities. All clinicians underwent local credentialing and privileging, while employees also underwent a professional standard board determination of rank.

By aligning with existing departments, administrative costs could be kept minimal, and waiting areas could be shared. Clinic implementation required simply hiring or contracting a provider, designating a treatment room, establishing parameters in the electronic medical record and scheduling system, providing an appropriate chiropractic table, sanitary items, and other modalities as appropriate. The salary ranges for clinicians ranged from $60,000 to $120,000[15] and was

Table 15.1 | Chiropractic Advisory Committee recommendations for the development and implementation of the chiropractic health program

General category	Recommendation	Truncated description
Qualifications for employment	Education requirement	Accredited chiropractic school/state licence approved school graduate
	Licensure requirement	Full unrestricted chiropractic licence from a state, territory, or U.S. commonwealth
	Other requirements	Meet physical, language, citizenship, and employment requirements of VA
Scope of practice	Scope of practice	Patient evaluation and care for neuro-musculoskeletal conditions within boundaries of state licensure, VHA privileges, and educational competency
Services to be provided (privileges)	Minimum initial privileges	(1) history, (2) neuro-musculoskeletal/physical examination, (3) order radiographs, (4) Determine appropriateness for chiropractic care, (5) provide chiropractic care (adjustment, mobilization/manipulation, manual therapy), (6) neuro-musculoskeletal care management, (7) referral when chiropractic care is not appropriate
	Other initial privileges	(1) order additional testing (imaging, laboratory, electro-physiological), (2) order/provide other treatment within scope of practice
	Additional privileges	After annual evaluation consistent with facility, training, and licensure
	Publication of information letter	VHA published information letter guiding facilities on recommended privileges approved by the secretary
Access to chiropractic care	Access to chiropractic care	In consultation with primary care or another VA provider

General category	Recommendation	Truncated description
Access to chiropractic care / cont'd	Continuity of care for newly discharged veterans	Should receive continuing chiropractic care following discharge from active duty
	Inpatient care recommendation	No admitting privileges, but may see inpatients upon VHA provider referral
	Chiropractic care in community-based outpatient clinics	Parent facility (medical centre) determines need and resource availability to provide such services
	Fee basis care	Authorized when patients are geographically remote from facility consistent with other VHA fee-basis care
	Occupational health programs	Chiropractors can be utilized in the occupational health program of VHA facilities
Referrals to and from doctors of chiropractic	Screening of patients	Identify "red flags" or contraindications to manual therapy (fracture, tumour, infection, progressive neurological deficit)
	Referral service agreements	Determine types of conditions appropriate for chiropractic care referral and pre-referral testing to share with specialty and primary care providers
	Referrals from doctors of chiropractic	Make referrals to other VHA services and providers as appropriate
Integration of chiropractic care into VHA	Coordination of care	Develop collaborative treatment regime with primary care and other VHA providers
	Co-management of care	Co-manage neuro-musculoskeletal patient care with primary care and other VHA providers

Placement of doctors of chiropractic within a health care team	Integrated to VHA system as health-care team partner
Site selection	Goal of chiropractic care in each VISN
Doctor of chiropractic staffing	Goal of enough chiropractors on staff at each facility to provide care without delay
Support staff	Clinical assistants and clerical staff will be needed
Space	Examination room large enough for a chiropractic table (2' × 7.5'), with space to move around the table, and a sink
Co-location with collaborating providers and services	Should be placed near collaborating services/providers
Equipment	Adjusting tables and examination equipment
Orientation	Standardized orientation programs for existing clinical and administrative staff and incoming chiropractors should be developed
Ongoing education of providers	Chiropractors should participate in facility interdisciplinary activities
Education of patients	VHA will provide standardized information on chiropractic care availability
Quality assurance	Chiropractic should be added to facility's quality assurance policy
Performance measures	Outcome/performance measures for chiropractic care should be developed by VHA

General category	Recommendations	Truncated desception
Integration of chiropractic care into VHA /cont'd	Evaluation of chiropractic care program	Formal evaluation of challenges/benefits of chiropractic care VHA should be completed within three years; annual progress reports should be directed to the secretary
	Medical staff voting privileges	Once credentialled and privileged, chiropractors should have full voting privileges
	Continuing education	Should be maintained as per licensure; VA should fund as per existing policy
	Oversight and consultation for the chiropractic program	A field advisory committee, and chiropractic advisor or director should be appointed
	Committee membership	Should be on appropriate facility, VISN, and national clinical/administrative committees, work group, and task forces
	Academic affiliations	VHA should provide educational/training experiences for senior chiropractic students and recent graduates
	Research	VHA with chiropractors, and education programs should conduct relevant clinical research on service-connected conditions/team integration of multidisciplinary providers

Source: Chiropractic Advisory Committee, "Recommendations of the Chiropractic Advisory Committee" (Washington, DC: U.S. Department of Veterans Affairs, 2003), 26.

determined through a standardized professional boarding process using an annual rate system consisting of five grades, each with ten steps.

All documentation within the VHA is managed using an award-winning (Innovations in American Government Award, Harvard University 2006) paperless electronic medical record (EMR) called the Computerized Patient Record System (CPRS), which is operated within the Veterans Health Information Systems and Technology Architecture (VistA). The VistA system, the CPRS graphical interface, and unlimited ongoing updates (nightly) are considered public domain software based on the Freedom of Information Act, and demonstration versions are available online for free download.[16] Regardless of geographic site, all patient documentation, from all the health-care providers within the VHA that interact with a given patient, are visible. Each patient's cover sheet automatically summarizes active problems/diagnoses, allergies/adverse reactions, postings, active medications, clinical reminders with dates due, recent lab results, vitals, and appointments/visits/admissions. Tabs clinicians can update containing highly detailed information within each patient's file include cover sheet, problems, medications, orders, notes, consults, surgery, discharge summaries, labs, and reports. Any provider may view or update the patient's common file within the system as needed. All changes, once signed by the inputting clinician, are immediately viewable by all other providers, and the system allows electronically secure communication between providers and facilities. Chiropractors brought on were integrated into the system and able to order devices, lab tests, and imaging on the basis of their clinical privileging. Chiropractors received all consult requests and were able to complete all patient notes immediately. The notes allowed for co-signature, facilitating the clinical involvement of trainees (student interns), or patient co-management. Customizable and modifiable templates can be created and utilized for increased efficiency of frequently documented items for new patient and follow-up notes. All previous diagnostic reports (imaging/lab tests) of patient consult requests can be screened prior to scheduling a patient consult to ensure the prospective patient is an appropriate candidate for chiropractic intervention.

Current and Ongoing Chiropractic Practice within the Veterans Health Administration

The chiropractic program is overseen nationally by the chief consultant of Rehabilitation Services, within the Office of Patient Care Services.[17] In 2007 a Veteran Affairs (VA) doctor of chiropractic (DC) was appointed the national director of chiropractic services to oversee policy and programmatic development. The director is responsible for providing clinical, administrative, and educational guidance to ensure that high-quality health care is accessible and efficiently provided to all eligible veterans. Congruent with recommendation 35 from the Chiropractic Advisory Committee,[18] a Field Advisory Committee (FAC) for chiropractic was created. The FAC is composed of field-based VHA DCs and medical doctors and serves as an advisory group for clinical and administrative issues relating to chiropractic care within VHA. The FAC reports to the national program director and serves as a communication channel to field-based practitioners and provides feedback to VA Central Office on matters of importance to doctors of chiropractic working within VHA.

On the basis of increased use by referring physicians and patient demand, the number of locations providing chiropractic care, and the number of onsite chiropractors has increased. As of October 2012, forty-four VA facilities have onsite chiropractic clinics, of which thirty-seven are located in medical centres and seven in CBOCs. These clinics are staffed by fifty-one chiropractors, of which thirty-five are full-time employees, nine are part-time employees, and seven are on shared appointments with affiliated academic institutions. Employees of the U.S. federal government are entitled to paid vacation, a benefits package, and pension plan.

While the VHA provides care for all honourably discharged veterans, the typical VHA chiropractic patient is a male (93%), over the age of fifty-five years (range 19–91) who is overweight.[19] The typical patient is a complex case (has multiple co-morbidities), most often with chronic progressive conditions. Veterans are a unique clinical population, as they present with no congenital anomalies that would have prevented them from joining the military. However, with injury and aging, there are many complicated special populations, including but not limited to cancer, traumatic brain injury, abdominal aortic aneurysm, post-spine surgery, post-amputation, poly-trauma, post traumatic stress disorder, and military sexual trauma. The most common conditions treated by chiropractors in a VHA clinic include low back pain (47.7%), and cervical spine pain (21.4%).[20] Less common complaints also addressed by chiropractors in VHA clinics include thoracic spine pain (9.8%), lower extremity pain (7.4%), headache (6.4%), and upper extremity pain (6.2%).[21]

Spinal manipulation (SM) is the most common chiropractic intervention delivered to veterans in a VHA clinic.[22] Spinal manipulation is typically a manually delivered high-velocity, low-amplitude thrust with the intent of moving targeted joints beyond their physiologic range of motion.[23] Performance-based objective outcome measures following SM include biomechanical changes (e.g., increased range of motion), neurological facilitation (e.g., increased grip strength), and enhanced perception performance (e.g., decreased reaction time).[24] Other common treatments delivered by VHA chiropractors are patient education (88% of chiropractors), exercise (76% of chiropractors), physical modalities (36% of chiropractors), acupressure (30% of chiropractors), and massage (27% of chiropractors).[25] Chiropractic care is considered a safe, effective, and cost-effective non-pharmacological/non-surgical intervention for myriad acute and chronic musculoskeletal complaints, particularly low back pain, with good levels of patient satisfaction.[26]

As a referral-based specialty, there is a wait time between a chiropractic referral request and first patient visit. There was a reported average wait time of twenty-

Table 15.2 | Incoming and outgoing consultation requests, 2008

Incoming consultation requests		Outgoing consultation requests	
Service	%	Service	%
Primary care	67.6	Primary care	34.8
Pain	9.4	Other	17.0
Physiatry	6.2	Pain	9.5
Orthopedic surgery	3.7	Physiatry	9.5
Neurology	3.6	Orthopedic surgery	7.9
Other	3.2	Neurology	5.3
Neurosurgery	2.0	Neurosurgery	4.3
Emergency	1.8	Podiatry	2.2
Rheumatology	1.4	Rheumatology	2.1
Podiatry	0.7	Emergency	1.1
Spinal cord injury rehabilitation	0.5	Spinal cord injury rehabilitation	0.2
Dentistry	0.1	Dentistry	0.0

Source: Cross-sectional survey study of 33 VA chiropractic providers nationwide

six days from the date of chiropractic consult request during fiscal year 2006.[27] Dunn and Passmore (2007) recognized that wait times occurred since demand for chiropractic care was greater than the availability of clinic resources, and devised six strategies to optimize VHA chiropractic clinic efficiency, maximize the ease of clinic access, and ethically allocate care in order to decrease wait times without compromising quality of care.[28] Referrals of patients to chiropractors for consultation come from the spectrum of health-care providers within the VHA system (see table 15.2). Upon the consultation request, accepted patients report for a consultation, which includes a detailed history, a physical examination, the communication of a diagnosis consistent with the International Classification of Diseases, and the report of findings, with potential treatment options and a prescribed course of care. Prior to the initiation of care, additional imaging or laboratory work may be required, and if the patient is an appropriate candidate for chiropractic intervention, informed consent procedures are adhered to. Chiropractic referrals that did not result in care initiation occurred in 17.51% of consult requests.[29] The informed consent process explains the known risks and benefits of chiropractic management. A new patient consultation may take from thirty to sixty minutes, depending on the complexity of the case. After initial treatment intervention, a series of follow-up visit are carried out, that typically take between fifteen and thirty minutes.

On average, the number of patient treatment visits is 6.44.[30] Re-evaluation appointments are scheduled at the discretion of the clinician, and the best available outcome measures are utilized to determine whether a patient's condition (1) has resolved and the patient can be discharged, (2) is responding to care, but has not yet resolved, (3) has not resolved, but has reached a plateau with intervention, or (4) is not responding to care and requires either an alternate treatment plan or referral to another health-care provider for a consult (refer to table 15.2).

The VHA utilizes an assortment of approaches to inform their patient population of the availability of chiropractic services. Some promotional methods are traditional, while others are progressive and involve the use of social media. The clinic is promoted onsite by the availability of VHA brochures describing what chiropractic is and the services provided. The Department of Veterans Affairs maintains a website, and since 2008 has maintained a Facebook page.[31] In fact all VA medical centres have Facebook pages, and many maintain blogs and Twitter and Flickr accounts in order to engage their clinic population and make them aware of activities and programs.[32] The Department of Veterans Affairs and the Veterans Health Administration also maintain YouTube accounts on which they make available videos describing and promoting their services. The VHA (using account VeteransHealthAdmin) has past episodes of their television program *The American Veteran* on YouTube. An episode promoting chiropractic services is available.[33]

The VHA strongly supports academic affiliation and training opportunities for clinician development.[34] From their inception, VHA chiropractic clinics have had academic affiliations. At present twenty VA facilities have affiliations with eleven chiropractic colleges across the country. As a result, since 2005 more than 750 chiropractic students have trained in VHA facilities during their student clerkship. Additionally, having an onsite chiropractor provides medical students, residents, and other trainees the opportunity to observe and do rotations within the clinic.

Research productivity and evidence-informed practices are a priority within the VHA.[35] Chiropractors within the VHA have made a concerted effort to demonstrate research productivity. Types of publication include but are not limited to commentaries, descriptive studies, case reports, narrative reviews, systematic reviews, and cross-sectional studies. Two federally funded randomized controlled trials have been completed and are in process of publication. A mixed methods health services study of program implementation also is underway. Journals in which VHA chiropractors have published VA research include *Military Medicine, Journal of Rehabilitation Research & Development* (JRRD), *Journal of Manipulative & Physiological Therapeutics* (JMPT), *Journal of the Canadian Chiropractic Association* (JCCA), *Journal of Chiropractic Education* (JCE), *Journal of Chiropractic Humanities* (JCH), *Journal of Chiropractic Medicine* (JCM), and *Manual Therapy* (table 15.3).[36] Prior to submission for publication, dissemination at peer-reviewed conferences is common, with the VHA supporting travel and registration costs in some instances.

Table 15.3 | VHA chiropractic research

Year	Journal	Design	Title	Authors
2005	JCE	Descriptive study	A Chiropractic Internship Program in the Department of Veterans Affairs Health Care System	A. S. Dunn*
2006	JMPT	Cross-sectional study	Chiropractic Consultation Requests in the Veterans Affairs Health Care System: Demographic Characteristics of the Initial 100 Patients at the Western New York Medical Center	A. S. Dunn,* J. J. Towle, P. McBrearty, S. M. Fleeson
2007	JCE	Survey	A Survey of Chiropractic Academic Affiliations within the Department of Veterans Affairs Health Care System	A. S. Dunn*
2007	JCH	Commentary	When Demand Exceeds Supply: Allocating Chiropractic Services at VA Medical Facilities	A. S. Dunn,* S. R. Passmore*
2008	Military Medicine	Cross-sectional study	Consultation Request Patterns, Patient Characteristics, and Utilization of Services within a Veterans Affairs Medical Center Chiropractic Clinic	A. S. Dunn,* S. R. Passmore*
2008	JMPT	Commentary	Chiropractic and Public Health: Current State and Future Vision.	C. Johnson, R. Baird, P. E. Dougherty,* G. Globe, B. N. Green, M. Haneline, C. Hawk, H. S. Injeyan, L. Killinger, D. Kopansky-Giles, A. J. Lisi,* S. Mior, M. Smith

Year	Journal	Design	Title	Authors
2009	Military Medicine	Cross-sectional study	A Cross-Sectional Analysis of Clinical Outcomes following Chiropractic Care in Veterans with and without Post-Traumatic Stress Disorder	A. S. Dunn,* S. R. Passmore,* J. Burke, D. Chicoine
2009	Manual Therapy	Case report	Positive Patient Outcome after Spinal Manipulation in a Case of Cervical Angina	S. R. Passmore,* A. S. Dunn*
2009	Military Medicine	Commentary	Chiropractic in U.S. Military and Veterans' Health Care	B. N. Green, C. D. Johnson, A. J. Lisi*
2009	JCE	Qualitative review	Managing Conflicts of Interest in Continuing Medical Education: A Comparison of Policies	A. J. Lisi*
2009	JCM	Case report	Chiropractic Management of Mechanical Low Back Pain Secondary to Multiple-Level Lumbar Spondylolysis with Spondylolisthesis in a United States Marine Corps Veteran: A Case Report	A. S. Dunn,* S. Baylis, D. Ryan
2009	JMPT	Descriptive study	An Analysis of the Integration of Chiropractic Services within the United States Military and Veterans' Health Care Systems	A. S. Dunn,* B. N. Green, S. Gilford
2009	JCCA	Review article	Chiropractic Practice in Military and Veterans Health Care: The State of the Literature	B. N. Green, C. D. Johnson, A. J. Lisi,* J. Tucker
2009	JRRD	Survey	Characteristics of Veterans Health Administration Chiropractors and Chiropractic Clinics	A. J. Lisi,* C. Goertz, D. J. Lawrence, P. Satyanarayana

Year	Journal	Type	Title	Authors
2010	JRRD	Case series	Management of Operation Iraqi Freedom and Operation Enduring Freedom Veterans in a Veterans Health Administration Chiropractic Clinic: A Case Series	A. J. Lisi*
2011	JRRD	Retrospective case series	Preliminary Analysis of Posttraumatic Stress Disorder Screening within Specialty Clinic Setting for OIF/OEF Veterans Seeking Care for Neck or Back Pain	A. S. Dunn,* R. Julian, L. R. Formolo,* B. N. Green, D. R. Chicoine
2011	JMPT	Retrospective case series	Chiropractic Management for Veterans with Neck Pain: A Retrospective Study of Clinical Outcomes	A. S. Dunn,* B. N. Green, L. R. Formolo,* D. R. Chicoine
2011	JRRD	Retrospective case series	Retrospective Case Series of Clinical Outcomes Associated with Chiropractic Management for Veterans with Low Back Pain	A. S. Dunn,* B. N. Green, L. R. Formolo,* D. R. Chicoine
2012	JMPT	Commentary	Chiropractic Care and Public Health: Answering Difficult Questions about Safety, Care through the Lifespan, and Community Action	C. D. Johnson, S. M. Rubinstein, P. Cote, L. Hestbaek, H. S. Injeyan, A. Puhl, B. Green, J. G. Napuli,* A. S. Dunn,* P. Dougherty,* L. Z. Killinger, S. A. Page, J. S. Stites, M. Ramcharan, R. A. Leach, L. D. Byrd, D. Redwood, D. Kopansky-Giles

Source: Adapted/updated from B. N. Green, C. D. Johnson, A. J. Lisi, and J. Tucker, "Chiropractic Practice in Military and Veterans Health Care: The State of the Literature," Journal of the Canadian Chiropractic Association 53, no. 3 (2009): 194–204.

* VHA chiropractor at the time of publication

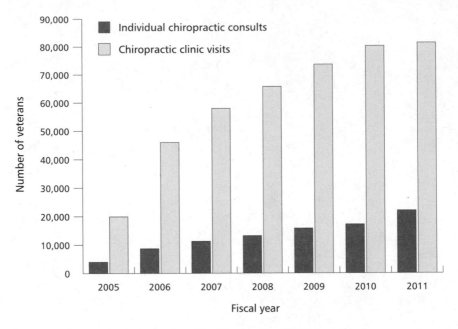

Figure 15.1 | VHA on-station nationwide chiropractic utilization

Research funding has been attained by VHA chiropractors from private philanthropic institutions (Samueli Institute), and publically supported granting agencies both internal (Veterans Affairs, Merit Grant program) and external to the VHA (Department of Health and Human Services, Human Resources and Service Administration Grant program).[37]

Integration of Chiropractic into the Veterans Health Administration System

The integration of chiropractic services into the VHA system can be assessed in expansion, utilization, and safety. Without further legislation, the practice of chiropractic within the VHA has grown from twenty-six to forty-four sites. If patients or facilities were unsatisfied with the integration of chiropractic services, there would be no precedent for such expansion. Chiropractic is a referral-based specialty within the VHA system. In fiscal year 2011, 22,007 patients were referred for chiropractic care, and since 2005 over 92,000 patients have completed consultations at the forty-four VHA chiropractic clinics (figure 15.1). If the referring clinicians saw no value to chiropractic care, they would not refer patients, and the chiropractic program as it exists would fail. The VHA maintains a highly integrated electronic medical record, and since 2005 there have been more than 425,000 treatment visits by chiropractors and no reports of major injuries or fatalities as a result of chiropractic intervention. The practice of chiropractic has demonstrated high levels of patient safety within the VHA.

Rationale for the Provision of Onsite Chiropractic Services

The delivery of chiropractic services onsite is valued by veterans[38] and VA primary care physicians.[39] Chiropractic services are part of the standard medical benefits package available to all enrolled veterans.[40] VHA first established on-station chiropractic clinics at select facilities in 2004 in response to veteran demand and congressional mandate. From fiscal year 2005 through 2011 VA has seen a 69% increase in the number of on-station chiropractic clinics, and the number of veterans seen by these clinics has increased five-fold. The use of chiropractic services within VHA is congruent with trends in other U.S. systems such as Medicare, all private insurance, and a growing number of Department of Defense facilities. Approximately 9% of the U.S. population uses chiropractic services.[41]

There is significant value associated with the integration of chiropractors onsite, within the health-care system. Chiropractors can deliver evidence-based, non-pharmacologic treatment options for management of musculoskeletal pain, which is highly prevalent in veteran populations. Use of chiropractic services has been associated with decreased opioid analgesic use[42] and decreased overall cost of care for non-surgical spinal conditions.[43] One full-time doctor of chiropractic (DC) can be expected to provide roughly 450 unique veteran consultations and roughly 2,000 follow-up visits per year. Management by DCs can decrease the number of return visits to primary care physicians (PCP) for spinal pain. VA PCPs express high satisfaction with chiropractic clinics and providers. Addition of a DC can improve overall access of other related disciplines facing a high musculoskeletal caseload.

Having the chiropractic provider onsite ensures that services provided are veteran-centred. Hiring chiropractors into onsite positions is a successful method to introduce chiropractic to a primary health team for reducing barriers to integration and collaboration.[44] Veterans at facilities that have included chiropractic services report high satisfaction with their facility's decision. When receiving on-station chiropractic care, veterans also express high satisfaction with care. Veterans at facilities that do not provide on-station chiropractic services express strong interest in receiving those services in the VA health system.

Summary

The integration of chiropractic services into the VHA occurred systematically. Legislation was proposed and passed. A committee of experts was formed to make recommendations on integration. Facilities began hiring clinicians as federal employees and created onsite chiropractic clinics. An internal field advisory committee formed to continue to shape best practices and integration. An electronic database and EMR tracked the activity and productivity of all clinics since their inception. Other professions within the VHA support the integration of chiropractic services, as evidenced by their patient referrals for onsite chiropractic care. Chiropractors have sustained productive clinics and been encouraged to maintain academic affiliations for chiropractic student training opportunities. Research is considered a priority with the VHA, and chiropractors within the system have made good use of resources to demonstrate research productivity. The expansion, utilization, and safety of chiropractic services within the VHA are a testament to successful integration. Integration to best serve a veteran population occurs through the provision of onsite chiropractic care within the publicly funded health-care system.

Conclusion

The successful integration of chiropractic services into the VHA did not occur by accident, but rather by design. Other countries or health-care systems interested in the integration of chiropractic services to better serve their clinical population should consider the process formulated by the United States Veterans Health Administration. The VHA integration of chiropractic may serve as a template for the components required for a successful integration, and a road map to monitor, document, and maintain productive service. The careful, calculated, and well planned integration of chiropractic care into a health-care system requires not only a short-term vision but also dedication in order to contribute in the long term to the health and well-being of those who matter most, the patients.

Notes

1 M. Anderson, "Lessons Learned from the Veterans Health Administration," *Healthcare Papers* 5, no. 4 (2005): 30–7.
2 Department of Veterans Affairs Health Care Programs Enhancement Act of 2001, Public Law 107-135, Program for Provision of Chiropractic Care and Services to Veterans (2000), 204.
3 The Department of Veterans Affairs Health Care Programs Enhancement Act of 2001, 204.
4 U.S. Department of Veterans Affairs, "VA Appoints Chiropractic Advisory Committee," news release, 12 August 2002, http://www.va.gov/opa/pressrel/pressrelease.cfm?id=488.
5 Ibid.
6 Ibid.
7 Ibid.
8 Ibid.

9 Ibid.

10 Department of Veterans Affairs Health Care Programs Enhancement Act of 2001, Public Law 107-135; U.S. Department of Veterans Affairs, "VA Appoints Chiropractic Advisory Committee."

11 Chiropractic Advisory Committee, "Recommendations of the Chiropractic Advisory Committee" (Washington, DC: U.S. Department of Veterans Affairs, 2003), 26.

12 Ibid.

13 U.S. Department of Veterans Affairs, "Veterans Health Administration: Locations," http://www2.va.gov/directory/guide/division_flsh.asp?dnum=1.

14 Department of Veterans Affairs Health Care Programs Enhancement Act of 2001. Public Law 107-135.

15 A. J. Lisi, C. Goertz, D. J. Lawrence, and D. J. Satyanarayana, "Characteristics of Veterans Health Administration Chiropractors and Chiropractic Clinics," *Journal of Rehabilitation Research and Development* 46, no. 8 (2009): 997–1002.

16 U.S. Department of Veterans Affairs, "CPRS Demo," 2012, http://www.ehealth.va.gov/EHEALTH/CPRS_Demo.asp.

17 U.S. Department of Veterans Affairs, "Rehabilitation Services," 2011, http://www.patientcare.va.gov/RehabilitationServices.asp.

18 Chiropractic Advisory Committee, "Recommendations of the Chiropractic Advisory Committee," 26.

19 A. S. Dunn and S. R. Passmore, "Consultation Request Patterns, Patient Characteristics, and Utilization of Services within a Veterans Affairs Medical Center Chiropractic Clinic," *Military Medicine Journal* 173, no. 6 (2008): 599–603.

20 Lisi et al., "Characteristics of Veterans Health Administration Chiropractors and Chiropractic Clinics."

21 Ibid.

22 Dunn and Passmore, "Consultation Request Patterns."

23 S. Dagenais and S. Haldeman, "Chiropractic," *Primary Health Care* 29, no. 2 (2002): 419–37.

24 S. R. Passmore and M. Descarreaux, "Performance Based Objective Outcome Measures and Spinal Manipulation," *Journal of Electromyography and Kinesiology* 22, no. 5 (2012): 697–707.

25 Lisi et al., "Characteristics of Veterans Health Administration Chiropractors and Chiropractic Clinics."

26 Dagenais and Haldeman, "Chiropractic."

27 Dunn and Passmore, "Consultation Request Patterns."

28 A. S. Dunn and S. R. Passmore, "When Demand Exceeds Supply: The Allocation of Chiropractic Services at VA Medical Facilities," *Journal of Chiropractic Humanities* 14, no. 1 (2007): 22–7.

29 Dunn and Passmore, "Consultation Request Patterns."

30 Ibid.

31 U.S. Department of Veterans Affairs, "Social Media Directory," http://www.va.gov/opa/socialmedia.asp

32 Ibid.

33 Veterans Health Administration, "Chiropractic Services," YouTube, 2009, http://www.youtube.com/watch?v=5OyTM4gAziU.

34 U.S. Department of Veterans Affairs, "Rehabilitation Services."

35 Ibid.

36 B. N. Green, C. D. Johnson, A. J. Lisi, and J. Tucker, "Chiropractic Practice in Military and Veterans Health Care: The State of the Literature," *Journal of the Canadian Chiropractic Association* 53, no. 3 (2009): 194–204.

37 Ibid.

38 L. M. Denneson, K. Corson, and S. K. Dobscha, "Complementary and Alternative Medicine Use among Veterans with Chronic Noncancer Pain," *Journal of Rehabilitation Research and Development* 48, no. 9 (2011): 1119–28.

39 J. F. Spelman, S. C. Hunt, K. H. Seal, and A. L. Burgo-Black, "Post Deployment Care for Returning Combat Veterans." *Journal of General Internal Medicine* 27, no. 9 (2012): 1200–09.

40 U.S. Department of Veterans Affairs, *Veterans Health Benefit Guide*, 2012, http://www.va.gov/healthbenefits/resources/publications/IB10-465_Veterans_Health_Guide2012_508.pdf.

41 P. M. Barnes, B. Bloom, and R. L. Nahin, "Complementary and Alternative Medicine Use among Adults and Children: United States, 2007," *National Health Statistics Reports* 10 (2008): 1–23.

42 Y. Rhee, M. S. Taitel, D. R. Walker, and D. T. Lau, "Narcotic Drug Use among Patients with Lower Back Pain in Employer Health Plans: A Retrospective Analysis of Risk Factors and Health Care Services," *Clinical Therapeutics* 29 (2007): S2603–12.

43 M. T. Vogt, C. K. Kwoh, D. K. Cope, T. A. Osial, M. Culyba, and T. W. Starz, "Analgesic Usage for Low Back Pain: Impact on Health Care Costs and Service Use," *Spine* 30, no. 9 (2005): 1075–81.

44 M. J. Garner, M. Birmingham, P. Aker, D. Moher, J. Balon, D. Keenan, and P. Manga, "Developing Integrative Primary Healthcare Delivery: Adding a Chiropractor to the Team," *Explore (NY)* 4, no. 1 (2008): 18–24.

16

Overcoming Systemic Obstacles to Veteran Transition to Civilian Life

ALLAN ENGLISH AND SYDNEY DALE-MCGRATH

Abstract

There are many obstacles to successfully reintegrating veterans into Canadian society. This study examines some systemic impediments to veteran transition to civilian life, an area that has not received much attention in the literature. The focus here is on one particularly important obstacle – divergent expectations about the goals of veteran care and transition policies among stakeholders in the transition process, especially between veterans and their families on the one hand and the public and governments on the other. It suggests strategies, based on harmonizing perceptions among stakeholders, which, if implemented, could increase the chances of creating more compassionate, effective, widely accepted, and fiscally responsible veteran reintegration programs.

Introduction

The transition from military to civilian life, especially for those who are injured, can be difficult. Lately, because of our almost ten-year involvement in combat operations in Afghanistan, this issue has become more pressing as "more than 8,000 Canadian Forces (CF) members were released for medical reasons" between 2006 and 2011. The financial cost for supporting them totalled about $500 million in the 2010–11 fiscal year alone.[1] The high cost of this support is, in part, caused by systemic obstacles to veteran transition to civilian life.[2]

A number of disciplines study concrete obstacles to successful transition; however, relatively little has been published about intangible systemic obstacles to veteran transition to civilian life. Nevertheless, a government study found that 25% of those released from the CF between 1998 and 2007 "reported a difficult transition to civilian life."[3] Some obstacles to Canadian veteran reintegration are unique to particular times and others are common to all times. There is evidence to suggest, however, that there are consistent and predictable systemic impediments to successfully reintegrating veterans into society.[4] This study, therefore, focuses on them and on identifying lessons from selected previous attempts to deal with these obstacles to help overcome them in the future. We will examine one particularly important systemic obstacle to transition – divergent expectations about the goals of veteran care and transition policies among stakeholders in the transition process, especially between veterans and their families on one hand and the public and governments on the other.

Since the First World War, the resources that Canada has been prepared to allocate to military and veteran health care have been strongly influenced by a dynamic social contract. The changing nature of this contract is influenced not only by the political climate and economic conditions, but also by perceptions of the military and the conflict in which the veterans participated.[5] This chapter argues that implementing strategies to create a more productive dialogue among stakeholders and the public can help to build the consensus required to produce compassionate, effective, widely accepted, and fiscally responsible programs for veteran transition to civilian life. We focus on the challenges in this area encountered during the First World War and its aftermath, because they provide the basic pattern for most subsequent challenges, and they parallel those identified in the current debates surrounding the New Veterans Charter (NVC) and the development of government policy for veteran reintegration in the twenty-first century.

First World War Challenges to Veteran Reintegration

The Great Challenge

Since the beginning of the twentieth century we have seen attitudes towards government-funded veterans' programs change, with the public believing at various times that these programs should be based on one or more of four principles: charity, rehabilitation, insurance, and/or entitlement.

For Canada, the First World War precipitated its earliest large-scale effort to reintegrate veterans into society. The 172,950 Canadian wounded were, and remain, unprecedented in our history, as innovations in military medicine meant that many more soldiers survived their injuries and illnesses than in previous wars and would face months or years of convalescence.[6] The issues that were raised and the lessons learned from reintegrating the injured, as well as the 250,000 members of the Canadian Expeditionary Force (CEF) who were repatriated after the war, have direct relevance to today's debates about the NVC, because today's challenges, even if not of the same magnitude as those at the beginning of the twentieth century, are perceived as large today.[7]

The policies developed by government for veterans during the conflict and in the postwar period of re-establishment laid the foundation for many of today's Canadian social benefits, including family allowances, old age pensions, and health care.[8] However, as we see today, the disillusionment of the postwar period coincided with the struggles of veterans in peacetime to secure benefits, pensions, and employment.[9]

During and after the First World War, Canadian society faced the unprecedented responsibility and challenges of large-scale veteran reintegration. One of the biggest challenges was dealing with the perceptual differences that developed concerning government policies for veteran care and re-establishment and the expectations of returned men and their advocates. As a result of these differing perceptions and expectations of veteran needs, the public, veterans and their families, and government disagreed on the appropriate goals of veteran care and transition policies during the war and the postwar period. However, these three groups did reconcile some of their divergent expectations and interests in the process of creating national policies, thereby improving their effectiveness.

Origins of Government-Funded Veteran Programs

During the Great War, the positive image of the citizen soldier and the dominant cultural interpretation of the conflict as justified helped to produce public demands for government support for the returned men.[10] The Canadian soldier was elevated in the public imagination from an anonymous figure to a recognizable and heroic individual.[11] Yet official treatment of the first casualties of the war who were transported back to Canada in January 1915, soldiers of the Princess Patricia's Canadian Light Infantry, did not meet Canadians' expectations. Upon their arrival in Halifax, the men were immediately stripped of their uniforms and shipped home without ceremony. Reports of this "insensitivity" immediately generated a public scandal, which influenced the new government policy towards returned men.[12] Prime Minister Robert Borden was quick to respond to demands for the respectful treatment of the growing number of "wounded heroes," a term widely used in the public discourse. A combination of private volunteers, public charities, and government bodies organized welcoming committees and entertainment for the discharged servicemen, and hundreds, sometimes thousands, of men and women, eager to "do their bit" for the troops, regularly gathered at local railway stations to welcome returning soldiers.[13] In 1917, Borden reflected popular sentiment with his pledge that "the government and the country [would] consider it their first duty to ... prove to the returned men its just and due appreciation of the inestimable value of the services rendered to the country and Empire."[14]

Public expectations also encouraged the government to take on responsibility for the treatment and rehabilitation of wounded veterans. In 1914, there was no national precedent for government-sponsored medical care, and the state had made few preparations for the monumental task of providing for wounded servicemen. Yet by 1916, Borden agreed that the "care of the disabled '[was] an obligation which should fall primarily on the State.'"[15] Over the course of the conflict, the government adopted the responsibility for the health and hospital care of ex-servicemen, and on 30 June 1915 it established the Military Hospitals Commission (MHC) to coordinate the care of disabled, wounded, and ill veterans of the CEF.[16]

Moreover, although the condition of shell shock was poorly understood and met with considerable ambivalence from the medical and lay community, civilians and government officials agreed that it was "intolerable" that any "suffering heroes" should be sent to recover with "mere lunatics." Therefore, the MHC opened a hospital at Cobourg dedicated to treating cases of "shell-shock."[17] This is just one example of government resources dedicated to veteran care, which was based on the view that these efforts would facilitate the prompt reintegration of returned men.[18]

The "Pension Evil" and Veteran Re-establishment

While the government developed an innovative veteran rehabilitation program, it also recognized its traditional obligation to provide pensions for veterans wounded in the line of duty. However, the government discouraged "paternalism" as well as "extravagant" expenditure on veterans.[19] This position was based on the American experience with pensions paid to its Civil War veterans, which were widely regarded as both too generous and a heavy financial burden – a situation labelled the "pension evil." To ensure that Canada did not repeat the U.S. experience, in June 1916 the federal government appointed the Board of Pension Commissioners (BPC) to administer pensions to veterans who had been permanently disabled because of their service.[20]

Conscious of the "pension evil," the BPC designed new benefits regulations for veterans of the Great War based on cost-effectiveness. Disability was henceforth classified under twenty categories by percentages, and disabled pensioners were to be recalled before the BPC for scrutiny annually, with their pensions subject to annual readjustment. Benefits were determined and awarded according to severity of the disability and its "attributability" to war service. By 1917, while Canada offered the most generous pension rates of all belligerents, its pension allocation system was extremely strict. Only 5% of claimants received the maximum pension rate, while the majority received below 25%.[21] This stringent policy was justified on the grounds that pensions were not designed to entitle veterans to an income for life; rather, they would constitute only a portion of disabled soldiers' earnings.

Cognizant of the costs of pensions, the government believed that the most pressing issue was the physical recovery of wounded soldiers so that they could return to productive employment. Its policies were based on the widely held belief that returned men would be able to immediately resume their "responsibilities ... of civil life by becoming wholly self-sufficient" and economically independent.[22] "Full re-establishment" soon became the central focus of veteran policy, and by the end of 1917 the commission provided training courses for almost 4,000 men.[23] The government was confident that these policies would assist veterans in resuming civilian employment and help to restore their initiative and independence, while avoiding the "pension evil."

Obstacles to Reintegration

In spite of these measures, real and imagined obstacles to reintegration soon appeared. Policies based on the assumption that providing employment and encouraging financial self-sufficiency for veterans were the most important objectives of re-establishment immediately met with practical problems. While most employers were ostensibly eager to hire returned men, the public and the government became concerned when many veterans were unable to resume steady work.

Soldiers' physical and psychological injuries complicated expectations of a seamless transition to civilian employment. Even men who attempted to return to their former occupations faced unforeseen challenges as a result of their injuries. Employers often misunderstood the complex nature of veterans' injuries and underestimated the attendant difficulties of readjustment.[24] The number of men physically unable to resume employment as a result of their injuries amounted to an overwhelming toll by the end of the war. For example, the Saskatchewan Returned Soldiers' Employment Commission found that by February 1918, of the 2,345 veterans in the province, about 40% remained unemployed, in large part because their injuries were severe.[25]

Moreover, the objectives of the government vocational training program conflicted with the practical needs of many veterans. In 1917, the MHC developed courses that ran from two to eight months, for six or seven hours a day. These intense courses were designed to prepare students for "the rigours of the workplace" so that the men would be able to compete in the job market. However, veterans often found that these courses were "too ambitious" and "too brief" for men who were only beginning to adjust to their injuries.[26] Therefore, by the winter of 1920, government-sponsored vocational training had ultimately failed to help the majority of veterans secure employment and achieve enduring economic independence.[27]

Mental health issues also prevented many men from resuming full-time work. While the medical diagnosis and treatment of "shell shock" evolved, these injuries were often stigmatized by the medical community and the public throughout the war and into the postwar period.[28] As a result, thousands of Canadian soldiers suffering from shell shock were denied access to vocational training.[29] It took some time before it was accepted that this "invisible" injury presented a unique set of challenges to re-establishment.[30]

Returned soldiers also faced the subtle challenges of reintegrating from what had become a culturally distinct veteran community, set apart by their experiences of warfare, into civilian society. Civilians had experienced warfare vicariously through widespread media coverage that idealized and sanitized the fighting; therefore, returned men found that only soldiers who had actually fought in the trenches were able to understand this experience and identify with one another.[31] The disparity between veteran and civilian perceptions has been called a cultural "no-man's land," and an impermeable barrier.[32] This cultural dissonance reinforced civilian anxieties that returned men had been fundamentally changed by their experiences overseas and become estranged from their families and peers who had remained on the home front. Veterans consequently came to self-identify as a distinct community, marked by their shared experience; as one soldier put it, "All of us [will] remain a separate, definite people" after the war.[33]

Veteran Advocacy and Government Response

Compelled, in part, by their feelings of isolation, veterans formed clubs where they could gather and share their experiences with fellow servicemen. The national assembly of veterans, the Great War Veterans Association (GWVA), was established in April 1917, and by the end of the year it had more than 25,000 members. Its membership requirements defined the strict parameters of this community, by initially restricting membership to those who had served overseas in the war and had experienced life in the trenches.[34] As returned men became "a significant minority" in their communities, they increasingly formed local and provincial organizations to lobby for their claims, which spread the views and discontents of Canadian veterans.[35]

In one example of advocacy on behalf of hundreds of thousands of demobilized veterans, the secretary-treasurer of the GWVA charged the BPC in 1921 with "a contemptible and cold-blooded conspiracy to deprive ex-Servicemen of rights" to which they were entitled. In response, the government launched a royal commission to investigate both pensions and civil re-establishment, under the direction of Lieutenant-Colonel J. L. Ralston, a veteran who was to become minister of national defence in the Second World War. Although the Ralston Commission ultimately found that the charge was unsupported, and the existing pension regime remained in place, the commission did launch a comprehensive three-year investigation into veterans' re-establishment, which served as a forum for stakeholders to express their views. The commission's hearings publicized the divergent goals of organized ex-servicemen and the government, and the subsequent dialogue marked an important step towards veteran consultation and government and veteran cooperation.[36]

Lessons of the First World War

The First World War brought about major change to how Canada treated its veterans. Almost unanimous public support for veterans inspired a shift from a largely charity-based approach to a rehabilitation approach with significant government leadership and funding.

Based on the primacy of the principle of rehabilitation and the fear of the entitlement-based "pension evil," the government funded programs that aimed to enable as many veterans as possible, even those with serious injuries, to re-enter the workforce in some capacity. Pensions were to be an income supplement only for those whose disabilities limited their ability to earn income. However, despite general support for this approach, veteran advocates drew attention to a number of real and imagined obstacles to successful veteran reintegration.

The first obstacle was that a significant number of veterans were either unemployed or unable to work full time because of the limitations imposed by their injuries, which were not well understood by civilians. This obstacle was compounded by a veteran culture based on horrifying experiences in the trenches that separated veterans from civilians who did not comprehend and could not empathize with veterans' experiences.

Nevertheless, veteran advocacy raised awareness of these and other issues, which were widely reported in the media. The Ralston Commission provided one of a number of forums for veterans and other stakeholders to exchange views, which promoted understanding and empathy. While these exchanges did not solve all the problems associated with veteran reintegration, they did allow stakeholders to share their perceptions of the issues, which ultimately led to an improvement in government policies and programs designed to help veterans transition to civilian life.

Today's Challenges for Veteran Reintegration

The New Veterans Charter

The New Veterans Charter became law in April 2005 with widespread support outside and inside Parliament. It also received "nearly unanimous" support from veterans' organizations and veterans, in part because it was described as "living" legislation that would be "a 'first step' in a process that would continue to produce changes to eventually create a respectful, caring and effective program that would meet all Veterans' and families' needs."[37] The need for the NVC was underlined by the fact that the Afghanistan mission, "the largest Canadian military operation since the Second World War," produced a new generation of veterans whose needs could not be addressed under the existing Pension Act, because it focused on "disability rather than on rehabilitation due to the structure of the financial benefits."

Much like legislation enacted after the First World War, the NVC aimed to "shift the philosophy of veteran support from one of compensation to one of wellness and rehabilitation," and "to facilitate the re-entry of veterans into civilian life in a way that promotes reintegration and independence."[38]

Despite the fact that there were over 21,000 NVC program "participants" in the four-year period ending 31 March 2010,[39] not long after the passage of the bill, some strongly criticized aspects of the legislation. Criticism focused mainly on the financial losses veterans had suffered with the implementation of the NVC when compared to the previous Pension Act benefits, as well as the inequities inherent in the "lump sum" disability award.[40] Some criticism was levelled at the ineffectiveness of certain NVC programs; for example, only 13% of over 4,000 participants completed "the vocational services component" of the Rehabilitation Program, a rate similar to such programs after the First World War.[41] Also like that in conflict, a significant reason for the differences in points of view on this question is the differences in perceptions among stakeholders about the nature of the problem and how it could be best addressed.

A Conceptual Framework

We propose here a framework as one way to conceptualize how differences among stakeholders in their perceptions of the treatment of veterans arise, as a first step towards mitigating the effects of these differences. We see three main factors that create systemic obstacles to establishing effective policies and programs for veteran transition to civilian life: public perceptions, non-government stakeholder perceptions, and government perceptions about the appropriate goals of veteran programs. All these perceptions can vary significantly, depending on a number of variables.

Key variables that affect perceptions are (1) cultural differences, (2) the nature of the veteran population, (3) perceptions of the causes of veteran disabilities, (4) perceptions of the military in society, (5) perceptions of how military personnel and veterans are being treated in relation to others in society, and (6) the role of stakeholders.

We know that cultural differences can cause divergent perceptions of the same situation, as we saw with case of First World War veterans. While Canadian military, and to a certain extent veteran, culture has varied in detail over time, it has retained fundamental characteristics that differentiate it from civilian culture.[42] For example, Canadian military culture has been characterized as being very goal-oriented, compared to a public service culture that is almost exclusively "process-oriented," and some veterans have had difficulty adjusting to workplaces that function differently from those in the military.[43] Cultural factors may, in part, explain a recurring theme in the history of veteran transition to civilian life – different perceptions of veteran needs. Clashing cultures can also lead to misunderstanding and perceived injustice. For example, in 1918, Sergeant E. R. R. Mills said, "When you go before a medical board, you are treated as a malingerer if you are a private ... in some cases I have heard them almost tell [veterans] to their faces that they were liars."[44] And recently, a number of CF veterans have complained of similar treatment before Veteran Review and Appeal Boards. [45]

The nature of the veteran population, especially its demographic characteristics related to age and types of disability, has important effects on perceptions and policies, as well as the expressed needs of veterans. For example, between 1914 and 1939 the demographics of the veteran population receiving benefits changed from a relatively young population with physical disabilities to an older population with a large proportion suffering from mental illnesses. After Canada's involvement in Afghanistan, many young veterans became part of a veteran population that had aged significantly since the end of the Second World War, and their needs were quite different from those of the older group.[46]

Perceptions of the causes of veteran disabilities are often linked to society's perception of the type of conflict in which injuries occurred. While there was widespread acceptance that veteran injuries in the First World War were legitimate, incurred in a "crusade" against a barbarous enemy, this was not the case in the "Decade of Darkness." In the 1990s, most people, including military personnel, believed that "legitimate" casualties were only those whose condition could be directly attributed to conventional combat.[47] In this era, it was assumed that there was a clear distinction between combat and non-combat missions, and all CF operations at the time were considered to be non-combat, what the U.S. military dismissively referred to as military operations other than war (MOOTW – pronounced "*moot*-wah"). Many believed that the nation had little or no responsibility for those injured on "non-combat" operations, when senior military leaders declared, "Real men don't do moot-wah."[48] This led to situations where even those who had suffered severe physical injuries received little official support. For example, Canadian Major Bruce Henwood, who lost both his legs below the knee as a result of his vehicle striking a mine in Croatia in 1995, was initially denied adequate compensation because his injuries were sustained on what was believed to be a benign peacekeeping mission.[49] In sum, perceptions of the conflict affect how veteran claims on national resources are viewed.[50]

Perceptions of how military personnel and veterans are being treated in relation to others in society also affect perceptions of whether or not the goals of veteran programs are appropriate. For example, between the First and Second World Wars, the annual cost of veteran programs and pensions was the second-largest government expense next to servicing the national debt, and during the Great Depression, when many Canadians suffered financially, some thought that veteran pensions were too liberal.[51] In today's difficult financial times, there are indications that some civilians have little sympathy for what are perceived to be overly generous veteran benefits.[52]

The roles of stakeholders also affect their perceptions. As one would expect, veteran groups generally advocate for better benefits; however, the extent and intensity of their advocacy varies according to the situation.[53] Government attitudes to benefits also vary according to economic and political conditions. As we have seen, at some times governments are quite receptive to generous benefits for veterans, at others, such as in times of fiscal crisis or low public support for benefits, they are not. In all cases, roles and circumstances combine to shape what any group perceives to be appropriate responses and satisfactory outcomes to veteran needs.

Mitigation Strategies

We have argued that differences in perceptions among stakeholders are the three main factors that create systemic obstacles to establishing effective policies and programs for veteran transition to civilian life. We therefore propose three ways to overcome those barriers: communication, understanding, and empathy.

Communication

The first way, communication, is one that everybody talks about but nobody does much about, to paraphrase Mark Twain. It took some time after the First World War for stakeholders to establish more effective communications among themselves. More recently, despite a series of changes to the "living" NVC in 2009 and 2010, vocal criticism of the NVC persists from some quarters. One reason for the criticism of the NVC is a lack of understanding of the NVC within the broader veteran community and among the Canadian public due to a lack of effective communication by Veterans Affairs Canada (VAC) about the goals and outcomes of the NVC.[54] Recently, VAC responses to the auditor general's criticisms of its programs were described as "several paragraphs of impenetrable gobbledygook on efforts to comply. It makes for difficult and discouraging reading, and must have a demoralizing impact on veterans and serving military members." Likewise, there appear to be communication difficulties within the bureaucracy, as the auditor general found that "quality of [program] delivery varies widely depending on individual field offices and the relationship between local DND [Department of National Defence] or Veterans Affairs officials."[55]

While ineffective official communications are one source of misunderstanding, certain actions by advocates can also create misunderstanding. Constant attacks on policies in the media often harden positions on both sides and may actually impede the stated goal of virtually all stakeholders – to help the veteran. It has been observed that extremely effective communication among stakeholders has occurred in certain committees where people met regularly, established bonds of trust, and were prepared to put aside their bureaucratic or advocate roles to listen to others.[56] The leadership in such meetings of those who were not stakeholders in the issues being discussed was essential to facilitating this process. Consultation in an informal setting, where information exchange was the main goal, supplemented public communications efforts, thereby making them more effective. This reduced the strident public media battles that can impede the next two mitigation strategies: understanding and empathy.

Understanding

The second way, increasing understanding, is achieved by a cognitive process in which we gain knowledge of various points of view and accept that others have valid beliefs that are different from our own. It is not necessary to agree with these views, but one should be able to accept that, on the basis of certain assumptions, they are valid. Achieving understanding allows different stakeholders to address the issue of divergent assumptions more directly to see how they might be minimized. Again, it has been observed that, in matters of military and veteran health, differing assumptions can be based on misinterpreting the actions or motives of other stakeholders. Sometimes, as indicated above, these misunderstandings can be corrected or reduced by getting to know others with different views in informal settings.

Empathy

The third way, creating empathy, can be achieved by attempting to appreciate what others experience emotionally in dealing with these issues. If one can gain insight into how it feels to work within another paradigm, one can be more sympathetic to the difficulties of others. For example, bureaucrats have been moved by veterans' accounts of the enormous challenges they face in trying to re-establish themselves in civilian life. There have also been instances where veteran advocates came to appreciate the tremendous emotional pressure some bureaucrats were under when they were prohibited by rules and regulations from "doing the right thing" for veterans. In both cases, each group came to see that others also had difficult challenges that affected their emotional state. In some cases, this led to modified behaviour or rules with the aim of addressing the legitimate concerns of veterans.

Unfortunately, many of these forums for informal exchanges no longer exist, and there is increased polarization of perceptions among stakeholders, to the detriment of providing compassionate, effective, and fiscally responsible support for veterans to transition to civilian life.

Conclusions

Canadian veteran health care and reintegration programs have been based on the principles of charity, rehabilitation, insurance, and/or entitlement, depending on the perceptions of the public, non-government stakeholders, and government officials. The First World War was the first time in our history that virtually all constituencies agreed that there was a need for large government-funded programs, based primarily on rehabilitation and secondarily on entitlement, to care for huge numbers of injured veterans and to reintegrate them into society. Our First World War experience established patterns for addressing the challenges of veteran health care and rehabilitation that continue to confront us today.

Public perceptions have been influenced by the cultural differences between civil and military society, perceptions of the causes of veteran disabilities, perceptions of the military in society, and perceptions of how military personnel and veterans are being treated in relation to others in society. While cultural differences have been a relatively constant influence on public perceptions, the other influences varied considerably, depending on the situation. Whenever the public had a high opinion of the military and veterans, their support for the allocation of resources to veteran care and reintegration was high. In fact during and immediately after the First World War, the public actually pressured the government for increased resources. However, at times when the military or its missions were not held in high regard, public support for veterans declined. In times of financial hardship, the public could even pressure the government to reduce veteran benefits if they were seen to be disproportionately high, compared to government benefits for civilians in need.

Non-government stakeholders, particularly veteran advocates, tend to focus on immediate issues, especially perceived injustices. While advocates provide indispensable services in raising public awareness of issues and representing veterans without a voice, their attention to immediate issues can obscure longer-term challenges.

Government policy towards veterans tends to be swayed by public opinion; however, governments must also balance public pressures with fiscal realities. When times are good, resources allocated to veteran care and reintegration tend to be high, and when they are bad, resources can be reallocated to other government priorities.

The nature of the veteran population is a factor that affects the perceptions of all. However, appreciation for the changing nature of the population often lags behind the actual changes, resulting in skewed perceptions about veteran needs in all parts of society. Therefore, when policies for veteran care and reintegration have been modified, it is frequently in reaction to growing awareness of gaps that have developed between existing programs and changing veteran needs.

In the past century, a common systemic obstacle to Canadian veteran transition to civilian life has been differing perceptions among stakeholders, resulting in divergent expectations about the goals of veteran care and transition policies. The outcome has sometimes been drawn-out conflict over what veterans require to meet their needs quickly and appropriately. We suggest that focusing on strategies to improve communication, understanding, and empathy among stakeholders can help to harmonize perceptions among stakeholders, thereby increasing the chances of building the consensus required to minimize divergent expectations, leading to more compassionate, effective, widely accepted, and fiscally responsible veteran reintegration programs. One way to augment formal consensus-building is the use of forums for informal exchanges, facilitated by those who are not stakeholders in the issues being discussed. In this way, we can help to create broad support for a national agenda to address veteran needs and for effective policies for veteran care and transition to civilian life.

Notes

1   Lee Berthiaume, "Government Pledge to Address Veterans' Problems Prompts Skepticism," *Postmedia News*, 23 October 2012, http://www.canada.com/ Government+pledge+address+veterans+problems+prompts+skepticism/7432510/ story.html.

2   Bruce Campion-Smith, "Wounded Afghan Vets Take Ottawa to Court over Compensation," *Toronto Star*, 30 October 2012, http://www.thestar.com/news/ canada/politics/article/1280067--wounded-afghan-vets-take-ottawa-to-court-over-compensation.

3   Canada, Veterans Affairs Canada (VAC), "Survey on Transition to Civilian Life: Report on Regular Force Veterans" (Charlottetown, PEI: VAC, 4 January 2011): 7–8.

4   Canada, Auditor General, "2012 Fall Report of the Auditor General of Canada," Chapter 4 – Transition of Ill and Injured Military Personnel to Civilian Life http://www.oag-bvg.gc.ca/internet/English/parl_oag_201210_04_e_37348.html; Canada, VAC, "Survey on Transition to Civilian Life," 9:77.

5   Allan English, "Not Written in Stone: Social Covenants and Resourcing Military and Veterans Health Care in Canada," in *Shaping the Future: Military and Veteran Health Research*, ed. Alice B. Aiken and Stephanie A. H. Belanger, 230–8 (Kingston, ON: Canadian Defence Academy, 2011).

6   Desmond Morton and Glenn Wright, *Winning the Second Battle: Canadian Veterans and the Return to Civilian Life 1915–1930* (Toronto: University of Toronto Press, 1987), 229; Desmond Morton, "'Noblest and Best': Retraining Canada's War Disabled 1915–1923," *Journal of Canadian Studies* 16 (1981): 80; Morton, "Military Medicine and State Medicine: Historical Notes on the Canadian Army Medical Corps in the First World War 1914–1919," in *Canadian Health Care and the State*, ed. David C. Naylor (Montreal and Kingston: McGill-Queen's University Press, 1992), 43.

7   Desmond Morton, *Fight or Pay: Soldiers' Families in the Great War* (Vancouver: UBC Press, 2004), 133; Allan Woods, "Medical Discharges from Military Increased Dramatically over a Decade in Afghanistan," *Toronto Star*, 3 February 2012, http://www.thestar.com/news/canada/politics/article/1126133--medical-discharges-from-military-increased-dramatically-over-a-decade-in-afghanistan.

8   Morton, "'Noblest and Best,'" 75; Lara Campbell, "'We Who Have Wallowed in the Mud of Flanders': First World War Veterans, Unemployment and the Development of

Social Welfare in Canada, 1929–1939," *Journal of the Canadian Historical Association* 11, no. 1 (2000): 125.

9 Sean Bruyea, "Can Veterans Trust Bureaucrats to Look After Their Interests? And What about Veterans Organizations Too Scared to Speak Out?," *Ottawa Citizen*, 8 February 2012, http://blogs.ottawacitizen.com/2012/02/08/can-veterans-trust-bureaucrats-to-look-after-their-interests-and-what-about-veterans-organizations-too-scared-to-speak-out/.

10 English, "Not Written in Stone," 231–2, 234.

11 Tim Cook, "Wet Canteens and Worrying Mothers: Alcohol, Soldiers and Temperance Groups in the Great War," *Histoire sociale / Social History* 35, no. 70 (2002): 314; Jonathan Vance, *Death So Noble: Memory, Meaning, and the First World War* (Vancouver: UBC Press, 1997), 115–16; Morton and Wright, *Winning the Second Battle*, ix.

12 Morton, *Fight or Pay*, 133; Desmond Morton, *When Your Number's Up: The Canadian Soldier in the First World War* (Toronto: Random House of Canada, 1993), 253.

13 Morton and Wright, *Winning the Second Battle*, 63.

14 English, "Not Written in Stone," 231–2.

15 Morton and Wright, *Winning the Second Battle*, 16–17.

16 Morton, *Fight or Pay*, 135–6.

17 Morton, "Military Medicine and State Medicine," 48; Morton and Wright, *Winning the Second Battle*, 39.

18 Robert Rutherdale, *Hometown Horizons: Local Responses to Canada's Great War* (Vancouver: UBC Press, 2004), 235.

19 Morton, "'Noblest and Best,'" 77.

20 Morton, *When Your Number's Up*, 255.

21 James Pitsula, *For All We Have and Are: Regina and the Experience of the Great War* (Winnipeg: University of Manitoba Press, 2008), 233–4; Desmond Morton, *A Military History of Canada*, 3rd ed. (Toronto: McClelland & Stewart, 1992), 166.

22 Morton, *When Your Number's Up*, 261.

23 Morton and Wright, *Winning the Second Battle*, 17, 81.

24 Morton, "'Noblest and Best,'" 80.

25 Pitsula, *For All We Have and Are*, 236.

26 Morton, *When Your Number's Up*, 259–60.

27 Morton, "'Noblest and Best,'" 80–2.

28 Morton, *Fight or Pay*, 151.

29 The Canadian Army treated 10,000 soldiers for "psychiatric reasons" during the war, half of whom were specifically labelled as "nervous." In reality, the number of men suffering from "shell shock" was likely much higher. Morton, "Military Medicine," 50.

30 Morton, "'Noblest and Best,'" 81; Morton and Wright, *Wining the Second Battle*, 133.

31 Rutherdale, *Hometown Horizons*, 225–30; Morton, *Military History of Canada*, 141; Eric J. Leed, *No Man's Land: Combat and Identity in World War I* (Cambridge: Cambridge University Press, 1979): 204–5; Vance, *Death So Noble*, 127.

32 Rutherdale, *Hometown Horizons*, 303.

33 Vance, *Death So Noble*, 127.

34 Morton, *Fight or Pay*, 157; Morton and Wright, *Winning the Second Battle*, 62.

35 Morton and Wright, *Winning the Second Battle*, 68, 155–7.

36 Morton, *When Your Number's Up*, 272–3.

37 Canada, VAC, "New Veterans Charter Evaluation – Phase II, Final: August 2010," i, http://www.veterans.gc.ca/pdf/deptReports/2010-08-NVCe-p2.pdf.

38 Alice Aiken and Amy Buitenhuis, *Supporting Canadian Veterans with Disabilities: A Comparison of Financial Benefits* (Kingston, ON: Defence Management Studies Program, School of Policy Studies, Queen's University, 2011), 3–5; Canada, VAC, "New Veterans Charter NVC Evaluation – Phase I, Final: December 2009," 11–13, http://www.veterans.gc.ca/pdf/deptReports/NCAC_phaseI_2009.pdf; Jordan Press, "Fresh from Dodging Taliban Bullets, Afghan Veterans Refocus Their Aim on Job Market," *Postmedia News*, 28 February 2012, http://www.canada.com/news/Fresh+from+dodging+Taliban+bullets+Afghan+veterans+refocus+their+market/6191311/story.html.

39 Canada, VAC, "New Veterans Charter NVC Evaluation – Phase III, Final: February 2011," 1, http://www.veterans.gc.ca/pdf/deptReports/2010-dec-NVC-eval-ph3/2010-dec-NVC-eval-ph3-e.pdf.

40 See, for example, John Labelle, "Canadian Politicians Pay Lip Service to Veterans: New Veteran Charter Cheats Vets and Their Families," *Ottawa Citizen*, 4 November 2012, http://blogs.ottawacitizen.com/2012/11/04/canadian-politicians-pay-lip-service-to-veterans-new-veteran-charter-cheats-vets-and-their-families/; Bruyea, "Can Veterans Trust Bureaucrats to Look After Their Interests?"

41 Canada, VAC, "New Veterans Charter NVC Evaluation – Phase III, Final: February 2011," i, 15.

42 Peter Kasurak, "Concepts of Professionalism in the Canadian Army, 1946–2000: Regimentalism, Reaction, and Reform," *Armed Forces & Society* 37, no. 1 (2011): 96.

43 "Veterans Joining Public Service Face Culture Shock: Few Supports in Place for Transition, Advocates Say," *CBC News*, 20 December 2011, http://www.cbc.ca/news/canada/ottawa/story/2011/12/19/ottawa-veterans-adjust-public-service.html.

44 Morton, *Fight or Pay*, 154; Morton and Wright, *Winning the Second Battle*, 76.

45 Murray Brewster, "Veterans Review and Appeal Board called Abusive, Demeaning by Ex-Soldiers," *Toronto Star*, 6 March 2012, http://www.thestar.com/news/canada/politics/article/1141605--veterans-review-and-appeal-board-called-abusive-demeaning-by-ex-soldiers.

46 Canada, VAC, "New Veterans Charter NVC Evaluation – Phase I, Final: December 2009," 1–2, 6–8; Canada, VAC, "Survey on Transition to Civilian Life," 24–9.

47 Allan English, "From Combat Stress to Operational Stress: The CF's Mental Health Lessons from the 'Decade of Darkness,'" *Canadian Military Journal* 4 (Autumn 2012): 9–17.

48 Fred Kaplan, "The Post-9/11 Military," *Slate*, 2 September 2011, http://www.slate.com/articles/news_and_politics/war_stories/2011/09/the_post911_military.html, citing the chairman of the US Joint Chiefs of Staff.

49 Canada, Standing Senate Committee on National Security and Defence, *Fixing the Canadian Forces' Method of Dealing with Death or Dismemberment*, Eighth Report (Ottawa: Senate of Canada, 10 April 2003), http://www.parl.gc.ca/Content/SEN/Committee/372/vete/rep/rep08apr03-e.htm.

50 Allan English, "Leadership and Operational Stress in the Canadian Forces," *Canadian Military Journal* 1, no. 3 (Autumn 2000): 33–8.

51 Morton, "Military Medicine and State Medicine," 38–66; Morton, *Military History of Canada*, 167.
52 David Pugliese, "Benefits for Canadian Military Families: Ongoing Problems and Various Viewpoints," *Ottawa Citizen*, 7 August 2012, http://blogs.ottawacitizen.com/2012/08/07/benefits-for-canadian-military-families-ongoing-problems-and-various-viewpoints/.
53 Bruyea, "Can Veterans Trust Bureaucrats to Look After Their Interests?"
54 Canada, Auditor General, *Report of the Auditor General of Canada to the House of Commons*, chapter 4: Transition of Ill and Injured Military Personnel to Civilian Life; Canada, VAC, "New Veterans Charter Evaluation – Phase II, Final: August 2010."
55 Kelly McParland, "Veterans Let Down by Bureaucratic Confusion," *National Post* 23 October 2012, http://fullcomment.nationalpost.com/2012/10/23/kelly-mcparland-veterans-let-down-by-bureaucratic-confusion/.
56 The observations in this section are based on the experiences of Allan English, who was a member of a number of committees related to DND, VAC, and RCMP mental health between 2004 and 2010.

17

Literature Review on Rural–Urban Differences in Well-being after Transition to Civilian Life

KIMBERLEY WATKINS

Abstract

Rural residence has been associated with certain socioeconomic disadvantages, such as lower income levels and employment rates, which have been shown to be related to poorer health. These limitations may hold implications for veterans. of the Canadian Forces (CF) because approximately 20% of CF veterans reside in rural regions. This study explores the literature on rural and urban differences in well-being among military veterans to determine whether one geographic group might be more at risk for difficulties in transition to civilian life. In the general population, urban dwellers tend to experience better physical health than their rural counterparts, but findings on mental health have been mixed. Veteran research has produced similar results, with urban veterans generally reporting better physical functioning, possibly due to reduced access to care. Research on the mental health of veterans, however, has not shown conclusive results, with some studies demonstrating an advantage for rural veterans in psychological well-being, and others indicating that veterans in rural regions are at an increased risk for mental health problems. The generalizability of the research is limited, however, by a lack of consistency in defining rural, and by a dearth of research on rural–urban differences among veterans of the CF.

Introduction

The Canadian population is becoming increasingly urbanized. In just five years (2001–06), metropolitan and urban areas experienced population growth rates of 6.9% and 4.0%, respectively, compared to just 1.0% in small towns and rural regions.[1] Furthermore, according to Statistics Canada's 2006 census, the vast majority of Canadians live in urban areas. Nonetheless, a notable percentage (20%) of

Canadians resides in rural areas, defined as locations outside areas of more than 1,000 residents and 400 residents per square kilometre.[2] The ratio of urban to rural residents varies greatly by province, with just 15% of Ontario and British Columbia residents inhabiting rural regions, but approximately half of the Territories' and Atlantic provinces' populations residing in rural settings.[3] It is important to note, however, that rural and urban are often defined differently. Some definitions classify more than 30% of Canada's population as rural dwellers.[4]

Location of residence has been associated with certain socioeconomic variables. For instance, rural residents have been shown to have less education and lower income levels and employment rates than their urban counterparts.[5] These disparities have been associated with poorer health status.[6] Rural U.S. residents are also more likely to cite cost as a barrier to accessing health services.[7] These discrepancies may hold important implications for veterans of the Canadian Forces (CF) and their care provider, Veterans Affairs Canada (VAC) because, similar to the general population, a notable proportion (approximately 20%) of CF veterans reside in rural regions.[8] In addition, the experiences of former CF members who are not VAC clients in accessing health services will be similar to those of the general population.

This study explores the literature on rural and urban differences in health and well-being among military veterans to determine whether one geographic group might be more at risk for difficulties in transition to civilian life. Rural–urban health differences in the general population will first be discussed, in order to provide a comparison for disparities among veterans. PsycINFO, PsycARTICLES, Google Scholar, and PubMed were searched using the keywords *military* or *veteran; rural; urban*; and *health*. To be included in the review, studies were required to have compared the health of rural and urban veterans, or assessed the impact of rural residence on veteran well-being. In total, twenty-eight articles, published between 1994 and 2012, were retained. Studies are presented in a narrative review, with results synthesized in accordance with the principal themes and trends.[9]

To provide a comparison group, rural and urban disparities in well-being in the general population are also summarized. The same databases mentioned above were searched, using the keywords *rural, urban*, and *health*. For the general population research, the findings of thirty-three studies, seven of which used Canadian samples, are summarized. This list is not exhaustive; there is a great deal of research on rural–urban health differences. Because the main focus of this review was on rural–urban differences among veterans, and general population research was simply for comparison, only a sample of studies found was included. Studies were selected primarily on the basis of following criteria: Canadian research; recently conducted research (for the most part, within the past decade); research on either mental health, physical health, or health service use; and research on older adults, to provide a more demographically comparable group to veterans and retiring military members.

Rural–urban health differences in the general population are first outlined, to provide context and comparison for veteran rural–urban disparities in well-being. Next, socioeconomic disparities between rural and urban veterans are examined. Rural veterans' reduced access to health services and lower likelihood of receiving specialized care are then described, followed by discussion of their generated health-care expenditures. Next, mental and physical health differences between rural and urban veterans are described. Finally, limitations of the research and directions for future research are detailed.

General Population Trends

The results of research on rural and urban health disparities in civilian samples have been mixed. In American and European research, rural and urban citizens have fared similarly on some measures of health, including health service use,[10] mental health service use,[11] perceived health or quality of life,[12] and prevalence of anxiety and depression.[13] In one Canadian study, participants from rural and urban communities were shown to have comparable morbidity and mortality rates on several illnesses.[14]

In general, however, research in this domain suggests that rural and urban residents differ in their health and health-related behaviours. Some Polish and American research has shown that urban dwellers may have a higher risk than rural residents of certain types of cancer.[15] For the most part, however, urban residents tend to experience better physical health. In Canadian and American studies, for instance, members of rural communities have been shown to be more likely to develop a pain-related condition,[16] to be overweight,[17] and to be limited in activities by poor health.[18] These differences may be attributed, in part, to urban residents' greater tendency to engage in preventive health behaviours (e.g., engaging in physical activity)[19] and, in Canada, to receive an influenza vaccination[20] and to wear a helmet while cycling.[21]

The advantage of urban versus rural residence in mental well-being, however, is less clear. Some Canadian, American, and European research has indicated that rural residents tend to have higher rates of depression,[22] cognitive impairment,[23] and suicide.[24] On the other hand, other research has suggested that individuals living in urban settings may be more likely to suffer from mental health symptoms[25] and disorders,[26] particularly depression.[27] They may also be more likely than rural residents to have difficulties with substance use[28] and to have higher alcohol-related mortality rates.[29] Rural community members, despite their residential location's lower population density, tend to report better social support than their urban counterparts,[30] which may contribute to the elevated psychological well-being that some studies have reported.

Limited access to specialized care may make it harder for rural residents to obtain appropriate treatment for their physical and mental health problems.

Individuals residing in Canadian rural settings are less likely to receive specialized services,[31] such as specialized treatment for stroke, osteoporosis, and diabetes.[32] Research in the United States has shown that rural dwellers are less likely to be given diet or exercise counselling and preventive procedures (e.g., cholesterol screening)[33] or to receive specialized treatment for chronic conditions like arthritis and hypertension.[34] British rural residents have also been shown to have a more advanced stage of cancer at diagnosis than urban dwellers, possibly because of reduced access to oncology services.[35] Lack of access to medical specialists may make rural U.S. residents more likely to seek care for specific health problems (such as memory difficulties)[36] from a general practitioner, which may lead to poorer treatment outcomes.

Limited access to health services may also make members of rural communities less likely than their urban counterparts to seek treatment for health problems. Rural residents have lower rates of health-care utilization[37] and are less likely to use after-hours telephone health services,[38] to see a health care professional over chronic pain,[39] and, in Canada, are less likely to have a regular family physician.[40] In terms of mental health treatment seeking, rural residents are less likely than urban dwellers to seek specialized treatment for depression[41] and, in Canada, to have contacted a mental health professional.[42] Care seeking for depression has also been shown to be negatively related to travel time.[43] In short, the direction of differences in psychological well-being is still unclear. Nonetheless, rural residents tend to have poorer physical health than their urban counterparts,[44] though residents of urban settings tend to receive more care for health-related issues. The disparity in treatment may account for some of the urban and rural differences in well-being in the general population.

Rural–Urban Differences in Military Veteran Research

The literature discussed here is based on U.S. veterans because, at the time of writing, there was no research on rural and urban differences in well-being among CF veterans. Rural and urban veterans – like the general population – tend to differ in their socioeconomic characteristics, such that urban veterans tend to have higher levels of education[45] and income[46] and are more likely to be employed than their rural counterparts.[47] Additionally, U.S. veterans below the Medicare age of eligibility living in non-metropolitan regions (i.e., counties encompassing towns with a population of 50,000 or less) are less likely than their urban counterparts to have health insurance.[48] Among U.S. veterans eligible for Medicare, rural residents are more likely to rely on it or on Veterans Affairs (VA) facilities for health coverage than on private insurance.[49] They are also more likely to have refrained from seeking needed medical treatment for financial reasons,[50] including the costs associated with travel (e.g., fuel prices).[51]

Indeed, for rural veterans, the physical distance from health services appears to be a substantial barrier to sufficient and appropriate treatment. In the United States, rural-dwelling veterans generally live farther from both private sector and VA health care facilities than veterans residing in urban communities.[52] As a result, they must incur the difficulties associated with travelling greater distances to receive treatment, particularly from high-quality health-care providers.[53] In addition to the financial costs of fuel, travel challenges include transport arrangements (because many veterans do not possess a driver's licence) and weather and infrastructure obstacles (e.g., lack of snow clearing of rural roadways).[54] These increased burdens on rural veterans appear to affect their decisions to seek or receive care, because use of these services tends to decline as distance from health-care facilities increases.[55] It should be noted, however, that the VA hospitals that do exist in rural regions – despite offering fewer specialized services – have been rated higher than urban hospitals in patient satisfaction, perhaps the result of a lower patient-to-provider ratio.[56]

In the research on U.S. veterans, rural dwellers tend to use health services less than veterans living in urban areas, whether as the result of travel challenges or other barriers. Urban veterans, for instance, are more likely to receive illness-detection procedures (e.g., echocardiograms)[57] and to obtain specialized care for mental health difficulties,[58] including individual or group psychotherapy,[59] crisis intervention and vocational assistance,[60] and inpatient addiction services (e.g., detoxification).[61] Homeless U.S. veterans in metropolitan areas are more likely to access VA health services than their non-metropolitan counterparts.[62] Urban U.S. veterans are also more likely than rural veterans to supplement VA services with other care sources[63] or to replace them with other health services when they are lacking or insufficient.[64] Meanwhile, rural veterans – likely as the result of limited access to suitable health services – are more likely to substitute existing veterans' services with less appropriate care. For example, U.S. veterans residing more than thirty miles from the nearest VA medical centre are more likely to visit a closer non-VA emergency department for health problems than they are to visit their VA service provider.[65] In addition to emergency services, rural veterans sometimes rely on other available sources of care, such as pharmacy services.[66]

Veterans with dementia living in rural communities are also more likely than their urban counterparts to receive inpatient treatment for chronic health problems that could be treated with outpatient care.[67] In other words, rural veterans are more likely to seek unnecessary hospitalization for certain conditions, which increases health-care costs. Of course, this may be due to barriers to accessing suitable outpatient services. Another U.S. study, however, found that the increased travel time from inpatient facilities for rural veterans was associated with a decreased likelihood of a potentially preventable early re-hospitalization after receiving treatment for congestive heart failure.[68] Mixed results were found in a sample of U.S. VA clients, with rural-dwelling veterans more likely to receive inpatient care and veterans from urban residences admitted for longer durations.[69] It is not clear whether rural or urban veterans are more likely to use inpatient services. In general, however, veterans living in urban areas tend to be more likely to seek mental and physical health care.

Despite their reduced care seeking, rural veterans tend to generate increased health service expenditures,[70] particularly older veterans,[71] though it should be noted that the research is on U.S. veterans only, and may not generalize to veterans of the CF. U.S. research has indicated that their greater health-care costs are due to poorer overall physical and mental functioning,[72] suggesting that rural veterans may be more likely to receive treatment for more health difficulties, even though they may be less likely than their urban counterparts to seek care at all. Rural veterans tend to report mental health status consistent with that of depression more often[73] and to report poorer mental health than urban veterans,[74] and they have been shown to be more likely to abuse alcohol.[75] Further, homeless veterans in rural areas are more likely than their urban counterparts to suffer from mental health problems and difficulties with alcohol use.[76]

Comparisons of rural and urban veterans' psychological well-being are mixed, however, in keeping with research on the general population. In light of the findings reported above, one would expect urban veterans to have better mental health status than rural ones. But the research on U.S. veterans has provided contradictory evidence. For example, a variety of psychiatric disorders, including depression, anxiety, and alcohol dependence, have been shown to be more common among urban than rural veterans.[77] These discrepancies, however, may reflect higher rates of diagnosis rather than greater actual incidence of psychological disorders, because urban residents are generally more likely to seek treatment for, and thus possibly be diagnosed with, mental health problems, such as depression.[78] In addition, among veterans with a psychological diagnosis, urban residents tend to have more severe symptoms.[79] Urban veterans are also more likely to be readmitted to a hospital shortly after discharge for a mental health problem[80] and tend to be less satisfied with the state of their social support.[81] In a sample of U.S. veterans with substance use problems, meanwhile, those from urban and rural regions did not differ in post traumatic stress symptoms associated with military experience.[82]

Findings that examined urban–rural physical well-being are less mixed. One study did link proximity of residence to a high-traffic roadway to greater odds of developing respiratory symptoms.[83] Nonetheless, military veteran research has generally indicated that rural residency is associated with poorer physical well-being. Rural veterans tend to report greater physical impairment and poorer overall physical functioning[84] and have a greater number of physical health problems[85] than their urban counterparts. They are also more likely to suffer from a physical health difficulty,[86] engage in risky health behaviours (such as smoking),[87] and to be readmitted to a hospital for a physical health problem soon after being discharged.[88] Rural veterans seeking treatment at a mobile clinic also rated their health quite poorly (significantly worse than that of private sector outpatients) and cited their physical health difficulties as impediments to participating in work and other activities.[89] Moreover, in one study of civilians with a traumatic brain injury (a growing concern among veterans of recent conflicts), the rural residents were more likely to be functionally dependent and were in poorer overall health.[90] Clearly, rural veterans are disadvantaged in their physical well-being, whether as the result of socioeconomic differences, barriers to accessing health care, or other reasons. The extent to which research with U.S. veterans can be generalized to rural–urban differences among veterans of the CF, however, is unclear.

Comment

There are some limitations and gaps in the research on rural–urban disparities in the health of military veterans. First, the definition of rural often varies from one study to the next.[91] Some studies[92] used a simple measure of population density (residents per square mile) to assess rural or urban status, while others[93] used census data via zip codes. Much of the research used a formal classification system, such as the U.S. Department of Agriculture's Rural-Urban Continuum Codes or Rural-Urban Commuting Area Codes.[94] However, the cut-off scores used to define rural and urban varied from one study to the next. Some studies restricted their analyses to participants in areas defined as "most urban" (i.e., residents of a metropolitan area with one million or more inhabitants) and "most rural" (i.e., residents of a completely rural region with a population of less than 2,500).[95] Others used a more liberal dichotomous separation of rural–urban status, with "urban" participants coming from areas with more than 50,000 citizens, and "rural" veterans defined as those from locations with fewer than 10,000 residents – veterans from less distinctly urban or rural regions excluded from analysis.[96] Still other studies elected to incorporate all eligible participants in their definitions of urban and rural by dividing a population into residents from areas with more or less than 50,000.[97] Finally, some researchers chose to add an extra category of residence to the urban and rural identifiers, such as suburban, highly rural, and micropolitan, resulting in systems of three[98] or four[99] categories.

This inconsistency in classifying urban versus rural status may limit the comparability of the findings. It has been shown that varying the definition of *rural* can alter the results in rural–urban disparities on measures of health.[100] In other words, substituting one study's definition of rural with that of another might produce notably different findings. These definitional discrepancies may account for the varied results found across studies in urban or rural advantage in mental health among veterans. A consistent categorization of "urban" and "rural" would have to be used to effectively review the literature and to identify trends in differences in well-being between rural and urban veterans.

Some findings from studies of the general population might guide future research on rural and urban disparities among military veterans. Research with adults[101] and older women,[102] for example, has shown that rural residents tend to weigh more than their urban counterparts and are also less likely to exercise.[103] Future research should explore whether these trends also exist in the veteran population, because being overweight, obese, and sedentary are associated with a number of health problems.[104] In addition, investigating health behaviours (such as physical activity) within the military veteran population might provide insight into the reasons for certain health discrepancies between rural and urban veterans. For instance, rural veterans, like members of the rural general population, may be less likely to engage in illness prevention. If so, this finding may provide an alternative explanation for the conclusion that rural veterans use health services less than their urban counterparts as the result of reduced access to care. Instead, rural veterans may be less likely to engage in prevention or detection (e.g., echocardiogram use)[105] located at health-care facilities because of other reasons for avoiding health behaviours detailed in theories of health behaviour engagement, such as subjective norms (i.e., the theory of planned behaviour)[106] or perceived susceptibility to certain illnesses (i.e., the health belief model).[107] While the majority of studies on rural and urban differences in veteran health have used large samples and quantitative data, qualitative research methods, such as interviews and focus groups, might provide a better perspective on the reasons rural veterans are less likely to engage in health behaviours and to seek treatment.

Finally, the literature on rural and urban health differences among military veterans is based on samples of U.S. veterans and thus may not be generalizable to CF veterans. The military experiences of U.S. and CF veterans likely differ because of U.S. participation in conflicts such as the Vietnam War, the Persian Gulf War and, most recently, Operation Iraqi Freedom. Exposure to theatres of combat such as these has been associated with poorer psychological well-being after leaving service.[108] Because the CF was not involved in these operations, veterans of the CF would not be susceptible to the mental health difficulties related to these experiences. Furthermore, after transitioning to civilian life, CF veterans receive their health care through Veterans Affairs Canada (VAC) or their provincial health insurance plan, while U.S. veterans are cared for by the VA or Medicare. Different health-care programs and compensation would almost certainly contribute to a variation in health-care usage and, consequently, health status. As a result, rural and urban health disparities need to be examined among veterans of the CF to determine whether they are similar to or different from those of U.S. military veterans. Although the experiences of CF veterans may differ from those of U.S. veterans in several ways, the present review of the literature could be used as a theoretical foundation from which to generate hypotheses in future research using health data of rural and urban CF veterans.

Summary

This literature review on rural–urban disparities in veteran well-being indicates that urban veterans tend to experience better physical health status than their rural counterparts, whether as the result of socioeconomic advantages, greater access to health services, or increased engagement in healthy behaviours. They are also more likely to seek treatment and receive care, possibly because they are closer to health care facilities. In terms of mental well-being, however, mixed results have been found: there is no consensus on rural or urban advantage in this domain. Future research would benefit from using a consistent classification system of "urban" and "rural," investigation of specific aspects of well-being and health behaviours, qualitative research methods, and studies of CF veterans.

Notes

1 Statistics Canada. "Chart 1: Urban-Rural Variation in Population Growth Across Canada, 2001 to 2006," 2008, http://www.statcan.gc.ca/pub/11-008-x/2007004/c-g/10313/4097923-eng.htm.

2 Statistics Canada, "Population, Urban and Rural, by Province and Territory," 2009, http://www.statcan.gc.ca/tables-tableaux/sum-som/l01/cst01/demo62a-eng.htm.

3 Ibid.

4 Valerie du Plessis, Roland Beshiri, and Ray D. Bollman, "Definitions of Rural," *Rural and Small Town Canada Analysis Bulletin* 3 (2001): 6–10.

5 Constanca Paul, Antonio M. Fonseca, Ignacio Martin, and Joao Amado, "Psychosocial Profile of Rural and Urban Elders in Portugal," *European Psychologist* 8, no. 3 (2003): 160–7, doi:10.1027//1016-9040.8.3.160; Janice C. Probst, Sarah B. Laditka, Charity G. Moore, Nusrat Harun, Paige Powell, and Elizabeth G. Baxley, "Rural-Urban Differences in Depression Prevalence: Implications for Family Medicine," *Family Medicine* 38, no. 9 (2006): 653–60; Kenneth G. Saag, Bradley N. Doebbeling, James E. Rohrer, Sheela Kolluri, Rachel Peterson, Mark E. Hermann, and Robert B. Wallace, "Variation in Tertiary Prevention and Health Service Utilization among the Elderly: The Role of Urban-Rural Residence and Supplemental Insurance," *Medical Care* 36, no. 7 (1998): 965–76.

6 Rachel T. Kimbro, Sharon Bzostek, Noreen Goldman, and German Rodriguez, "Race, Ethnicity, and the Educational Gradient in Health," *Health Affairs* 27, no. 2 (2008): 361–72, doi:10.1377/hlthaff.27.2.361; Catherine E. Ross and John Mirowsky. "Does Employment Affect Health?," *Journal of Health and Social Behavior* 36, no. 3 (1995): 230–43; Peter Saunders, "Income, Health, and Happiness," *Australian Economic Review* 29, no. 4 (1996): 353–66, doi:10.1111/j.1467-8462.1996.tb00941.x; Karien Stronks, H. van de Mheen, J. van den Bos, and J. P. Mackenbach, "The Interrelationship between Income, Health, and Employment Status," *International Journal of Epidemiology* 26, no. 3 (1997): 592–600; Olaf von dem Knesebeck, Pablo E. Verde, and Nico Dragano, "Education and Health in 22 European Countries," *Social Science & Medicine* 63, no. 5 (2006): 1344–51.

7　Dan G. Blazer, Lawrence R. Landerman, Gerda Fillenbaum, and Ronnie Horner, "Health Services Access and Use among Older Adults in North Carolina: Urban vs Rural Residents," *American Journal of Public Health* 85, no. 10 (1995): 1384–90.

8　Mary Beth MacLean, Linda Van Til, Debra Kriger, Jill Sweet, Alain Poirier, and David Pedlar, *Well-Being of Canadian Forces Veterans: Canadian Community Health Survey 2003* (Charlottetown: Veterans Affairs Canada, in press).

9　Bart N. Green, Claire D. Johnson, and Alan Adams, "Writing Narrative Literature Reviews for Peer-Reviewed Journals: Secrets of the Trade," *Journal of Chiropractic Medicine* 5 (2006): 101–17, doi:10.1016/S0899-3467(07)60142-6.

10　Blazer et al., "Health Services Access," 1386–7.

11　Neale R. Chumbler, Marisue Cody, Brenda M. Booth, and Cornelia K. Beck, "Rural-Urban Differences in Service Use for Memory-Related Problems in Older Adults," *Journal of Behavioral Health Services & Research* 28, no. 2 (2001): 212–21, doi:10.1007/BF02287463.

12　Olli Nummela, Tommi Sulander, Antti Karisto, and Antti Uutela, "Self-Rated Health and Social Capital among Aging People across the Urban-Rural Dimension," *International Journal of Behavioral Medicine* 16 (2009): 189–94, doi:10.1007/s12529-008-9027-z; Paul et al., "Psychosocial Profile," 164–6.

13　Karin Dahlberg, Yvonne Forsell, Kerstin Damstrom-Thakker, and Bo Runeson, "Mental Health Problems and Healthcare Contacts in an Urban and Rural Area: Comparisons of Two Swedish Counties," *Nordic Journal of Psychiatry* 61 (2007): 40–6, doi:10.1080/08039480601129333.

14　Alain Vanasse, J. Courteau, A. A. Cohen, M. G. Orzanco, and C. Drouin, "Rural-Urban Disparities in the Management and Health Issues of Chronic Diseases in Quebec (Canada) in the early 2000s," *Rural and Remote Health* 10 (2010): 1548.

15　Michalina Krzyzak, Dominik Maslach, Marzena Juczewska, Wieslaw Lasota, Daniel Rabczenko, Jerzy T. Marcinkowski, and Andrzej Szpak, "Differences in Breast Cancer Incidence and Stage Distribution between Urban and Rural Female Population in Podlaskie Voivodship, Poland in years 2001–2002," *Annals of Agricultural and Environmental Medicine* 17 (2010): 159–62; Sara McLafferty and Fahui Wang, "Rural Reversal? Rural-Urban Disparities in Late-Stage Cancer Risk in Illinois," *Cancer* 115, no. 12 (2009): 2755–64, doi:10.1002/cncr.24306.

16　Pamela K. Hoffman, Brian P. Meier, and James R. Council, "A Comparison of Chronic Pain between an Urban and Rural Population," *Journal of Community Health Nursing* 19, no. 4 (2002): 213–24, doi:10.1207/S15327655JCHN1904_02; Janice C. Probst, Charity G. Moore, Elizabeth G. Baxley, and John J. Lammie, "Rural-Urban Differences in Visits to Primary Care Physicians," *Family Medicine* 34, no. 8 (2002): 609–15; Dean A. Tripp, Elizabeth G. Van Den Kerkhof, and Margo McAlister, "Prevalence and Determinants of Pain and Pain-Related Disability in Urban and Rural Settings in Southeastern Ontario," *Pain Research & Management* 11, no. 4 (2006): 225–33.

17　Jeffrey Sobal, Richard P. Troiano, and Edward A. Frongillo Jr, "Rural-Urban Differences in Obesity," *Rural Sociology* 61, no. 2 (1996): 289–305, doi:10.1111/j.1549-0831.1996.tb00621.x; Sara Wilcox, Cynthia Castro, Abby C. King, Robyn Housemann, and Ross C. Brownson, "Determinants of Leisure Time Physical Activity in Rural Compared with Urban Older and Ethnically Diverse Women in the

United States," *Journal of Epidemiology and Community Health* 54 (2000): 667–72, doi:10.1136/jech.54.9.667.

18 Probst et al., "Rural-Urban Differences in Depression Prevalence," 654–8.

19 S. E. Parks, Robyn A. Housemann, and Ross C. Brownson, "Differential Correlates of Physical Activity in Urban and Rural Adults of Various Socioeconomic Backgrounds in the United States," *Journal of Epidemiology and Community Health* 57 (2003): 29–35, doi:10.1136/jech.57.1.29.

20 Lyn M. Sibley and Jonathan P. Weiner, "An Evaluation of Access to Health Care Services along the Rural-Urban Continuum in Canada," *BMC Health Services Research* 11 (2011): 20, doi:10.1186/1472-6963-11-20.

21 Sande Harlos, Lynne Warda, Norma Buchan, Terry P. Klassen, Virginia L. Koop, and Michael E. K. Moffatt, "Urban and Rural Patterns of Bicycle Helmet Use: Factors Predicting Usage," *Injury Prevention* 5 (1999): 183–8, doi:10.1136/ip.5.3.183.

22 Samia Mechakra-Tahiri, Maria V. Zunzunegui, Michel Préville, and Micheline Dubé, "Social Relationships and Depression among People 65 Years and Over Living in Rural and Urban Areas of Quebec," *International Journal of Geriatric Psychiatry* 24 (2009): 1226–36, doi:10.1002/gps.2250; Probst et al., "Rural-Urban Differences in Depression Prevalence," 654–8.

23 Belina Nunes, Ricardo D. Silva, Vitor T. Cruz, Jose M. Roriz, Joana Pais, and Maria C. Silva, "Prevalence and Pattern of Cognitive Impairment in Rural and Urban Populations in Northern Portugal," *BMC Neurology* 10 (2010): 42, doi:10.1186/1471-2377-10-42.

24 Aleck S. Ostry, "The Mortality Gap between Urban and Rural Canadians: A Gendered Analysis," *Rural and Remote Health* 9 (2009): 1286; Gopal K. Singh and Mohammad Siahpush, "Increasing Rural-Urban Gradients in US Suicide Mortality, 1970–1997," *American Journal of Public Health* 92, no. 7 (2002): 1161–7, doi:10.2105/AJPH.92.7.1161.

25 Dahlberg et al., "Mental Health Problems and Healthcare Contacts," 413; Paul et al., "Psychosocial Profile," 164–6; Eugene S. Paykel, R. Abbott, R. Jenkins, T. Brugha, and H. Meltzer, "Urban-Rural Mental Health Differences in Great Britain: Findings from the National Morbidity Survey," *International Review of Psychiatry* 15 (2003): 97–107, doi:10.1080/0954026021000046001.

26 Viviane Kovess-Masfety, Jordi Alonso, Ron de Graaf, and Koen Demyttenaere, "A European Approach to Rural-Urban Differences in Mental Health: The ESEMeD 2000 Comparative Study," *Canadian Journal of Psychiatry* 50 (2005): 926–36; J. Peen, R. A. Schoevers, A. T. Beekman, and J. Dekker, "The Current Status of Urban-Rural Differences in Psychiatric Disorders," *Acta Psychiatrica Scandinavica* 121 (2010): 84–93, doi:10.1111/j.1600-0447.2009.01438.x.

27 Kovess-Masfety et al., "ESEMeD 2000 Comparative Study," 929–31; Kate Walters, Elizabeth Breeze, Paul Wilkinson, Gill M. Price, Chris J. Bulpitt, and Astrid Fletcher, "Local Area Deprivation and Urban-Rural Differences in Anxiety and Depression among People Older than 75 Years in Britain," *American Journal of Public Health* 94, no. 10 (2004): 1768–74; Jian L. Wang, "Rural-Urban Differences in the Prevalence of Major Depression and Associated Impairment," *Social Psychiatry and Psychiatric Epidemiology* 39 (2004): 19–25, doi:10.1007/s00127-004-0698-8.

28 Dahlberg et al., "Mental Health Problems and Healthcare Contacts," 41–3; Paykel et al., "Urban-Rural Mental Health Differences," 97–107.
29 Sally Erskine, Ravi Maheswaran, Tim Pearson, and Dermot Gleeson, "Socioeconomic Deprivation, Urban-Rural Location and Alcohol-Related Mortality in England and Wales," *BMC Public Health* 10 (2010): 99, doi:10.1186/1471-2458-10-99.
30 Paul et al., "Psychosocial Profile," 164–6; Paykel et al., "Urban-Rural Mental Health Differences," 99–104.
31 Sibley and Weiner, "Evaluation of Access to Health Care," 20.
32 Vanasse et al., "Rural-Urban Disparities," 1548.
33 Probst et al., "Rural-Urban Differences in Visits to Physicians," 610–12.
34 Saag et al., "Variation in tertiary prevention," 969–73.
35 Neil C. Campbell, A. M. Elliott, L. Sharp, L. D. Ritchie, J. Cassidy, and J. Little, "Rural and Urban Differences in Stage at Diagnosis of Colorectal and Lung Cancers," *British Journal of Cancer* 84, no. 7 (2001): 910–14, doi:10.1054/ bjoc.2001.1708.
36 Chumbler et al., "Rural-Urban Differences in Service Use," 215–16.
37 Dahlberg et al., "Mental Health Problems and Healthcare Contacts," 41–3; Sharon L. Larson and John A. Fleishman, "Rural-Urban Differences in Usual Source of Care and Ambulatory Service Use: Analyses of National Data Using Urban Influence Codes," *Medical Care* 41, no. 7 (2003): III 65–III 74; Tripp et al., "Prevalence and Determinants of Pain and Disability," 227–30.
38 Joanne Turnbull, David Martin, Val Lattimer, Catherine Pope, and David Culliford, "Does Distance Matter? Geographical Variation in GP Out-of-Hours Service Use: An Observational Study," *British Journal of General Practice* 58 (2008): 471–7, doi:10.3399/ bjgp08X319431.
39 Hoffman et al., "Comparison of Chronic Pain," 217–20.
40 Sibley and Weiner, "Evaluation of Access to Health Care," 20.
41 Kathryn Rost, Mingliang Zhang, John Fortney, Jeff Smith, and G. Richard Smith Jr, "Rural-Urban Differences in Depression Treatment and Suicidality," *Medical Care* 36, no. 7 (1998): 1098–107.
42 Wang, "Rural-Urban Differences in the Prevalence of Depression and Associated Impairment," 21–3.
43 John C. Fortney, Carol E. Kaufman, David E. Pollio, Janette Beals, Carrie Edlund, Douglas K. Novins, AI-SUPERPFP Team, "The Impact of Geographic Accessibility on the Intensity and Quality of Depression Treatment," *Medical Care* 37 (1999): 884–93.
44 Probst et al., "Rural-Urban Differences in Depression Prevalence," 654–8.
45 Todd A. MacKenzie, Amy E. Wallace, and William B. Weeks, "Impact of Rural Residence on Survival of Male Veterans Affairs Patients after Age 65," *Journal of Rural Health* 26 (2010): 318–24, doi:10.1111/j.1748-0361.2010.00300.x; Somaia Mohamed, Michael Neale, and Robert A. Rosenheck, "VA Intensive Mental Health Case Management in Urban and Rural Areas: Veteran Characteristics and Service Delivery," *Psychiatric Services* 60, no. 7 (2009): 914–21, doi:10.1176/appi.ps.60.7.914; Amy E. Wallace, Richard Lee, Todd A. Mackenzie, Alan N. West, Steven Wright, Brenda M. Booth, Kara Hawthorne, and William B. Weeks, "A Longitudinal Analysis of Rural and Urban Veterans' Health-Related Quality of Life," *Journal of Rural Health* 26 (2010): 156–63, doi:10.1111/j.1748-0361.2010.00277.x; Alan West and William B.

Weeks, "Physical and Mental Health and Access to Care among Nonmetropolitan Veterans Health Administration Patients Younger Than 65 Years," *Journal of Rural Health* 22 (2006): 9–16, doi:10.1111/j.1748-0361.2006.00014.x; Alan N. West and William B. Weeks. "Health Care Expenditures for Urban and Rural Veterans in Veterans Health Administration Care," *Health Services Research* 44 (2009): 1718–34, doi:10.1111/j.1475-6773.2009.00988.x.

46 Jeffrey A. Cully, John P. Jameson, Laura L. Phillips, Mark E. Kunik, and John C. Fortney, "Use of Psychotherapy by Rural and Urban Veterans," *Journal of Rural Health* 26 (2010): 225–33, doi:10.1111/j.1748-0361.2010.00294.x; MacKenzie et al., "Impact of Rural Residence," 319–21; Wallace et al., "Longitudinal Analysis," 158; William B. Weeks, Lewis E. Kazis, Yujing Shen, Zhongxiao Cong, Xinhua S. Ren, Donald Miller, Austin Lee, and Jonathan B. Perlin. "Differences in Health-Related Quality of Life in Rural and Urban Veterans," *American Journal of Public Health* 94, no. 10 (2004): 1762–7, doi:10.2105/AJPH.94.10.1762; West and Weeks, "Physical and Mental Health," 11–13; West and Weeks, "Health Care Expenditures," 1721–31.

47 Mohamed, Neale, and Rosenheck, "VA Intensive Mental Health Case Management," 916–18; Weeks et al., "Differences in Health," 1764–5; William B. Weeks, Amy E. Wallace, Stanley Wang, Austin Lee, and Lewis E. Kazis, "Rural-Urban Disparities in Health-Related Quality of Life within Disease Categories of Veterans," *Journal of Rural Health* 22, no. 3 (2006): 204–11, doi:10.1111/j.1748-0361.2006.00033.x; West and Weeks, "Physical and Mental Health," 11–13.

48 West and Weeks, "Physical and Mental Health," 11–13.

49 West and Weeks, "Health Care Expenditures," 1721–31.

50 West and Weeks, "Physical and Mental Health," 11–13.

51 Benjamin L. Schooley, Thomas A. Horan, Pamela W. Lee, and Priscilla A. West, "Rural Veteran Access to Healthcare Services: Investigating the Role of Information and Communication Technologies in Overcoming Spatial Barriers," *Perspectives in Health Information Management* (Spring 2010): 3–6.

52 Weeks et al., "Differences in Health," 1764–5; Weeks et al., "Rural-Urban Disparities," 206–7.

53 Alan N. West, William B. Weeks, and Amy E. Wallace, "Rural Veterans and Access to High-Quality Care for High-Risk Surgeries," *Health Services Research* 43, no. 5 (2008): 1737–51, doi:10.1111/j.1475-6773.2008.00876.x; William B. Weeks, Amy E. Wallace, Alan N. West, Hilda R. Heady, and Kara Hawthorne, "Research on Rural Veterans: An Analysis of the Literature," *Journal of Rural Health* 24, no. 4 (2008): 337–44, doi:10.1111/j.1748-0361.2008.00179.x.

54 Schooley et al., "Rural Veteran Access to Healthcare Services," 3–6.

55 James F. Burgess Jr and Donna A. DeFiore, "The Effect of Distance to VA Facilities on the Choice and Utilization of VA Outpatient Services," *Social Science & Medicine* 39, no. 1 (1994): 95–104; Kathleen Carey, Maria E. Montez-Rath, Amy K. Rosen, Cindy L. Christiansen, Susan Loveland, and Susan L. Ettner, "Use of VA and Medicare Services by Dually Eligible Veterans with Psychiatric Problems," *Health Services Research* 43, no. 4 (2008): 1164–83, doi:10.1111/j.1475-6773.2008.00840.x; Denise M. Hynes, Kristin Koelling, Kevin Stroupe, Noreen Arnold, Katherine Mallin, Min-Woonh Sohn, Frances M. Weaver, Larry Manheim, and Linda Kok, "Veterans' Access to and Use of Medicare and Veterans Affairs Health Care," *Medical Care* 45, no. 3 (2007):

214–23, doi:10.1097/01.mlr.0000244657.90074.b7; Kingston Okrah, Mary Vaughan-Sarrazin, Peter Kaboli, and Peter Cram, "Echocardiogram Utilization among Rural and Urban Veterans," *Journal of Rural Health* 28 (2012): 211–20, doi:10.1111/j.1748-0361.2011.00380.x; Schooley et al., "Rural Veteran Access to Healthcare Services," 3–6; Susan K. Schmitt, Ciaran S. Phibbs, and John D. Piette, "The Influence of Distance on Utilization of Outpatient Mental Health Aftercare Following Inpatient Substance Abuse Treatment," *Addictive Behaviors* 28 (2003): 1183–92, doi:10.1016/S0306-4603(02)00218-6; William B. Weeks, David M. Bott, Rebecca P. Lamkin, and Steven M. Wright, "Veterans Health Administration and Medicare Outpatient Health Care Utilization by Older Rural and Urban New England Veterans," *Journal of Rural Health* 21, no. 2 (2005): 167–71, doi:10.1111/j.1748-0361.2005.tb00077.x.

56   William B. Weeks, Elizabeth M. Yano, and Lisa V. Rubenstein, "Primary Care Practice Management in Rural and Urban Veterans Health Administration Settings," *Journal of Rural Health* 18 (2002): 298–303, doi:10.1111/j.1748-0361.2002.tb00890.x; Weeks et al. "Research on Rural Veterans," 338–40.

57   Okrah et al., "Echocardiogram Utilization," 214–16.

58   Weeks et al., "Veterans Health Administration," 167–71.

59   Cully et al., "Use of Psychotherapy," 228–9.

60   Mohamed, Neale, and Rosenheck, "VA Intensive Mental Health Case Management," 916–18.

61   Amy E. Wallace, Alan N. West, Brenda M. Booth, and William B. Weeks, "Unintended Consequences in Regionalizing Specialized VA Addiction Services," *Psychiatric Services* 58, no. 5 (2007): 668–74, doi:10.1176/appi.ps.58.5.668.

62   Adam J. Gordon, Gretchen L. Haas, James F. Luther, Michael T. Hilton, and Gerald Goldstein, "Personal, Medical, and Healthcare Utilization among Homeless Veterans Served by Metropolitan and Nonmetropolitan Veteran Facilities," *Psychological Services* 7, no. 2 (2010): 65–74, doi:10.1037/a0018479.

63   Hynes et al., "Veterans' Access to and Use of Medicare," 217.

64   Wallace et al., "Unintended Consequences," 670–2.

65   Schooley et al., "Rural Veteran Access to Healthcare Services," 3–6.

66   West and Weeks, "Health Care Expenditures," 1721–31.

67   Joshua M. Thorpe, Courtney H. Van Houtven, Betsy L. Sleath, and Carolyn T. Thorpe. "Rural-Urban Differences in Preventable Hospitalizations among Community-Dwelling Veterans with Dementia," *Journal of Rural Health* 26 (2010): 146–55, doi:10.1111/j.1748-0361.2010.00276.x.

68   Kyle J. Muus, A. Knudson, M. G. Klug, J. Gokun, M. Sarrazin, and P. Kaboli, "Effect of Post-Discharge Follow-up Care on Re-admissions among US veterans with Congestive Heart Failure: A Rural-Urban Comparison," *Rural and Remote Health* 10 (2010): 1447.

69   Ethan M. Berke, Alan N. West, Amy E. Wallace, and William B. Weeks, "Practical and Policy Implications of Using Different Rural-Urban Classification Systems: A Case Study of Inpatient Service Utilization among Veterans Administration Users," *Journal of Rural Health* 25, no. 3 (2009): 259–66, doi:10.1111/j.1748-0361.2009.00228.x.

70   Amy E. Wallace, William B. Weeks, Stanley Wang, Austin F. Lee, and Lewis E. Kazis, "Rural and Urban Disparities in Health-Related Quality of Life among Veterans with Psychiatric Disorders," *Psychiatric Services* 57, no. 6 (2006): 851–6, doi:10.1176/appi.ps.57.6.851; Weeks et al., "Rural-Urban Disparities," 206–7.

71 West and Weeks, "Health Care Expenditures," 1721–31.
72 Wallace et al., "Rural and Urban Disparities," 853–4; Weeks et al., "Rural-Urban Disparities," 206–7.
73 Nelda P. Wray, Thomas W. Weiss, Carol E. Christian, Terri Menke, Carol M. Ashton, and John C. Hollingsworth, "The Health Status of Veterans Using Mobile Clinics in Rural Areas," *Journal of Health Care for the Poor and Undeserved* 10, no. 3 (1999): 338–48.
74 Wallace et al., "Rural and Urban Disparities," 853–4; Weeks et al., "Differences in Health," 1764–5; Weeks et al., "Rural-Urban Disparities," 206–7.
75 Mohamed, Neale, and Rosenheck, "VA Intensive Mental Health Case Management," 916–18.
76 Gordon et al., "Personal, Medical, and Healthcare Utilization," 67–9.
77 Weeks et al., "Differences in Health," 1764–5; Weeks et al., "Research on Rural Veterans," 338–40.
78 Fortney et al., "Impact of Geographic Accessibility and Treatment," 888–90.
79 Cully et al., "Use of Psychotherapy," 228–9.
80 William B. Weeks, Richard E. Lee, Amy E. Wallace, Alan N. West, and James P. Bagian. "Do Older Rural and Urban Veterans Experience Different Rates of Unplanned Readmission to VA and non-VA Hospitals?," *Journal of Rural Health* 25, no. 1 (2009): 62–9, doi:10.1111/j.1748-0361.2009.00200.x.
81 Mohamed, Neale, and Rosenheck, "VA Intensive Mental Health Case Management," 916–18.
82 David L. Nash, Jamie Wilkinson, Bryce Paradis, Stephanie Kelley, Ahsan Naseem, and Kathleen M. Grant, "Trauma and Substance Use Disorders in Rural and Urban Veterans," *Journal of Rural Health* 27, no. 2 (2011): 151–8, doi:10.1111/j.1748-0361.2010.00326.x.
83 Eric Garshick, Francine Laden, Jaime E. Hart, and Amy Caron, "Residence Near a Major Road and Respiratory Symptoms in U.S. Veterans," *Epidemiology* 14, no. 6 (2003): 728–36, doi:10.1097/01.ede.0000082045.50073.66.
84 Wallace et al., "Rural and Urban Disparities," 853–4; Wallace et al., "Longitudinal Analysis," 158; Weeks et al., "Differences in Health," 1764–5; Weeks et al., "Rural-Urban Disparities," 206–7; West and Weeks, "Physical and Mental Health," 11–13; West and Weeks, "Health Care Expenditures," 1721–31.
85 Okrah et al., "Echocardiogram Utilization," 214–16; Weeks et al., "Differences in Health," 1764–5; Weeks et al., "Rural-Urban Disparities," 206–7; Weeks et al., "Research on Rural Veterans," 338–40.
86 Gordon et al., "Personal, Medical, and Healthcare Utilization," 67–9; Mohamed, Neale, and Rosenheck, "VA Intensive Mental Health Case Management," 916–18.
87 MacKenzie et al., "Impact of Rural Residence," 319–21.
88 Weeks et al., "Do Older Rural and Urban Veterans," 65–6.
89 Wray et al., "Health Status of Veterans," 342–3.
90 Mario Schootman and Laurence Fuortes, "Functional Status Following Traumatic Brain Injuries: Population-Based Rural-Urban Differences," *Brain Injury* 13, no. 12 (1999): 995–1004.
91 Weeks et al. "Research on Rural Veterans," 340.
92 Gordon et al., "Personal, Medical, and Healthcare Utilization," 67.

93 Hynes et al., "Veterans' Access to and Use of Medicare," 216; Muus et al., "Effect of Post-Discharge Follow-up Care," 1447.

94 Cully et al., "Use of Psychotherapy," 227; MacKenzie et al., "Impact of Rural Residence," 319; Mohamed, Neale, and Rosenheck, "VA Intensive Mental Health Case Management," 915; Okrah et al., "Echocardiogram Utilization," 213; Wallace et al., "Rural and Urban Disparities," 852–3; Wallace et al., "Unintended Consequences," 669–70; Wallace et al., "Longitudinal Analysis," 157; Weeks et al., "Differences in Health," 1763; Weeks et al., "Veterans Health Administration," 168–9; Weeks et al., "Rural-Urban Disparities," 205–6; West and Weeks, "Physical and Mental Health," 10; West et al., "Rural Veterans and Access," 1739.

95 Cully et al., "Use of Psychotherapy," 227.

96 Wallace et al., "Rural and Urban Disparities," 852–3; Wallace et al., "Unintended Consequences," 669–70; Weeks et al., "Rural-Urban Disparities," 205–6.

97 West and Weeks, "Physical and Mental Health," 10; Weeks et al., "Veterans Health Administration," 168–9.

98 Okrah et al., "Echocardiogram Utilization," 213; Wallace et al., "Longitudinal Analysis," 157; Weeks et al., "Differences in Health," 1763; West et al., "Rural Veterans and Access," 1739.

99 MacKenzie et al., "Impact of Rural Residence," 319; Mohamed, Neale, and Rosenheck, "VA Intensive Mental Health Case Management," 915; Thorpe et al., "Rural-Urban Differences in Preventable Hospitalizations," 148.

100 Berke et al. "Practical and Policy Implications," 259–66.

101 Sobal et al., "Rural-Urban Differences in Obesity," 295–9.

102 Wilcox et al., "Determinants of Leisure Time Physical Activity," 669–71.

103 Parks et al., "Differential Correlates of Physical Activity," 32–4.

104 Health Canada, *Canadian Guidelines for Body Weight Classification in Adults* (Ottawa: Health Canada Publications Centre, 2003): 6–7; Public Health Agency of Canada, "The Benefits of Physical Activity," http://www.phac-aspc.gc.ca/alw-vat/intro/key-cle-eng.php.

105 Okrah et al., "Echocardiogram Utilization," 214–16.

106 Icek Ajzen, "The Theory of Planned Behaviour," *Organizational Behavior and Human Decision Processes* 50 (1991): 179–211, doi:10.1016/0749-5978(91)90020-T.

107 Irwin M. Rosenstock, Victor J. Strecher, and Marshall H. Becker, "Social Learning Theory and the Health Belief Model," *Health Education and Behavior* 15, no. 2 (1988): 175–83, doi:10.1177/109019818801500203.

108 Joseph A. Boscarino, "Posttraumatic Stress Disorder, Exposure to Combat, and Lower Plasma Cortisol among Vietnam Veterans: Findings and Clinical Implications," *Journal of Consulting and Clinical Psychology* 64, no. 1 (1996): 191–201, doi:10.1037/0022-006X.64.1.191; Jillian F. Ikin, Malcolm R. Sim, Mark C. Creamer, Andrew B. Forbes, Dean P. McKenzie, Helen L. Kelsall, Deborah C. Glass, Alexander C. McFarlane, Michael J. Abramson, Peter Ittak, Terry Dwyer, Leigh Blizzard, Kerry R. Delaney, Keith W. A. Horsley, Warren K. Harrex, and Harry Schwarz, "War-Related Psychological Stressors and Risk of Psychological Disorders in Australian Veterans of the 1991 Gulf War," *British Journal of Psychiatry* 185 (2004): 116–26, doi:10.1192/bjp.185.2.116.

18

Transition-Focused Treatment: An Uncontrolled Study of a Group Program for Veterans

DANIEL W. COX, TIMOTHY G. BLACK, MARVIN J. WESTWOOD, AND ERIC K. H. CHAN

Abstract

Major depression is the most common psychiatric disorder among Canadian Forces members and is exacerbated by reduced social support. Social support being an important protective factor indicates interpersonally focused mental health programs as potentially helpful for reducing psychiatric distress. This chapter examines the impact of the Veterans Transition Program (VTP) – a group-based approach – on reducing depression among Canadian veterans with mild, moderate, or severe depressive symptoms. Thirty-nine veterans attended all phases of the VTP and completed a pre- and post-test measure of depression (i.e., Beck Depression Inventory–II). Participants were categorized into three groups that were organized by depressive symptom severity. Significant improvement was found for all three groups ($p < .001$) and all effect sizes were large. Results indicate that following the VTP, veterans have reduced depressive symptoms, and change occurs regardless of initial symptom severity. These findings encourage future research on the effects of the VTP.

Introduction

In a recent survey of Canadian veterans, approximately one-quarter reported a difficult adjustment to civilian life.[1] Further, the most difficult adjustment was reported by veterans released for medical reasons, followed by those who were widowed, separated, or divorced. While there are many barriers to successful transition, chief among them are the psychiatric disorders associated with veteran status.[2] In the Canadian Forces (CF), major depression is the most prevalent psychiatric disorder, with rates approximately three times greater than post traumatic stress disorder (PTSD).[3] Depression's relationship with suicidality further increases the importance of understanding and treating the disorder. In studies of

CF members, depression was identified as the psychiatric disorder most predictive of suicide ideation *and* suicide attempts.[4] Together, these findings indicate that depression is one of the strongest barriers to transition among Canadian veterans, and thus an important outcome for veteran mental health programs to attend to.

While much of the research on the mental health impact of trauma on military members and veterans has focused on PTSD, researchers have also identified trauma as a predictor of depression. In studies of CF members, combat, peacekeeping, and witnessing atrocities or massacres has been correlated with major depression.[5] Further, the members' number of lifetime traumas predicts depression.[6] These findings are consistent with previous research using international samples and samples from across the lifespan.[7]

Social support is one of the strongest mediating factors in the relationship between trauma and depression.[8] The importance of social support is particularly relevant for veterans. Because they experience large amounts of social cohesion while serving[9] and often lose this support when they leave the CF, difficulties with transition are exacerbated.[10] While individual therapy is commonly used with veterans to treat psychiatric barriers to transition, group modalities treat psychiatric concerns while attending to the loss of community.[11] Several studies found that participation in group psychotherapy increased participants' perceived social support outside of the group.[12] Further, this increase in social support is greater for group than individual psychotherapy[13] and mediates depressive symptom reduction.[14] Cumulatively, these findings suggest that the interpersonal nature of group psychotherapy improves participants' perceived social support outside of the group, which reduces depressive symptoms.

The current study investigates the pre- to post-impact of the Veterans Transition Program (VTP) – a group-based approach for reducing barriers to transition – on decreasing depressive symptoms in Canadian veterans. While previous investigations have demonstrated the value of the VTP, they are limited by sample heterogeneity.[15] The current study goes beyond those by examining the impact of the VTP on veterans with mild, moderate, or severe depressive symptoms.

Methods

Participants

Veterans were referred to the VTP by fellow veterans or health-care professionals. The inclusion criterion was having a traumatic experience that was causing distress. Exclusion criteria included active psychotic symptoms, active suicidality, and refusal to abstain from drug and alcohol use during treatment.

The total sample, which has been reported in another publication,[16] consisted of fifty-six male veterans. The present analyses included only the thirty-nine veterans whose depression scores indicated mild, moderate, or severe depression – creating a more homogenous sample than previously analyzed. Participants were a mean age of 41.6 years (SD = 14.23). Twenty were married or in a common-law relationship, twelve were single, six were divorced or separated, and one was widowed. Among participants, thirty-one were Caucasian, six were First Nations, one was Arab, and one was Latin American.

Measure

The Beck Depression Inventory-II is a twenty-one-item (4-point scale) self-report measure of depressive symptoms.[17] Participants rate how they felt during the past two weeks, including today. Responses are summed for total depression scores, with greater scores indicating greater severity. Scores are categorized as follows: fourteen to nineteen indicate mild depression, twenty to twenty-eight indicate moderate depression, and twenty-nine to sixty-three indicate severe depression.

Procedure

Participants completed the BDI–II at the beginning of the first day and at the end of the last day of the Veterans Transition Program (VTP), a group-based, transition-focused treatment program for veterans of the Canadian Forces who are struggling with transitioning to civilian life.[18] The VTP assists veterans in identifying, addressing, and removing emotional, relational, and career-related barriers to successful transition. Group members consist of six to eight veterans, and the group is facilitated by two registered psychologists or one psychologist and one medical doctor with training in group counselling. In addition, two paraprofessionals who are veterans who had been through the VTP and had since completed a certificate program training them on basic therapeutic skills are in each group.

The VTP occurs over ten days in a retreat setting, where participants and facilitators live, eat, and sleep in shared quarters. The ten days are divided into three phases with approximately one month between each phase.

Phase One: Group Building and Life Review (4 Days)

The first phase focuses on introducing group members to each other, orienting members to the format and content of the program, establishing guidelines for participation (i.e. group norms), and addressing questions and concerns. Facilitators employ a number of techniques and exercises to establish adequate group cohesion. Group members learn and practise active listening skills with fellow group members through guided reflection by group facilitators on their proudest moment in the military. The main activity during this phase is a structured and guided process called life review, focusing on two main themes: major branching points in my life and my experiences of unnatural or abnormal events. In life review, each veteran writes a two-page reflection on the theme via a worksheet with guiding questions. Each veteran reads his or her reflection to the group, and group members respond to the reading by letting the reader know which aspect of the story affected them the most and why. The leaders reinforce active listening and help participants articulate their responses.

Life review is the focus of approximately three of the four days, providing many opportunities for members to practise active listening skills, disclose personal experiences in a structured way, and develop cohesion. The end of phase one includes personal goal setting for the weeks between phases one and two. Participants are taught to set realistic and attainable goals, which they verbally present to the group as a means of ensuring goal commitment and follow-through.

Phase Two: Therapeutic Enactment (4 Days)

The focus of phase two is removing barriers to transition via therapeutic enactment (TE).[19] While a full description of TE is beyond the scope of this chapter, following is a summary. Building on the life reviews from phase one, each group member identifies a target traumatic event that is causing substantial distress. Then – one group member at a time – those traumatic events are enacted, like a scene in a play. Prior to the TE, an extended planning and preparation phase occurs. The facilitators engage in focused dialogue with the participant to identify (1) what happened that should not have happened and (2) what needs to happen now for the person to move beyond the event. Once these two foci have been identified, the facilitators plan each step of the TE with the veteran, according to what the veteran feels would work best and in accordance with the therapeutic possibilities and limits identified by the facilitators. Then the TE is enacted in the group, with fellow group members assuming roles to assist the veteran doing the TE. Once the TE is done, the group processes the TE together, with group members providing feedback (as in phase one) to the participant about the part of the enactment that affected them the most. As in phase one, the end of phase two includes member goal-setting and goal presentation to the group.

Phase Three: Integration, Goal Consolidation, and Closing (2 Days)

During phase three, group members report their progress towards the goals they identified throughout the VTP and set final goals for themselves. Members reflect on what they are taking from all the exercises, skills practised, and interactions. Finally, facilitators discuss referrals to community resources for emotional, physical, family, and relationship concerns.

Data Analyses

All thirty-nine veterans completed all phases of the VTP as well as the pre- and post-assessment. Among all BDI–IIs, three items were left blank by respondents

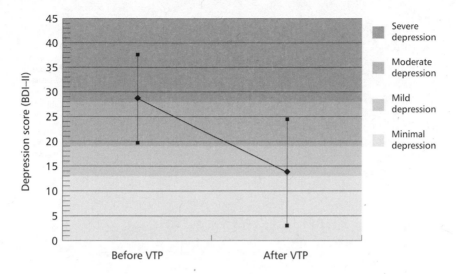

Figure 18.1 | BDI–II change among veterans with mild, moderate, or severe pre-VTP depression scores ($n = 39$).

(0.003% missing data). Following Tabachnick and Fidell's guidelines,[20] data were imputed via the expectation maximization algorithm. The normality assumption was then evaluated – based on skewness and kurtosis values. The data did not depart from normality.

Three analyses were conducted using paired-sample t tests to evaluate BDI–II score change from pre- to post-treatment. First, all veterans with mild, moderate, or severe BDI–II scores were analyzed ($n = 39$). Second, veterans with moderate or severe BDI–II scores were analyzed ($n = 33$). Third, veterans with severe BDI–II scores were analyzed ($n = 17$). Further, Cohen's d standardized mean difference effect sizes were computed.[21] Effect sizes of 0.2, 0.5, and 0.8 represent small, medium, and large effect sizes, respectively.

Results

Among veterans categorized as mildly, moderately, or severely depressed, BDI–II scores significantly dropped from pre- ($M = 28.65$; $SD = 8.95$) to post-treatment ($M = 13.74$; $SD = 10.72$), $t(38) = 9.71$, $p < .001$, $d = 1.55$) (figure 18.1). Among veterans categorized as moderately or severely depressed, BDI–II scores significantly dropped from pre- ($M = 30.89$; $SD = 7.81$) to post-treatment ($M = 14.66$; $SD = 11.12$), $t(32) = 9.72$, $p < .001$, $d = 1.69$) (figure 18.2). Among veterans categorized as severely depressed, BDI–II scores significantly dropped from pre- ($M = 36.80$; SD

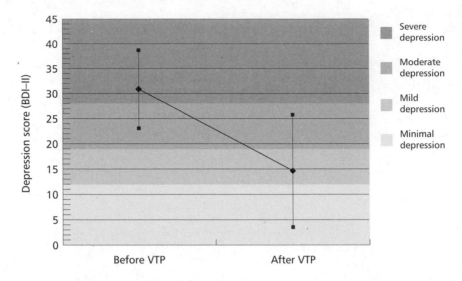

Figure 18.2 | BDI–II change among veterans with moderate or severe pre-VTP depression scores (*n* = 33)

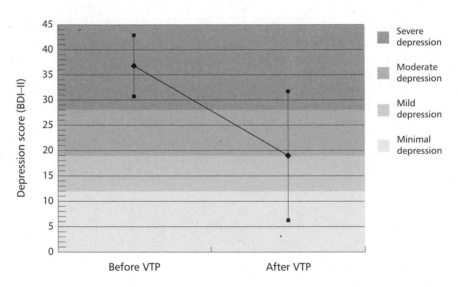

Figure 18.3 | BDI–II change among veterans with severe pre-VTP depression scores (*n* = 17)

= 6.09) to post-treatment (M = 18.99; SD = 12.72), $t(16)$ = 6.66, p < .001, d = 1.62) (figure 18.3).

Discussion

The present study demonstrates that veterans with mild, moderate, and severe depressive symptoms experience symptom reduction from pre- to post-VTP. These findings build on the previous literature demonstrating the impact of the VTP.[22]

While research indicates the difficulty Canadian veterans have transitioning to civilian life,[23] there are few programs that aid veterans in that process. Further, the treatments that attend to veterans' psychiatric concerns often occur in one-on-one settings, despite impoverished social support being a significant predictor of psychiatric distress and impaired transition.[24] We identify the VTP as *transition-focused treatment*, an approach that integrates transition and treatment by incorporating psychological interventions with peer support to reduce psychiatric barriers to care (e.g., depressive symptoms) to help veterans transition into civilian life. Our findings provide depth to understanding the VTP's impact. All three categories of depressive symptom severity analyzed had significantly reduced depressive symptoms. Further, pre-VTP depression score means of all three groups fell into the severely depressed range. Following the VTP, they were all categorized as mildly depressed – indicating clinically significant change.[25] These data support the ability of a transition-focused treatment approach for reducing psychiatric (i.e., depressive) symptoms.

This study has several limitations that promote future research. First, there is no control group. While our findings are encouraging, it is unknown how much of the change is due to treatment versus some other variable or set of variables. Having a control group would improve the internal validity of VTP evaluation. Future studies including a control group would more clearly indicate if the VTP is the causal ingredient in symptom reduction. Second, while the improvements observed are statistically significant and clinically meaningful, it is unknown how or if they persist over time. Efforts are being made to obtain these data, and their collection and analysis will further aid in understanding the value of the VTP. Also, our assessment of depression is based on the BDI–II, a psychometrically sound, yet limited, measure of depression.[26] A more sophisticated diagnostic tool, such as the structured clinical interview for DSM–IV, would allow a more accurate diagnostic understanding of veterans in the VTP and their change on depressive symptoms and diagnosis. Finally, on the basis of theory and previous research, we argued that group-based psychotherapy (i.e., the VTP) will increase participants' perceived social support, which will reduce depressive symptoms. However, we did not measure perceived social support. In the future, conducting a mediational analysis assessing how participants' changes in perceived social support influence depressive symptoms would improve our understanding of the VTP's active ingredients.

This study also had several strengths. First, the primary outcome variable was depressive symptoms. While depression is noted as the most common psychiatric disorder among CF members [27] and a consequence of military-related trauma,[28] it is often neglected in veteran treatment studies that instead focus on post traumatic stress disorder. Also, while previous analyses have evaluated the VTP, samples used were diagnostically heterogeneous.[29] The present sub-analyses increased the homogeneity of the VTP sample by including only participants whose pre-depression scores were mild, moderate, or severe. We then created even more homogeneous samples by restricting the range of inclusion to moderate and severe, followed by solely severe depression levels. These analyses provide greater depth of understanding about the impact of the VTP on veterans.

Notes

1 Jim Thompson, Mary Beth MacLean, Linda Van Til, Kerry Sudom, Jill Sweet, Alain Poirier, Jonathan Adams, Vaughn Horton, Catherine Campbell, and David Pedlar, "Survey on Transition to Civilian Life: Report on Regular Force Veterans," Veterans Affairs Canada and Department of National Defence, 4 January 2011, http://publications.gc.ca/collections/collection_2011/acc-vac/V32-231-2011-eng.pdf.

2 James R. Rundell and Robert J. Ursano, "Psychiatric Responses to War Trauma," in *Emotional Aftermath of the Persian Gulf War: Veterans, Families, Communities, and Nations,* ed. Robert J. Ursano and Ann E. Norwood, 43–81 (Washington, DC: American Psychiatric Publications, 1996).

3 Jitender Sareen, Shay-Lee Belik, Murray Stein, and Gordon J. G. Asmundson, "Correlates of Perceived Need for Mental Health Care among Active Military Personnel," *Psychiatric Services* 61, no. 1 (2010): 50–7; Jitender Sareen, Brian J. Cox, Tracie O. Afifi, Murray B. Stein, Shay-Lee Belik, Graham Meadows, and Gordon J. G. Asmundson, "Combat and Peacekeeping Operations in Relation to Prevalence of Mental Disorders and Perceived Need for Mental Health Care: Findings from a Large Representative Sample of Military Personnel," *Archives of General Psychiatry* 64, no. 7 (2007): 843–52.

4 Shay-Lee Belik, Murray B. Stein, Gordon J. G. Asmundson, and Jitender Sareen, "Are Canadian Soldiers More Likely to Have Suicidal Ideation and Suicide Attempts Than Canadian Civilians?," *American Journal of Epidemiology* 172, no. 11 (2010): 1250–8; Charles Nelson, Kate S. Cyr, Bradley E. Corbett, Elisa Hurley, Shannon Gifford, Jon D. Elhai, and J. Donald Richardson, "Predictors of Posttraumatic Stress Disorder, Depression, and Suicidal Ideation among Canadian Forces Personnel in a National Canadian Military Health Survey," *Journal of Psychiatric Research* 45, no. 11 (2011): 1483–8.

5 Sareen et al., "Combat and Peacekeeping Operations"; Jitender Sareen, Shay-Lee Belik, Tracie O. Afifi, Gordon J. G. Asmundson, Brian J. Cox, and Murray B. Stein, "Canadian Military Personnel's Population Attributable Fractions of Mental

Disorders and Mental Health Service Use Associated with Combat and Peacekeeping Operations," *American Journal of Public Health* 98, no. 12 (2008): 2191–8.

6 Nelson et al., "Predictors of Posttraumatic Stress."

7 G. A. Fava, F. Munari, L. Pavan, and R. Kellner, "Life Events and Depression: A Replication," *Journal of Affective Disorders* 3, no. 2 (1981): 159–65; Linda N. Freeman, Hartmut Mokros, and Elva O. Poznanski, "Violent Events Reported by Normal Urban School-Aged Children: Characteristics and Depression Correlates," *Journal of the American Academy of Child & Adolescent Psychiatry* 32, no. 2 (1993): 419–23; Vivian Kraaij, Ella Arensman, and Philip Spinhoven, "Negative Life Events and Depression in Elderly Persons: A Meta-Analysis," *Journals of Gerontology Series B: Psychological Sciences and Social Sciences* 57, no. 1 (2002): 87–94; Andreas Maercker, Tanja Michael, Lydia Fehm, Eni S. Becker, and Jürgen Margraf, "Age of Traumatisation as a Predictor of Post-Traumatic Stress Disorder or Major Depression in Young Women," *British Journal of Psychiatry* 184, no. 6 (2004): 482–7; Scott Vrana and Dean Lauterbach, "Prevalence of Traumatic Events and Post-Traumatic Psychological Symptoms in a Nonclinical Sample of College Students," *Journal of Traumatic Stress* 7, no. 2 (2006): 289–302.

8 Nelson et al., "Predictors of Posttraumatic Stress."

9 Harold Braswell and Howard I. Kushner, "Suicide, Social Integration, and Masculinity in the US Military," *Social Science & Medicine* 74, no. 4 (2012): 530–6.

10 Ronald J. Koshes, "The Care of Those Returned: Psychiatric Illnesses of War," in *Emotional Aftermath of the Persian Gulf War: Veterans, Families, Communities and Nations*, ed. Robert Ursano and Ann Norwood, 393–414 (Arlington, VA: American Psychiatric Publication, 1996); Marvin J. Westwood, Timothy G. Black, Stefan Kammhuber, and Alexander C. McFarlane, "Case Incident 18: The Transition from Veteran Life to the Civilian World," in *Case Incidents in Counseling for International Transitions*, ed. Nancy Arthur and Paul Pederson, 297–311 (Alexandria, VA: American Counseling Association, 2008).

11 Irving D. Yalom, *The Theory and Practice of Group Psychotherapy* (New York: Basic Books, 2005).

12 Miri Cohen and Abraham Kuten, "Cognitive-Behavior Group Intervention for Relatives of Cancer Patients: A Controlled Study," *Journal of Psychosomatic Research* 61, no. 2 (2006): 187–96; Brent Mallinckrodt, "Social Support and the Effectiveness of Group Therapy," *Journal of Counseling Psychology* 36, no. 2 (1989): 170–5; John S. Ogrodniczuk, Anthony S. Joyce, and William E. Piper, "Changes in Perceived Social Support after Group Therapy for Complicated Grief," *Journal of Nervous and Mental Disease* 191, no. 8 (2003): 524–30.

13 Eunice Chen, Stephen W. Touyz, Pierre J. V. Beumont, Christopher G. Fairburn, Rosalyn Griffiths, Phyllis Butow, Janice Russell, David E. Schotte, Robert Gertler, and Christopher Basten, "Comparison of Group and Individual Cognitive-Behavioral Therapy for Patients with Bulimia Nervosa," *International Journal of Eating Disorders* 33, no. 3 (2003): 241–54.

14 Ogrodniczuk, Joyce, and Piper, "Changes in Perceived Social Support," 524–30.

15 Marvin J. Westwood, Daniel W. Cox, Stuart M. Hoover, Eric K. H. Chan, Carson A. Kivari, Michael R. Dadson, and Bruno D. Zumbo, "The Evaluation of a Group Intervention for Veterens Who Experienced Military-Related Trauma," under

review; Marvin J. Westwood, Holly McLean, Douglas Cave, William Borgen, and Paul Slakov, "Coming Home: A Group-Based Approach for Assisting Military Veterans in Transition," *Journal for Specialists in Group Work* 35, no. 1 (2010): 44–68.

16 Westwood et al., "Evaluation of a Group Intervention."

17 Aaron T. Beck, Robert A. Steer, and Gregory K. Brown, *Manual for the Beck Depression Inventory – II* (San Antonio, TX: Psychological Corporation, 1996).

18 Westwood et al., "Coming Home: A Group-Based Approach."

19 Marvin J. Westwood and Patricia Wilensky, *Therapeutic Enactment: Restoring Vitality through Trauma Repair in Groups* (Vancouver, BC: Group Action, 2005).

20 Barbara G. Tabachnick and Linda S. Fidell, *Using Multivariate Statistics*, 5th ed. (Boston: Allyn and Bacon, 2007).

21 Jacob Cohen, *Statistical Power Analysis in the Behavioral Sciences*, 2nd ed. (Hillsdale, NJ: Erlbaum, 1988).

22 Westwood et al., "Evaluation of a Group Intervention"; Westwood et al., "Coming Home: A Group-Based Approach."

23 Thompson et al., "Survey on Transition," 70–2.

24 Nelson et al., "Predictors of Posttraumatic Stress"; Westwood et al., "Case Incident 18."

25 Neil S. Jacobson and Paula Truax, "Clinical Significance: A Statistical Approach to Defining Meaningful Change in Psychotherapy Research," *Journal of Consulting and Clinical Psychology* 59, no. 1 (1991): 12–19.

26 Beck, Steer, and Brown, *Manual for the Beck Depression Inventory – II.*

27 Sareen et al., "Correlates of Perceived Need"; Sareen et al., "Combat and Peacekeeping Operations."

28 Ibid.; Nelson et al., "Predictors of Posttraumatic Stress"; Sareen et al., "Canadian Military Personnel's Population."

29 Westwood et al., "Evaluation of a Group Intervention"; Westwood et al., "Coming Home: A Group-Based Approach."

19

The Paradox of Military Training: Survival on the Streets among Homeless Veterans

SUSAN L. RAY, KAREN E. HAINES, AND MARIE S. S. LONGO

Abstract

This secondary analysis of the first national study on homelessness among veterans of the Canadian Forces (CF) and Allied Forces (AF) explores homeless veterans' survival on the streets as both helped and hindered by their military training. An interpretive phenomenological approach was used as the methodology for the study. Although all fifty-four transcripts from the primary study were reviewed, fifteen were chosen because these participants spoke extensively about their lives on the streets. Military training as a double-edged sword for homeless veterans is the overarching analytical interpretation that emerged. Common sub-themes were identified until an understanding of homeless veterans' survival on the streets was attained. The three sub-themes illustrate the paradox.

Sub-theme one: Although their military training prepares them for survival on the streets such as sleeping rough, they may keep their distance from others and may therefore have difficulty in accessing services.

Sub-theme two: The training to "fight" if directed onto civilian society can result in difficulties obtaining and retaining employment, difficulties in relationships, and difficulties with the law.

Sub-theme three: Difficulties developing an autonomous adult identity as normal development can be interrupted by military training that precludes independent decision-making, which is a required adult coping ability.

Health-care service providers need to recognize, validate, and respond to the effects – positive and negative – of life in the armed forces for homeless veterans in order to provide the best care. Building upon their strengths attained during their military training and education about conflict resolution, assertiveness, and the provision of counselling to build an adult identity post-military are some of the implications from this study.

Introduction

Over the generations, young recruits have entered the military to serve their country, further educational goals, develop a promising career, or use it as a stepping stone to better prepare for adult responsibilities of civilian life.[1] The military offers promise to young recruits, but the challenges of training and serving at home and in wartime or on peacekeeping missions are intense, complex, and often violent and may result in long-lasting physical and psychological consequences.[2] Recent changes from peacekeeping to peace-making and deployment of CF troops have led to an increase in traumatic experiences.[3] As a result, there is increased potential for higher numbers of homeless veterans with undiagnosed and untreated psychiatric disorders.[4] It is estimated that 30% of CF veterans transitioning to civilian life have an operational stress injury (OSI), described as "any persistent psychological difficulty that has resulted from military service," such as post traumatic stress disorder (PTSD), addiction, or other mental health problems.[5] Many of these returning veterans have undiagnosed addictions and mental health problems and suffer in silence.[6]

Transitioning from military life to civilian life includes interpersonal, emotional, and social challenges.[7] A younger generation of veterans with different expectations, a greater volume of operational injuries, new emerging injuries, and the cumulative impact of years of increased and sustained military operations on members and their families suggest that transitional needs are and will be significantly different from what have been offered in the past.[8] Even though there are relatively few young veterans in the Canadian homeless population, there are already signs of potential trouble. Without adequate transitional services, many young veterans returning to civilian life will spiral into poverty and homelessness.[9] At this time, little is known about homelessness among the CF and AF veterans. The purpose of this secondary analysis of the first national study on homelessness among veterans of the CF and AF[10] is to deepen our understanding of the experience of homeless veterans' survival on the streets as both helped and hindered by their military training.

Literature Review on Homeless Veterans

The literature review includes international studies on the numbers of homeless veterans; demographics including psychiatric co-morbidity; homeless veterans and violence; and the first national study on homelessness among CF and AF veterans. International research indicates that the number of homeless people in the veteran community is quite significant. In the United States, for example, veterans comprise 11% of the total male population aged eighteen and over, but account for more than 26% of the male homeless population.[11] In Australia, researchers estimate that at least 3,000 homeless veterans, representing 3% of the homeless population, are living on the streets.[12] Researchers in the United Kingdom suggest that

6% of London's homeless population served in the military with approximately 3,600 veterans sleeping in shelters, hostels, or on the streets.[13]

Increased awareness within the media has revealed that many CF veterans who once served our country no longer have a home. Findings from the first national study inferred that, on the basis of the available international research related to homelessness, the number of homeless veterans in Canada ranges from 3% to 26% of the homeless population.[14]

Demographics Including Psychiatric Co-Morbidity on Homeless Veterans

Most of the research literature on homeless veterans is from the United States, with most of the studies from the 1980s Vietnam War era. Compared to the homeless civilian population, homeless veterans are older and more likely to be white, have served time in jail, have problems related to alcohol abuse, and are more likely to have been hospitalized for a psychiatric or a substance abuse problem.[15] Re-analyzed data from three surveys conducted during the late 1980s found that homeless veterans were more likely to be better educated, and more often previously or currently married, but were not different on indicators of residential instability, current social functioning, physical health, mental illness, or substance abuse.[16] Thus, the factors related to veteran homelessness in the Vietnam War era appear inconclusive.

More recent articles from the United States indicate a continuing complex number of influences that predispose veterans to homelessness, including post-military psychiatric disorder, especially depression, schizophrenia,[17] and PTSD,[18] poverty, alcohol and substance use, social isolation,[19] low socio-economic status at the time of service entry,[20] service in the Vietnam war,[21] and involvement with the criminal justice system.[22]

In developing a "Five Year Plan to End Homelessness among Veterans" by 2015, the U.S. Department of Veterans Affairs (DVA) has committed to help veterans transition to civilian life.[23] A sample of more than one million veterans accessing the DVA mental health services determined that the demographic characteristics of being male, aged forty to sixty-four years, Black or other minority group, and having an income below $7,000 per year predicted post-military homelessness.[24] Although the study results demonstrate that 9.7% of veterans in this sample were considered homeless, veterans who served in Afghanistan and Iraq were protected from homelessness. This result was interpreted as an effective outcome of the DVA's outreach to aid veterans' access to services.

Homeless Veterans and Violence

In a 2009 study of 2,012 recently booked arrestees in Arizona, 132 of the arrestees were homeless veterans.[25] Only 16% of the veteran arrestees reported military service after the Iraq or Afghanistan wars, with the majority serving more than ten years ago. Most of the veterans were charged after violent offences and demonstrated substantially higher rates of opiate and crack cocaine use. Even though the sample was a small portion of the arrestees in an Arizona county jail, as many as 8,000 military veterans might have been arrested there. Therefore, it appears that a greater number of veterans might be arrested in the United States after using violence than have been recognized. These researchers conclude that a relationship between violence and military service is mediated by PTSD, other mental illnesses, traumatic brain injury, and illicit drug use.[26]

The tenets of the violent veteran model suggest military training provides soldiers with survival skills, primarily through use of violence, but these skills are not "untaught" upon discharge from the military.[27] Over the years, however, empirical support for the violent veteran model has been mixed. Recent research supporting the model suggests that trauma and combat exposure, PTSD symptoms, substance abuse, and post-deployment adjustment problems may be positive predictors of incarceration for veterans.[28] However, using data from the National Vietnam Veterans Readjustment Study,[29] researchers concluded that veterans who exhibited antisocial behaviour after deployment tended to have long histories of conduct problems before entering the military (e.g., pre-existing conditions). In a mixed-method study of veterans who had been deployed to Iraq and Afghanistan, veterans who subsequently developed military-related PTSD had increased rates of intimate partner violence.[30]

First National Study on Homelessness among CF and AF Veterans

The results of the first national study on homelessness among CF and AF veterans indicated that although homelessness may have occurred many years after military service, homeless veterans struggle during the transition into civilian life.[31] Issues such as alcohol abuse, drug addiction, and mental illness arise during or after military discharge and lead to veterans' living on the streets. Despite the significant findings and recommendations from this first national study, a major issue emerged that was left unexplored. The veterans described military training as both helping and hindering their transition to civilian life. Therefore, a secondary analysis that utilizes existing data was conducted to explore this issue in greater depth in order to provide further insights into how best to care for this population.

Methodology

An interpretive phenomenological approach was used as the methodological framework guided by the life-world existentials of lived body (corporeality), lived space (spatiality), lived human relation (relationality or communality), and lived time (temporality).[32] This approach is used when little is known about the research topic. The significance of an interpretive phenomenological approach rests with the opportunity to provide a richer and deeper understanding of the experience of homelessness among CF and AF veterans.

There are five distinct types of secondary analysis: *retrospective interpretation*, in which an existing database is tapped to develop themes that emerged but were not fully analyzed in the original study; *armchair induction*, in which inductive methods of textual analysis, such as hermeneutical inquiry, are applied to existing data sets, such as those constructed by another researcher; *amplified sampling*, in which comparison of several distinct and theoretically representative databases permits broader analysis than the original studies could consider; *cross validation*, in which analysis of existing data sets is used to confirm or discount patterns or themes beyond the sample with which the researcher has had personal involvement; and *analytic expansion*, in which the researcher conducts a secondary interpretation in order to put new questions to the primary material that was originally collected to address different research questions.[33] The type of secondary analysis for this study was an *analytic expansion*, as new research questions were posed.

Methods

In the primary study,[34] data were collected from 2010 to 2011, via one tape-recorded, in-depth interview with fifty-four homeless veterans from five Canadian cities. All fifty-four participants were male, with an average age of fifty-five years. On average, they had served in the CF for six years and had been released twenty-seven years ago from the CF. Eighty-seven per cent had served in the Regular CF and 13% in the Reserves. Forty-four per cent were either separated or divorced and 37% were single. The majority (42.6%) had a high school education and 74% identified themselves as Caucasian Canadian. On average they had experienced their first episode of homelessness eleven years ago and had spent a total of seven years homeless. Seventy per cent were in shelters, 26% were presently housed, and 4% were of no fixed address (NFA).

The interviewing style used in the primary study enhanced the richness of the data available to address the research questions for the secondary analysis. The veterans were not constrained with a rigid set of interview questions; instead, they were allowed to emphasize what was important to them in their experience. Thus, the veterans were able to give rich descriptions of their experience of homelessness that shed some light on the aim of our work in this secondary analysis: to deepen our understanding of homeless veterans' survival on the streets.

Data Analysis

Although all fifty-four transcripts from the primary study were reviewed, this secondary data analysis includes fifteen transcripts, selected because these participants spoke extensively about their experience of military life and homelessness.

Six interactive steps for interpretive phenomenological inquiry and analysis of data were employed: (1) orienting oneself to the phenomenon of interest and ex-plicating assumptions and pre-understandings, (2) investigating experiences as lived through conversational interviews, rather than as we conceptualize it, (3) re-flecting upon and conducting thematic analysis, which characterizes the phenom-enon and interpretation through conversations, (4) describing the phenomenon through the art of writing and rewriting (rethinking, reflecting, recognizing), which aims at creating depthful writing, (5) maintaining a strong and oriented relation to the fundamental question about the phenomenon, and (6) balancing the research context by considering parts and wholes.[35]

In secondary analysis, it is appropriate for the primary researcher to obtain in-terpretation validation by another person such as secondary researchers.[36] Veri-fication of meaning was ensured by having the primary researcher confirm with the secondary researchers the overarching analytical interpretation and the three sub-themes found in the data. As the sub-themes evolved, the primary researcher returned to the transcripts several times to verify meaning and to find exemplary quotes. The fifteen transcriptions were analyzed as in the six interactive steps to identify the sub-themes until an understanding of homeless veterans' survival on the streets as helped and hindered by their military training was attained.

Limitations

Interpretive phenomenological methodology is a type of qualitative inquiry and thus the findings cannot be generalizable to other homeless veterans and the larger military population. Transferability refers to the degree to which the results of qualitative research can be transferred to other contexts or settings.[37] The reader makes the judgment on how "transferable" the results are to a different context. The research design of a secondary analysis is a limitation because the data were not collected originally to address the specific aims of this study. In addition, a secondary analysis prevents the second step ("conversational interviews" and then returning to the participants) in data analysis from being followed.[38] Thus, the verification of the findings is limited to the primary researcher confirming the overarching analytic interpretation and the sub-themes with the secondary researchers.

Findings

Military training as a double-edged sword for homeless veterans is the overarching analytical interpretation that emerged from the analysis. The double-edged sword is described as "something that has, or can have, both favorable and unfavorable consequences."[39] Three sub-themes emerged from the overarching analytical in-terpretation of the double-edged sword: (1) military training prepares veterans for survival on the streets, (2) military training prepares one to defend oneself with aggression, if necessary, and (3) a military identity can interrupt development of an adult identity, and they illustrate the paradox that emerged. A paradox is "a statement that is seemingly contradictory or opposed to common sense and yet is perhaps true."[40] The paradox of the double-edged sword that emerged from this secondary analysis is that the positive aspects of military life that many place great value on – ability to survive in adverse situations, ability to defend oneself physically, security, structure, family-like bonds with others in the military brotherhood, camaraderie, and predictability in what must often be rather unpredictable situations – can become negative aspects upon release from the military when making the transition to civilian life. The sub-themes are not linear but overlap to form the overarching analytical interpretation of the whole. Each sub-theme found within the analysis will be illustrated with excerpts followed by an interpretation.

Sub-Theme One: Military Training Prepares Veterans for Survival on the Streets

Excerpt 1. "You need discipline to take orders. And even though discipline is valued because you have to hold your tongue and mentally tolerate things, it's good in a way too, because it helps you bypass a lot of crap … the reality of the street."

Excerpt 2. "I will never forget the sound of the 50-calibre machine guns opening up on Hell Highway … But when you take somebody out from the bush and put them into a city like Toronto, they're gone. Because these guys know how to live out in the land … And if they don't want you to find them, you aren't ever going to find them."

Excerpt 3. "The military training will stay with me all my life. I try to think before I speak, I try to choose the proper words and stuff like that before I speak. Especially because you don't want to hurt someone by using certain words. I swear once in a while, I try not to. But we're all human beings. We do get angry, we have feelings … I've been trained, like I said, in the army, and you know we know what to do; we just go along with the flow."

The excerpts reveal that veterans' experiences of homelessness are to some extent conditioned by their military experiences. The veteran in the first excerpt described how mental toughness gained from his Canadian military training was beneficial to survival on the streets, such as the personal resources of competitiveness, confidence, and staying positive.[41] The results suggest how mental skills are positively related to resilience and may have implications for the development of mental strength, specifically adaptive responses to adversity on the streets.

Our understanding or perception of our world is a mystery; however, the life-world existentials of body, relationship, time, and space ground our perception of what we experience in the world in ourselves, and in relation to others.[42] The veteran in the first excerpt refers to the discipline exacted by military training on the soldier's body and mind; it helps to build an ability to withhold reacting or responding verbally and to tolerate more, perhaps, than civilians would. In the reality of the lived space in the streets, military training appears to help veterans live above distasteful events and can be interpreted as a positive consequence. The training increases veterans' chances of survival by helping them to perceive and tolerate their life situation and withholding a negative response, and thus maintaining safety.

The second excerpt conveys an AF veteran's experience of lived combat. In considering the belief that perception is experienced by the body in the moment[43] and not after the event is over, the soldier "heard" the guns firing as the noise entered his ears before he interpreted all that the sound meant or lived with its full impact in his life. Hearing the guns go off and connecting the sound to his knowing that the bullets are killing people lives within his body; it touches his human relationships and is with him in the lived space he shares with his community.

In the third excerpt, the homeless veteran's military training has conditioned how he relates to others in the civilian world. He explains what happens inside his body; he attempts to explain his humanness, identified by emotions and feelings. Military training guides how he conducts himself relationally, and, reflecting on the existential of lived relationality, he chooses words carefully and suppresses in his body the thoughts and feelings that might cause discomfort to others.[44] By just going "along with the flow," a veteran's potential for survival on the streets is greater than if he were to disagree with or express anger to others. Although short-term survival is enhanced by carefully choosing the words to say, the long-term effect of unexpressed anger or stress on the human body can result in physical illness.[45]

Despite ongoing wear and tear on the body from the stress of trauma,[46] the veterans quoted in these excerpts describe military training as leading to a highly advanced ability to live on the land outside of social interaction or support. Although military training prepares soldiers for survival on civilian streets, they may keep their distance from other homeless people who have not had these experiences, and this may hinder or make it difficult for homeless veterans to access services. In addition, veterans may be too proud to ask for help from others, including healthcare providers.

Sub-Theme Two: Military Training to Defend Oneself with Aggression If Necessary

Excerpt 4. "Once a soldier gets in trouble in the streets, the Canadian police say, 'Oh you're a soldier tough guy' … and push, push, push. And you go being what you do not want to be … I am discriminated against in every situation … so I am at war no matter how you look at it. I said I have 165 counts of assault … There is one that never got reported. With police officers, I have three attempted murders … and it has happened in jail … It was very hard to keep my anger under control."

Excerpt 5. "At the very least you come out of the forces with an attitude. They instil this attitude into you that's no good in the workplace. I don't want anybody over my shoulder. I won't put up with it ... You know you trust me to do the job, or just f— off, basically. The biggest part, the hardest part, is the frustration."

Excerpt 6. "Military mentality ... that doesn't jive well with the rest of the world ... My hackles get up when I hear people speaking with Russian accents on the street or speaking Russian ... because when I was a kid they were targets. If I don't shoot them they're going to shoot me ... My family has been full of military people for generations. Every one of them has had trouble adjusting to the civilian world."

The training to fight, if directed onto civilian society, can result in trouble with the law, including time served in jail, difficulties in relationships, and obtaining and retaining employment. Reflecting the negative side of the double-edged sword, the soldier in the fourth excerpt describes an almost impossible existence after release from the military. His contacts with police are highlighted by anger, aggression, and violence, including 165 counts of assault, attempted murder against police, and jail time served. Military training leaves lasting effects on veterans, and confrontation or being pushed by others may exacerbate an aggressive response. If individuals are suffering from PTSD, their ability to maintain self-control in emotionally charged situations may be compromised, and reactive anger may be the result.[47] Lived experience integrates the body, mind, world, and time, which can be interpreted in this veteran's experience of his world.[48] Sensed and communicated through his embodied experience of anger exploding from inside him, the veteran renders a bleak verbal sketch of the perceived hopelessness and lack of choice that lives within him.

The veteran quoted in the fifth excerpt describes becoming irritated in the workplace. He carries frustration and impatience with authority and does not want anyone looking over his shoulder. This discomfort might reflect his experience in military service or be an indication of needing additional space to feel trusted and at ease within an unfamiliar civilian work environment. However, it might also indicate a veteran's struggle with the nerve-wracking after-effects of traumatic experiences, particularly if the veteran is experiencing PTSD. In addition, the veteran maybe frustrated by working in a "process-oriented" civilian workplace rather than the "result-oriented" military culture.

In the sixth excerpt, living with a "military mentality" has presented difficulties for the veteran in the civilian world. His early life experience of understanding Russian individuals as targets has carried over into his present life as a civilian. Through personal and military relationships he learned to defend his body against "others," who, in this case, are people who speak Russian or are of Russian descent. The veteran embodies the belief that if he does not use aggression by shooting the Russians, who live in close proximity to him, first, they will shoot him. He confirms that all of his family members with military experience have struggled with adjustment to civilian life. The damage and after-effects of trauma are known to pass between generations and can affect the relationships of the youngest to oldest within immediate and extended families.[49]

Sub-Theme Three: Military Identity When Serving Interrupts the Development of an Adult Identity

Excerpt 7. "I was actually homeless when I was, like, fifteen or sixteen, because I kept running away from home, from my adopted family ... And my buddy said, "Well, your dad is always beating you, so he understands some of the discipline ... I asked my dad for consent to join ... I just turned seventeen ... when I joined the military."

Excerpt 8. "I went from high school to the army ... All you know is the army. So it was, like, you get out and well, what am I? ... For three months I did not know what to do. You know, I got to deal with this repercussion of not eating that well anymore ... my parents didn't teach me any cooking ... In the military everything is provided ... so to have that taken away ... If you're not used to it, it could cripple you."

Excerpt 9. "They were good parents, considering that they raised a big family in the sixties. They did what they could with what they had. I felt, sort of like, when you've got a family that size, there is always one that is, sort of like, ignored."

Many homeless veterans reported enlisting in the military as teenagers,[50] and although the military offered them an identity during service (such as sailor, soldier), the military identity may have interrupted the development of their adult identity after their release to civilian life. Emerging adulthood encompasses the late teenage years, from eighteen to the late twenties.[51] For these homeless veterans, difficulty developing an autonomous and secure identity during the transition to adulthood may follow early entry to the military, because learning to adapt to military life may preclude completing the emerging adult developmental stage.[52] The ability to reach adult autonomy and independent decision-making is most significant in this process within military life, because it may be blocked and discouraged when training new recruits by insisting they obey orders and not question those in authority.

However, some homeless veterans have struggled with childhood trauma of physical, sexual, and emotional abuse, adoption, neglect, and poverty, which also may have delayed or arrested their psychological development and the development of a strong adult self-identity.[53] The lived body and lived relational existentials are echoed in Excerpts 7 and 9 by veterans who experienced childhood physical and emotional neglect.[54] The body and mind hold the after-effects of abuse that occurs at a young age and affects the victim's perception of the world and relationships.[55]

In Excerpt 8, the veteran discloses his perception of how difficult civilian life becomes without the structure of the military. Soldiers' needs for clothing, housing, equipment, and sustenance are met by the powerful military parent, without expecting those in service to attend to these common adult responsibilities on their own.

In Excerpt 9, a child's experience of feeling ignored or neglected, as an outsider to a supportive, caring relationship can be heard. The child was not supported emotionally in his closest relationships while growing up, preventing him from feeling safe and supported, and from developing a strong sense of self.

Discussion

The paradox of military training is a double-edged sword with both favourable and unfavourable consequences for homeless veterans. Training prepares veterans for survival, a favourable outcome. However, if the training to fight is directed onto civilian society, difficulties in obtaining and retaining employment, difficulties in relationships, and trouble with the law, including time served in jail, can result. The military offers a ready-made identity that can appear favourable to young recruits; however, completing the emerging adult developmental task of growing a strong and autonomous individual adult identity[56] may be interrupted during their military service.

Sub-Theme One

While many of the triggers for homelessness among veterans are similar to those commonly reported by other homeless people, it is clear that a military background influences how veterans experience homelessness, and often in profoundly favourable and unfavourable ways. Veterans consider themselves better equipped to endure and are less fearful of the hardships of street life. However, they are also less inclined to seek or accept help because of their tendency to elevate the perceived "shame" of their situation. These factors, together with a greater propensity to drink heavily – which many claim was initiated or exacerbated by the military lifestyle – combine to make veterans more susceptible to sustained or repeated instances of homelessness.

Sub-Theme Two

Soldiers are trained to defend themselves if necessary during deployments to survive. However, after the years of military service are over, ex-service personnel are expected to conform to the new civilian world expectations placed on them that require relational skills outside the realm of aggression. Military training may leave many veterans with the message to fight ingrained in their psyches and can compound the challenge not to use aggression in civilian life. When PTSD, other mental illnesses, or substance use is present in the homeless veteran's life, violence, arrest, and time served in jail are frequent outcomes.[57] The criminal justice system involvement of homeless veterans is an unfavourable outcome of the fight to survive within the expectations of the civilian world when burdened with the after-effects of military experience.

Sub-Theme Three

The military offers a ready-made identity for young recruits, and many may have enlisted before they developed a mature, adult identity.[58] In human developmental stages, adolescence has been identified as a time to develop one's identity.[59] If this stage is not successfully worked through and completed, confusion about the teen's role and purpose in life can result. With encouragement, reinforcement, and support, youth can emerge from this stage with a strong sense of identity, independence, and personal control; however, if they remain unsure of their own beliefs and desires, they will feel insecure and confused about themselves and the future. The lack of a secure sense of identity leaves individuals unfavourably dependent on external structure that, in military members, is the structure of the military establishment. It has been argued that "emerging adulthood" is a recent, culturally relevant shift in industrialized countries that has replaced the teenage "identity versus role confusion" stage.[60] Emerging adulthood occurs during the late teenage years to age thirty and provides youth with an extended time to explore and develop their self-identity outside of permanent adult commitments. The development of technology and greater wealth has enabled more youth to gain higher levels of education, and shifts in cultural values have allowed youth more time to choose a life partner and enter the workforce later than in earlier generations.[61] However, it is important to note in a discussion of the U.S. military and the transition to adulthood that military life is career and family oriented, and that this orientation assists the majority of young recruits toward responsible adult membership in their families and the wider community.[62]

In this secondary analysis, ten homeless veterans revealed histories of one or more forms of sexual, physical, or emotional abuse, adoption, neglect, or poverty during childhood. These experiences can lead to developmental arrest that can result in greater difficulty developing a healthy and strong individual adult identity.[63] To compound the difficulties of emerging into adulthood for these military veterans, those who experienced childhood abuse have been robbed of a sense of free choice and personal agency, which are necessary lived experiences in the development of a coherent and stable sense of autonomous identity.[64]

Implications for Practice, Education, and Research

These differences of experience and perception for homeless people with a military background contain messages for providers of services to homeless people. Service providers must recognize, validate, and respond to the positive and negative effects of life in the armed forces in order to provide the best care. The need to build on veterans' strengths attained during their military training and education about conflict resolution and assertiveness are some of the implications emerging from this study. The Royal Canadian Legion (RCL) and health-care agencies that specifically serve people with a military services background are particularly well placed to enable increased understanding of, and response to, veterans' attitudes and needs.

Social service programs have been launched within Canada in an attempt to respond to the homeless veteran population.[65] However, they have yet to be evaluated in research. More veterans are returning from deployments, requiring that service providers gain an advanced understanding of factors related to homelessness, of ways to build therapeutic relationships, and of ways to advocate for homeless veterans with decision-makers at political levels. Inspired by the DVA[66] program, a pilot program was launched by Veterans Affairs Canada partnered with the RCL.[67] Outreach workers in Toronto assist and coordinate resources to homeless veterans. Another implication for further consideration is the need to assist military veterans transitioning to civilian life to develop a strong and autonomous adult identity prior to leaving military service.

In conclusion, the paradox of military training as a double-edged sword that emerged from these secondary analysis data sharpened our understanding of both the favourable and unfavourable effects of military training on homeless veterans. The military identity can delay the need to grow through emerging adulthood, as young recruits join the military family and brotherhood of camaraderie. The structured military lifestyle can be poor preparation for the complex aspects of civilian life: housing, retraining, and education, etc. When the homeless veterans in this study left the military, they were left floundering without a strong sense of individual adult identity and often feel isolated and alone in the civilian world.

These difficulties can trigger the use of aggression learned in training and strengthened on deployments, which can place veterans – in particular, homeless veterans – at risk for involvement with the criminal justice system. Health-care providers need to build on veterans' strengths attained during their military training and provide education about conflict resolution and assertiveness, as well as provide education and counselling to assist veterans in building an adult identity outside of the military. This study clearly presents findings to inform future directions to better support homeless veterans transitioning to civilian life. The paradox of military training needs to be understood and addressed in order to provide the best care to those who served our country.

Notes

1 R. Kelty, D. R. Segal, and M. Kleykamp, "The Military and the Transition to Adulthood," *Future of Children* 20, no. 1 (2010): 181–207.

2 R. Dallaire, *Shake Hands with the Devil: The Failure of Humanity in Rwanda* (Toronto: Random House, 2003); C. Nelson, K. St Cyr, B. Corbett, E. Hurly, S. Gifford, J. D. Elhai, and J. D. Richardson, "Predictors of Postraumatic Stress Disorder, Depression, and Sucidal Ideation among Canadian Forces Personnel in a National Canadian Military Health Survey, *Journal of Psychiatric Research* 45 (2011): 1483–8.

3 Ibid., 1486.

4 S. L. Ray, "The Experience of Contemporary Peacekeepers Healing from Trauma," *Nursing Inquiry* 16, no. 1 (2009): 53–63.

5 Statistics Canada, CCHS *Supplement: Briefing Document* (Ottawa: Statistics Canada, 2003).

6 Ray, "Experience of Contemporary Peacekeepers," 54; S. L. Ray, "Contemporary Treatment Approaches for Trauma from the Perspective of Peacekeepers," *Canadian Journal of Nursing Research* 14, no. 2 (2009b): 114–82.

7 S. L. Ray, "Contemporary Treatment Approaches for Trauma from the Perspective of Peacekeepers," 55.

8 S. L. Ray, W. Ta'an, M. Bamford, C. Forchuk, and N. Acosta, "A Downward Spiral: Homelessness among Canadian Forces and Allied Forces Veterans," *Esprit de Corps* 18, no. 10 (2011): 42–59.

9 Ibid., 45.

10 Ibid.

11 M. Cunningham, M. Henry, and W. Lyons, *Vital Mission: Ending Homelessness among Veterans* (Washington, DC: National Alliance to End Homelessness, Homelessness Research Institute, 2007).

12 C. Chamberlain and D. MacKenzie, *Australian Census Analytic Program: Counting the Homeless* (Canberra: Australian Bureau of Statistics, 2006).

13 S. Johnsen, A. Jones, and J. Rugg, *The Experience of Homeless Ex-Service Personnel in London* (York, UK: University of York Research Report, 2008).

14 Ibid., 46.

15 M. J. Robertson, "Homeless Veterans: An Emerging Problem?," in *The Homeless in Contemporary Society*, ed. R. D. Bingham, R. E. Green, and S. B. White, 64–81 (Thousand Oaks, CA: Sage Publications, 1987); D. Roth, B. G. Toomey, and R. J. First, "Gender, Racial, and Age Variations among Homeless Persons," in *Homelessness: A National Perspective. Topics in Social Psychiatry*, ed. M. Robertson and M. Greenblatt, 199–211 (New York: Plenum, 1992); R. K. Schutt, T. Meschede, and J. Rierdan, "Distress, Suicidal Thoughts, and Social Support among Homeless Adults," *Journal of Health and Social Behavior* 35, no. 2 (1994): 134–42.

16 R. Rosenheck and P. Koegel, "Characteristics of Veterans and Nonveterans in Three Samples of Homeless Men," *Hospital & Community Psychiatry* 44, no. 9 (1993): 858–63.

17 T. Ghose, A. J. Gordon, S. Metraux, and A. C. Justice, "Mental Illness and Homelessness among Veterans," *Psychiatric Services* 62 (2012): 1514–15.

18 R. C. Tessler, R. Rosenheck, and G. Gamache, "Comparison of Homeless Veterans with Other Homeless Men in a Large Clinical Outreach Program," *Psychiatric Quarterly* 73, no. 2 (2002): 109–19.

19 Cunningham, Henry, and Lyons, *Vital Mission: Ending Homelessness among Veterans*, 10; Tessler, Rosenheck, and Gamache, "Comparison of Homeless Veterans," 111.

20 E. L. Edens, W. Kasprow, J. Tsai, and R. A. Rosenheck, "Association of Substance Use and VA Service-Connected Disability Benefits with Risk of Homelessness among Veterans," *American Journal on Addictions* 20 (2011): 412–19.

21 M. D. White, P. Mulvey, A. M. Fox, and D. Choate, "A Hero's Welcome? Exploring the Prevalence and Problems of Military Veterans in the Arrestee Population," *Justice Quarterly* 29 (2012): 258–86; B. A. Williams, J. McGuire, R. G. Lindsay, J. Baillargeon, I. S. Cnzer, S. J. Lee, and M. Kushel, "Coming Home: Health Status and Homelessness Risk of Older Pre-Release Prisoners," *Journal of General Internal Medicine* 25 (2010): 1038–44.

22 Edens et al., "Association of Substance Use," 415; White et al., "Hero's Welcome?," 260; Williams et al., "Coming Home," 1041.

23 United States Veterans Affairs, Public and Intergovernmental Affairs, *Five Year Plan Unveiled at Summit* (Washington, DC: United States Veterans Affairs, 2009).

24 Ibid., 105.

25 White et al., "Hero's Welcome?," 265.

26 Ibid., 272.

27 D. Archer and R. Gartner, "Violent Acts and Violent Times: A Comparative Approach to Postwar Homicide Rates," *American Sociological Review* 11, no. 6 (1976): 937–63.

28 J. McGuire, R. A. Rosenheck, and W. J. Kasprow, "Health Status, Service Use, and Costs among Veterans Receiving Outreach Services in Jail or Community Settings," *Psychiatric Services* 42 (2003): 201–7; A. J. Saxon, T. M. Davis, K. L. Sloan, K. M. Miles, E. McFall, and D. R. Kivlahan, "Trauma Symptoms of Posttraumatic Stress Disorder and Associated Problems among Incarcerated Veterans," *Psychiatric Services* 52 (2001): 959–64; T. Yager, R. Laufer, and M. Gallops, "Some Problems Associated with War Experience in Men of the Vietnam Generation," *Archives of General Psychiatry* 41 (1984): 327–33.

29 A. F. Fontana and R. Rosenheck, "The Role of War Zone Trauma and PTSD in the Etiology of Antisocial Behavior," *Journal of Nervous and Mental Disease* 193 (2005): 203–9.

30 E. P. Finley, M. Baker, M. J. Pugh, and A. Peterson, "Patterns and Perceptions of Intimate Partner Violence Committed by Returning Veterans with Post-Traumatic Stress Disorder," *Journal of Family Violence* 25 (2010): 737–43.

31 Ray et al., "Downward Spiral," 44.

32 M. Merleau-Ponty, *Phenomenology of Perception* (New York: Routledge, 1962); M. van Manen, *Researching Lived Experience*, 3rd ed. (London, ON: Althouse, 1998).

33 J. Heaton, *Reworking Qualitative Data* (Thousand Oaks, CA: Sage Publications, 2004); S. Thorne, "Pearls, Pith and Provocation: Ethical and Representational Issues in Secondary Analysis," *Qualitative Health Research* 8, no. 4 (1998): 547–55.

34 Ray et al., "Downward Spiral," 44.

35 Van Manen, *Researching Lived Experience*, 30.

36 V. Szabo and V. R. Strang, "Secondary Analysis of Qualitative Data: Methods of Clinical Inquiry," *Advances in Nursing Science* 20, no. 2 (1997): 66–74.

37 Y. S. Lincoln and E. G. Guba, *Naturalistic Inquiry* (Newbury Park, CA: Sage Publications, 1985).

38 Thorne, "Pearls, Pith and Provocation," 549.

39   *Merriam-Webster Dictionary*, 20th ed., s.v. "double-edged sword."

40   Ibid., s.v. "paradox."

41   M. A. Pickering, J. Hammermeister, C. Ohlson, B, Holliday, and G. Ulmer, "An Exploratory Investigation of Relationships among Mental Skills and Resilience in Warrior Transition Unit Cadre Members," *Military Medicine* 175, no. 4 (2010): 213–19.

42   Merleau-Ponty, *Phenomenology of Perception*, 83.

43   Ibid., 84.

44   Ibid., 85.

45   G. Mate, *When the Body Says No: The Cost of Hidden Stress* (Toronto: Vintage, 2004).

46   Ibid., 85.

47   White et al., "Hero's Welcome?," 275.

48   Merleau-Ponty, *Phenomenology of Perception*, 164.

49   B. A. Van der Kolk and W. d'Andrea, "Towards a Developmental Trauma Disorder Diagnosis for Childhood Interpersonal Trauma," in *The Impact of Early Life Trauma on Health and Disease*, ed. R. Lanius, E. Vermitten, and C. Pain, 57–68 (New York: Cambridge University Press, 2010).

50   Ray et al., "Downward Spiral," 44.

51   J. J. Arnett, "Emerging Adulthood: What Is It, and What Is It Good For?," *Society for Research in Child Development* 1, no. 2 (2007): 68–73.

52   Ray et al., "Downward Spiral," 45.

53   Van der Kolk and d'Andrea, *Impact of Early Life Trauma*, 60.

54   Merleau-Ponty, *Phenomenology of Perception*, 167.

55   Van der Kolk and d'Andrea, *Impact of Early Life Trauma*, 65.

56   Arnett, "Emerging Adulthood," 72.

57   White et al., "Hero's Welcome?," 280.

58   S. J. Swartz, J. E. Cote, and J. J. Arnett, "Identity and Agency in Emerging Adulthood: Two Developmental Routes in the Individuation Process," *Youth & Society* 37 (2005): 201–29.

59   E. H. Erikson, *Identity and the Life Cycle: Selected Papers* (New York: International Universities Press, 1959).

60   Ibid., 64.

61   Arnett, "Emerging Adulthood," 73.

62   Kelty, Segal, and Kleykamp, *Future of Children*, 204.

63   Van der Kolk and d'Andrea, *Impact of Early Life Trauma*, 66.

64   Ibid., 67.

65   Veterans Affairs Canada, "New Homeless Initiative for Greater Toronto Area," *Salute!* 702 (2010): 5–10; Royal Canadian Legion, *Operation Leave the Streets Behind* (Ottawa: Royal Canadian Legion, 2011); G. Parent, *Government of Canada Announces a New Pilot Project to Support Veterans in Canada* (Ottawa: Veterans Affairs Canada, 2012); Wounded Warriors, "Mission Statement," http://woundedwarriors.ca/mission/; Veterans Emergency Transition Services, "About Vets," http://vetscanada.org/about-us/2012; Veterans Affairs Canada, "New Homeless Initiative."

66   United States Veterans Affairs, *Five Year Plan*, 1807–20.

67   Royal Canadian Legion, *Operation Leave the Streets Behind*, 78.

20

Pilot Project on Incarcerated Former Military Personnel in Three Ontario Detention Centres, 2011–2012

ISABELLE COTÉ

Abstract

There is limited research on incarcerated former military personnel in Canada and no systematic identification of former military personnel at any level of the Canadian criminal justice system. In March 2011, a pilot project on this population was approved by the Ministry of Community Safety and Correctional Services in three Ontario detention centres. The objectives of this study were to determine over a one-year period (April 2011 to March 2012) the number and characteristics of incarcerated former military personnel and identify factors associated with their incarceration. Inmates reporting a military history volunteered to participate. Demographic variables and military history, including number of years in the military, the country for which they served, rank, branch of service, member of the Regular Force or the Reserve Force, history of deployment to a war zone, and/or involvement in operational missions, nature of discharge, and reasons for leaving the military were obtained through a semi-structured interview. History of previous incarcerations, treatment for psychiatric problems, street-drug use and/or alcohol consumption were acquired by reviewing the admission notes of the facilities. The current offences of the participants were accessed through the Offender Tracking Information System. Nineteen male inmates in three provincial correctional facilities reported military service. The average length of service was five years. Almost all identified veteran inmates had previous incarcerations. The timing of their first offence relative to their military service varied. Current offences were more serious in those inmates who had no history of deployment, while those who had a history of deployment and/or involvement in operational missions were more likely to have been diagnosed with a psychiatric problem. All veteran inmates reported at least one risk factor for incarceration (e.g., previous incarceration, mental illness, homelessness, substance and/or alcohol abuse). This study demonstrates that inmates with self-reported military history were incarcerated in provincial correctional facilities in 2011–12. The latency period between service and incarceration may be difficult to predict. Military history should be part of intake screening upon admission to all correctional facilities in Canada to aid custodial personnel to better characterize and address the unique needs of incarcerated veterans.

Background

With the long and sustained missions in Iraq and Afghanistan, the media turned their attention to the consequences of the mental health of returning troops. They also reported on the issue of military personnel and veterans being involved in the criminal justice system. Such titles could be found in the written press: "The Number of Canadian Soldiers Jailed in Edmonton's Military Prison Has Doubled since 2001."[1] "Number of [U.K.] Military Veterans in Jail Has More Than Doubled in Six Years."[2]

The notion that military personnel or former military personnel are involved in committing crimes is not new. Gilles de Rais, a leader in the French army and a companion-in-arms of Joan of Arc engaged in a series of child murders starting in 1432. He retired from military life in 1434–35 but the killings, possibly numbering in the hundreds, continued until 1440, when he was brought to trial and condemned to death.[3]

Fast forwarding to more recent times, scholarly articles on incarcerated Vietnam-era veterans began appearing in the 1970s and 1980s.[4] In the mid-1980s, the U.S. Bureau of Justice Statistics started conducting surveys of jail and prison inmates and their prior military service.[5] Since then, post-military antisocial behaviour has continued to be an important area of research in the United States. Since the early 2000s, a number of different organizations in the United Kingdom have also reported on the prevalence of incarcerated veterans.[6]

Research has shown that substance-use disorder, severe mental illness, homelessness, past criminal justice-system involvement, and disadvantageous socio-demographic characteristics are risk factors for incarceration.[7] Studies done on veterans indicate that military service or aspects of military service could also be considered a risk factor. It is now well recognized that war-zone exposures may have considerable negative physical, emotional, and behavioural consequences, including misconduct.[8] Certain factors such as exposure to combat,[9] post traumatic stress disorder (PTSD), and/or other post-combat mental health disorders,[10] diagnoses of alcohol and drug abuse and dependence,[11] difficulty making the transition from the military to civilian society,[12] and selection factors in the recruiting process across different service eras[13] may increase the risk of incarceration in the veteran population. Other factors such as being a member of a minority group, not being married, having less education, and being younger have also been found to be risk factors for incarceration among veterans.[14]

According to the U.S. Bureau of Justice Statistics 2004 Survey of Inmates in State and Federal Correctional Facilities, 10% of state prisoners reported prior service in the U.S. Armed Forces, down from 20% in 1986.[15] In this survey, veterans in state and federal prison were almost exclusively male (99%). The average length of military service of veterans in prison was about four years; one in five reported combat duty. Veterans of the Iraq-Afghanistan eras comprised 4% of veterans in both state and federal prisons. Among adult males, the incarceration rate of veterans (630 prisoners per 100,000) was less than half that of non-veterans (1,390 prisoners per 100,000). Over half (57%) of veterans were serving time for a violent offence, including 15% for homicide and 23% for sexual assault, compared to 47% for non-veterans. Veterans had shorter criminal records than non-veterans in state prison but reported longer prison sentences and expected to serve more time in prison than non-veterans. The median age of veterans in state prison was forty-five years, compared to thirty-three years for non-veterans. Veterans were much better educated than other state prisoners. Veterans (30%) were more likely than non-veterans (24%) to report a recent history of mental health services. There was little difference in the mental health histories of combat veterans compared to non-combat veterans in state prison.

In the United Kingdom, the Defence Analytical Services and Advice (DASA) of the Ministry of Defence and the Ministry of Justice estimated in September 2010 that 3.5% of all those currently in custody in England and Wales served in the British Armed Forces.[16] Of these, 99.6% were male. The most common offence categories for veterans in prison were violence against the person (33%), and sexual offences (25%). DASA estimated that 51% of ex-servicemen in prison were over the age of forty-five years and 29% were over the age of fifty-five years, compared to 9% of the general prison population being aged fifty years or older. These statistics suggested that many ex-servicemen in prison had offended a considerable time after their date of discharge from the military.[17]

In Canada, the only published data available on former military personnel in prison consist of a review extending a study undertaken by the Addictions Research Centre of the Correctional Service Canada (CSC) on the prevalence of veterans in CSC.[18] This latter study was requested by the Office of the Veterans Ombudsman Canada in order to gain a better understanding of the number of federally incarcerated offenders who had served in the Canadian military.[19] Since about one in thirty Canadians has served in the armed forces, it was predicted that veterans would account for approximately 3% of CSC offenders.[20] In their review, a veteran was defined as any person who reported prior service in the Canadian Forces (CF), regardless of the type of military discharge. A total of 2,054 male offenders from the Atlantic, Ontario, and Pacific regions responded to questions about military service from 11 February 2009 to 11 May 2010. Of this sample, 2.8% reported having served in the Canadian military. Of the self-reported military veterans in the study, 48% served less than one year, 36% served between one and five years, and about 14% reported serving in the Canadian Forces for more than five years. Applying this 2.8% to the 2010/2011 figures by Statistics Canada on the number of people remanded or sentenced in provincial or territorial correctional facilities[21] would mean that an estimated 685 incarcerated veterans would be sentenced or remanded in these facilities.

No Canadian studies have examined demographics, physical and mental health needs, offence-related characteristics, length of sentence, and risk of recidivism of incarcerated veterans. There is no formal identification of ex-serviceman at any level of the criminal justice system in Canada. Unless an arrestee decides to reveal his or her history of military service or unless a police officer, probation officer, correctional officer, nurse, or health worker in a jail or a penitentiary asks the offender the question, this information remains unknown.

In March 2011, a pilot study on the number of ex-military personnel incarcerated in three Ontario detention centres in which the researcher works as a consulting psychiatrist was ethically approved by the Research Committee of the Ontario Ministry of Community Safety and Correctional Services (MCSCS). The correctional facilities included the Niagara detention centre (capacity 260, males only), the Hamilton-Wentworth detention centre (capacity 414, males and females), and the Brantford jail (capacity 90, males only).[22] In contrast to federal penitentiaries, the primary function of provincial/territorial jails and detention centres is to hold accused persons awaiting trial, sentencing, or other court proceedings. Jails and detention centres also hold those who have been given short sentences.[23]

The aims of this pilot study were to determine the number and characteristics of incarcerated former military personnel, in particular those who were deployed to a war zone or had been involved in operational missions, over a one-year period, and to identify factors associated with veterans' incarceration. To our knowledge, this is the first study in Canada to examine such matters. In this study, a veteran is defined as any person who has reported prior service in a country's armed forces, regardless of the type of military discharge.

Methods

Participants

In order to recruit subjects, posters announcing a study on people with a history of military service and now facing legal problems were placed in the admission areas and health care units of the Niagara detention centre, the Hamilton-Wentworth detention centre, and the Brantford jail as well as in each holding unit of each facility. Any inmate who expressed an interest in participating in the research was asked to complete and sign a written request to participate. These request forms were made available in the admission's areas, health care units, and cellblocks. Completed request forms were forwarded to the health care unit to the attention of the researcher. With the cooperation of the nursing and correctional staff, arrangements were made by the researcher to contact and interview the inmate after obtaining consent. Potential participants had to self-identify as being a veteran of any country's Armed Forces. Excluded from the study were those who were under the age of 16 years when they were in the military, those who had not actually served, those who had worked for the military as civilians, and those who provided unreliable, inconsistent, and/or implausible information.

Data Collection and Measures

The data collection included a semi-structured interview. The researcher asked each inmate who volunteered to participate in the study questions about military history, including the number of years in the military, the country for which each served, rank, branch of service, member of the Regular Force or the Reserve Force, nature of discharge, and reasons for leaving the military. All were also asked whether they had deployed to a war zone and/or had been involved in an operational mission, and if so, which country was involved. Since none of the information could be validated with official records of the respective armed forces and/or Veterans Affairs in question, the interview provided an opportunity for the researcher to assess the inmate's knowledge of military matters (or lack thereof) to evaluate the plausibility of the information provided.

Once an inmate was identified as having a military history, the Health Care Record – Part A (Health Assessment) completed on admission of the inmate to the facility by a nurse was reviewed by the researcher for date of birth, history of previous incarceration(s), history of treatment for psychiatric problems and diagnosis, street-drug use and/or alcohol consumption (current and past), and suicidal ideation reported on admission. The Offender Tracking Information System (OTIS), the database system used by the Ontario MCSCS to record information about adult offenders (both inmates and probationers)[24] was also reviewed by the researcher to get the inmates' official offence history, including current offence(s) and year of first recorded offence.

Results

From April 2011 to March 2012, twenty-six inmates identified themselves as having served in the military. Of these, seven (27%) were excluded from the study mostly because of implausible or inconsistent information. Of the remaining nineteen who met the inclusion criteria, seventeen (89%) were Caucasians and two (11%) were Aboriginals. All participants were men; no female inmates from the detention centre housing both men and women identified themselves as having a history of military service. The average age of veteran inmates was forty-seven years (range 27 to 70 years).

Table 20.1 | Characteristics of inmates with a history of military service

	Not deployed (n = 13)	Deployed (n = 6)
Previous incarceration	12 (92%)	4 (67%)
Treatment for psychiatric problems/diagnoses	4 (31%)	5 (83%)
Street-drug SSE (past and/or current)	7 (54%)	5 (83%)
Alcohol consumption (past and/or current)	9 (69%)	5 (83%)
Suicidal ideation on admission	0 (0%)	0 (0%)

Thirteen (67%) served in the CF, four (22%) in the U.S. armed forces, one in the Polish armed forces, and one in the Portuguese armed forces (compulsory service). The average duration of service was five years (range 6 months to 27 years). Two (11%) served less than one year, twelve (63%) served between one and five years, and five (26%) served for more than five years. Of those inmates who had stayed in the military beyond the first six months of basic training, the average age at which they joined their respective armed forces was nineteen years (range 16 to 25 years). Five (26%) reported receiving benefits from Veterans Affairs.

Most participants (16, 84%) had a history of previous incarcerations. For their current incarceration, the most common offences were those against the person, including assault and sexual assault (47%), those against the administration of law and justice (42%), and against rights of property (37%). The average length of time between being released from the military and first recorded incarceration in Ontario was sixteen years (range 0 to 49 years). The average length of time between being released from the military to current incarceration was twenty-four years (range 5 to 49 years).

Most veteran inmates (17, 89%) described street-drug use (e.g., cannabis, steroids, crack cocaine, phencyclidine, and peyote) and/or alcohol consumption. No one in the current study was designated as suicidal on admission to a detention centre. However, one inmate with PTSD became suicidal during his detention and required additional mental health care during his incarceration.

Of the thirteen CF veterans, reported ranks were privates and corporals and the branch of service was mostly army of the Regular Force. Reasons given for leaving the military included service no longer required, not wanting to adhere to military life, getting into legal trouble, and having physical problems. Two (15%) inmates expressed regrets about leaving the CF. One attributed his involuntary release from the military as a result of government cutbacks as his reason for developing an addiction to alcohol and crack cocaine and his current arrest three years after becoming homeless.

Six (32%) inmates reported deployment to a war zone and/or involvement in operational missions from the 1970s onwards. Countries involved included Cyprus, Vietnam, South Asia, Bosnia, Lebanon, Grenada, and Iraq; none reported deployment to Afghanistan. The majority (5, 83%) reported receiving benefits from Veterans Affairs (3 in Canada and 2 in the United States). The length of time between being released from the military to first recorded offence in Ontario for the six inmates ranged from one to thirty-seven years. The length of time between being released from the military to current incarceration ranged from eight to thirty-seven years. One inmate was admitted to a detention centre five times during the study period.

Veteran inmates who had not been deployed were compared to inmates reporting experiences in war zones and/or operational missions (see table 20.1).

Categories of current offences for those who did not report deployment included offences against the administration of law and justice, against the person, against rights of property, firearms and other weapons, wilful and forbidden acts, and sentencing. The nature of the current offences for those who reported experiences in war zones or operational missions included offences against the administration of law and justice, against the person, and against rights of property. Although many of the offences were similar between the two groups, the inmates with no history of deployment had more serious offences than the group who had deployed. However, those who had deployed were more likely to have been diagnosed with a psychiatric condition prior to their current incarceration and to have received treatment for it than those who had not deployed. Five of the six inmates who had deployed and/or had been involved in operational missions reported being given the diagnosis of PTSD as a direct result of their military activities.

Discussion

This is the first descriptive study in Canada to examine the characteristics of provincial inmates with a history of military service and the first study to include veterans of other countries' armed forces.

The average age of the inmate participants was similar to U.S. and U.K. incarceration studies of veterans.[25] The mean age of forty-seven years was older than the general population of provincial inmates in Ontario. In a study of 522 mentally ill inmates in Ontario correctional facilities, the sample's mean age was 35 years.[26] In another study of 363 inmates, who had been incarcerated in one of four provincial correctional facilities in the Greater Toronto Area for at least five consecutive nights and were scheduled for release within one week, the sample's mean age was 36.7 years.[27] Study participants were also older than the average federal inmate in Canada.[28]

Most men enter the military at a young age, but late entries in Canada have become more common since the mid-1980s.[29] Research has suggested that age at which an individual enters the military is associated with different effects across the life course, with late mobilization putting men at greater risk of negative trajectories on physical health due in part to postwar work-life disadvantages.[30] In our sample, all of the incarcerated veterans had entered the military either in their late adolescence or early twenties, thus minimizing the effects of service on life disruption. It is unknown to what extent their military service had any influence on their latent criminal propensity.

This study shows that the population of veteran inmates detained in Ontario's detention centres is diverse, ranging from men who had never seen combat to men who had fought wars in Vietnam and Iraq and/or had been involved in difficult operational missions. Other studies have not included veterans who served in armed forces of other countries[31] but one-third of study participants served outside Canada. Almost all had volunteered for military service; one man was obligated to serve one year in his country's armed forces. The average duration of military service of the participants was quite similar to that reported in the 2004 survey of inmates in U.S. state and federal prison.[32] Reasons for discharges differed; some voiced difficulties transitioning to civilian life and regretted leaving.

Veteran inmates in this study reported the same risk factors for incarceration as those reported in the literature for non-veteran inmates, including prior criminal conviction, mental illness, homelessness, and substance abuse. Some participants had extensive criminal backgrounds, while others had no prior conviction. Some had committed their first offence while in the military, some shortly after leaving the military, and others became involved in the criminal justice system decades later. Likewise DASA found a long gap between military discharge and custody for many ex-servicemen in the United Kingdom who became offenders.[33]

In a review of sixty-two surveys from twelve countries, Fazel and Danesh found that prisoners were several times more likely to have psychosis and major depression, and about ten times more likely to have antisocial personality disorder, than the general population.[34] Mental health problems are by far the most significant cause of morbidity in prisons.[35] Almost half of the study participants reported having been diagnosed with a mental disorder at some point prior to their current incarceration. The number of those who had experienced mental health problems pre-military, during military service, and/or post-military was unknown. The veteran inmates who had deployed to war zones and/or had been involved in operational missions were almost all diagnosed with PTSD. It was not possible to determine whether PTSD was an added risk factor in the commission of their crimes.

Incarcerated veterans have been noted to be at the intersection between two populations with documented elevations in suicide rate: prisoners and veterans. Although it has been hypothesized that incarcerated veterans face a high suicide risk, the true suicide rate among incarcerated veterans is unknown.[36] None of the study participants presented with suicidal ideation on admission to any of the three correctional facilities; however, one became suicidal during his incarceration.

As the number of modern-day veterans in the general population grows as a result of Canada's involvement in international missions,[37] correctional facilities will likely see a rise in the number of incarcerated former military personnel, assuming that the number of incarcerated veterans is related to their prevalence in the general population.[38] If veteran status was included as part of intake screening upon admission to correctional facilities, this would aid custodial personnel to better characterize this population and identify potential needs that differentiate it from the incarcerated non-veteran population. Because there is increased risk of suicide, professionals treating inmates should routinely inquire about veteran status.[39] Information about military history would further assist correctional personnel in designing appropriate treatment and helping link offenders to community rehabilitative services upon release. It would also aid in connecting veteran inmates with the services developed by the Department of National Defence and/ or Veterans Affairs Canada (VAC). The establishment of collaborative work between correctional institutions and VAC would facilitate addressing various needs of this population.

Conclusion

The incarcerated veteran population in Ontario's detention centres is diverse but shows risk factors for incarceration similar to those for non-veterans. The offending history of veterans cannot be attributed solely to their previous military service. Since the latency period between military service and custody varied, systematic screening of provincial and federal inmates in Canada would promote collaboration between correctional institutions and vac to address the needs of the veteran inmates and design optimal correctional plans.

Limitations and Future Directions

This study had a number of limitations. Convenience sampling of volunteers may limit the representativeness of the sample to the general population of provincial inmates in Ontario. The sample size was small, which further restricts generalization of results. The data relied on inmates' self-report, and the military history of the offenders in the sample could not be validated with official records. Further research is required to better understand factors leading to incarceration of former military personnel.

Notes

1   "Rise in Soldiers in Prison Not Tied to Afghanistan: Army," *Edmonton Journal*, 1
    April 2008, http://www.canada.com/edmontonjournal/news/cityplus/story.html
    ?id=eaf2a319-78e4-41ba-8bd1-88ab550408cf.

2 R. Ford, "Number of Military Veterans in Jail 'Has More Than Doubled in Six Years,'" *Times*, 25 September 2009, http://www.timesonline.co.uk/tol/news/uk/crime/article6848238.ece.

3 "Gilles de Rais," Wikipedia, http://en.wikipedia.org/wiki/Gilles_de_Rais, accessed 3 September 2011.

4 J. Landolfi and D. P. Leclair, "Profile of Vietnam Era Veterans Incarcerated in Massachusetts Correctional Institutions" (Boston: Massachusetts Department of Correction, 1976); J. I. Walker, "Vietnam Combat Veterans with Legal Difficulties: A Psychiatric Problem?," *American Journal of Psychiatry* 138, no. 10 (1981): 1384–5; B. Pentland and G. Rothman, "Incarcerated Vietnam-Service Veteran: Stereotypes and Realities," *Journal of Correctional Education* 33, no. 1 (1982): 10–14.

5 C. J. Mumola, "Veterans in Prison or Jail," U.S. Department of Justice, January 2000, http://bjs.ojp.usdoj.gov/content/pub/pdf/vpj.pdf.

6 Howard League for Penal Reform, *Report of the Inquiry into Former Armed Service Personnel in Prison*, 2011, http://www.howardleague.org/fileadmin/howard_league/user/pdf/Veterans_inquiry/Military_inquiry_final_report.pdf.

7 D. A. McNiel, R. L. Binder, and J. C. Robinson, "Incarceration Associated with Homelessness, Mental Disorder, and Co-Occurring Substance Abuse," *Psychiatric Services* 56, no. 7 (2005): 840–6; S. K. Erickson, R. A. Rosenheck, R. L. Trestman, J. D. Ford, and R. A. Desai, "Risk of Incarceration between Cohorts of Veterans with and without Mental Illness Discharged from Inpatient Units," *Psychiatric Services* 59, no. 2 (2008): 178–83; G. A. Greenberg and R. A. Rosenheck, "Jail Incarceration, Homelessness, and Mental Health: A National Study," *Psychiatric Services* 59, no. 2 (2008): 170–7.

8 R. L. Campise, S. K. Geller, and M. E. Campise, "Combat Stress," in *Military Psychology: Clinical and Operational Applications*, ed. C. H. Kennedy and E. A. Zillmer, 215–40 (New York: Guilford, 2006).

9 H. S. Resnick, D. W. Foy, C. P. Donahoe, and E. N. Miller, "Antisocial Behavior and Post-Traumatic Stress Disorder in Vietnam Veterans," *Journal of Clinical Psychology* 45, no. 6 (1989): 860–6; D. H. Barrett, H. S. Resnick, D. W. Foy, D. Dansky, W. D. Flanders, and N. E. Stroup, "Combat Exposure and Adult Psychosocial Adjustment among U.S. Army Veterans Serving in Vietnam, 1965–1971," *Journal of Abnormal Psychology* 105, no. 4 (1996): 575–81; G. A. Greenberg, R. A. Rosenheck, and R. A. Desai, "Risk of Incarceration among Male Veterans and Nonveterans: Are Veterans of the All Volunteer Force at Greater Risk?," *Armed Forces & Society* 33, no. 3 (2007): 337–50.

10 A. Fontana and R. Rosenheck, "The Role of War-Zone Trauma and PTSD in the Etiology of Antisocial Behavior," *Journal of Nervous and Mental Disease* 193, no. 3 (2005): 203–9; B. R. Karney, R. Ramchand, K. Chan Osilla, L. Barnes Caldarone, and R. M. Burns, "Predicting the Immediate and Long-Term Consequences of Post-Traumatic Stress Disorder, Depression, and Traumatic Brain Injury in Veterans of Operation Enduring Freedom and Operation Iraqi Freedom," in *Invisible Wounds of War: Psychological and Cognitive Injuries, Their Consequences, and Services to Assist Recovery*, ed. T. L. Tanielian and L. H. Jaycox, 119–66 (Santa Monica: Rand Corporation, 2008).

11 Erickson et al., "Risk of Incarceration."

12 M. J. Boivin, "Forgotten Warriors: An Evaluation of the Emotional Well-Being of
    Presently Incarcerated Vietnam Veterans," *Genetic, Social, and General Psychology
    Monographs* 113, no. 1 (1987): 109–25; Greenberg, Rosenheck, and Desai, "Risk of
    Incarceration among Male Veterans and Nonveterans," 170–7.
13 G. A. Greenberg and R. Rosenheck, "Mental Health and Other Risk Factors for Jail
    Incarceration among Male Veterans," *Psychiatric Quarterly* 80, no. 1 (2009): 41–53.
14 Ibid., 41–3.
15 M. E. Noonan and C. J. Mumola, "Veterans in State and Federal Prison, 2004,"
    U.S. Department of Justice, May 2007, http://bjs.gov/content/pub/pdf/vsfp04.pdf,
    accessed 25 May 2008.
16 Defence Analytical Services and Advice, *Estimating the Proportion of Prisoners in
    England and Wales Who Are Ex-Armed Forces – Further Analysis* (London: Ministry
    of Defence, 2010).
17 Howard League for Penal Reform, *Report of the Inquiry*.
18 P. Bensimon and R. Ruddell, "Veterans in Canadian Correctional Systems," last mod-
    ified November 2010, http://www.csc-scc.gc.ca/text/rsrch/briefs/b46/b46-eng.shtml.
19 S. Farrell, J. Gileno, and B. A. Grant, "Canadian Military Service of Federal Male
    Offenders," *Research Snippet*, no. 09-1, 2009.
20 Bensimon and Ruddell, "Veterans in Canadian Correctional Systems."
21 Statistics Canada, "Adult Correctional Services, Average Counts of Offenders, by
    Province, Territory and Federal Programs, 2010/2011," http://www.statcan.gc.ca/
    tables-tableaux/sum-som/l01/cst01/legal31a-eng.htm.
22 Ontario Ministry of Community Safety and Correctional Services, "Correctional
    Services, Adult Offenders, Facilities," http://www.mcscs.jus.gov.on.ca/english/
    corr_serv/ adult_off/facilities/det_centres.htm.
23 Standing Senate Committee on Social Affairs, Science and Technology. *Out of the
    Shadows at Last: Transforming Mental Health, Mental Illness and Addiction Services
    in Canada*, 2006. http://www.parl.gc.ca/Content/SEN/Committee/391/soci/rep/
    rep02may06-e.htm.
24 G. P. Brown, "Seriously Mentally Ill Inmates in Ontario Correctional Facilities:
    Prevalence, Mental Health Care Needs, and Implications for Correctional and Mental
    Health Care Policy" (presentation, Human Services and Justice Co-ordinating
    Committee Conference, Niagara Falls, Ontario, 26–28 October 2009).
25 Noonan and Mumola, "Veterans in State and Federal Prison, 2004"; DASA,
    "Estimating the Proportion of Prisoners in England and Wales."
26 Brown, "Seriously Mentally Ill Inmates in Ontario Correctional Facilities."
27 A. Kellen, J. Freedman, S. Novac, L. Lapointe, R. Maaranen, and A. Wong, "Homeless
    and Jailed: Jailed and Homeless" (Toronto: John Howard Society of Toronto, August
    2010).
28 Public Safety Canada, "Corrections and Conditional Release Statistical Overview,"
    2012, http://www.publicsafety.gc.ca/res/cor/rep/2011-ccrso-eng.aspx#c5.
29 A. C. Okros, personal communication, 16 November 2012.
30 G. H. Elder, M. J. Shanahan, and E. Colerick Clipp, "When War Comes to Men's
    Lives: Life-Course Patterns in Family, Work and Health," *Psychology and Aging* 9, no.
    1 (1994): 5–16.

31 Noonan and Mumola, "Veterans in State and Federal Prison, 2004"; DASA, "Estimating the Proportion of Prisoners in England and Wales"; Bensimon and Ruddell, "Veterans in Canadian Correctional Systems."

32 Noonan and Mumola, "Veterans in State and Federal Prison, 2004."

33 DASA, "Estimating the Proportion of Prisoners in England and Wales."

34 S. Fazel and J. Danesh, "Serious Mental Disorder in 23,000 Prisoners: A Systematic Review of 62 Surveys," *Lancet* 359 (2002): 545–50.

35 L. Birmingham, "The Mental Health of Prisoners," *Advances in Psychiatric Treatment* 9 (2003): 191–201.

36 H. S. Wortzel, I. A. Binswanger, A. C. Anderson, and L. E. Adler, "Suicide among Incarcerated Veterans," *Journal of the American Academy of Psychiatry and the Law* 37, no. 1 (2009): 982–91.

37 Treasury Board of Canada Secretariat, "Veterans Affairs Canada," 2009, http://www.tbs-sct.gc.ca/rpp/2010-2011/inst/dva/dva01-eng.asp#a01.

38 Bensimon and Ruddell, "Veterans in Canadian Correctional Systems."

39 Wortzel et al., "Suicide among Incarcerated Veterans," 982–91.

Abbreviations

ABC	Activities-Specific Balance Confidence Scale
ACE	adverse childhood event
ADHA	attention deficit hyperactivity disorder
ADL	activities of daily living
AF	Allied Forces
AGS	auxiliary gas supply
ALS	amyotrophic lateral sclerosis
ANOVA	analysis of variance
AUDIT	The Alcohol Use Disorders Identification Test
AWS TECH	air weapons systems technician
BAI	Beck Anxiety Inventory
BDI–II	Beck Depression Inventory–II
BG	bubble grade
BGPR	precordial bubble grade
BOLD	blood oxygen level dependant
BPC	Board of Pension Commissioners
BT	bottom time
CAPS	Clinician-Administered PTSD Scale
CAREN	computer assisted rehabilitation environment
CBF	cerebral blood flow
CBOC	community-based outpatient clinic
CCHL	Canadian College of Health Leaders
CCNO	critical care nursing officer
CEF	Canadian Expeditionary Force
CF	Canadian Forces
CFHSvcs	Canadian Forces Health Services
CFHSvcsGp	Canadian Forces Health Services Group
CFNO	Canadian Forces nursing officer
CHAMP	comprehensive high activity mobility predictor
CHCA	Canadian Home Care Association

CIMVHR	Canadian Institute for Military and Veteran Health Research
$CMRO_2$	metabolic rate of oxygen consumption
CO_2	carbon dioxide
CPRS	Computerized Patient Record System
CPT	cognitive processing therapy
CSC	Correctional Services Canada
CT	conventional computed tomography
CUMA	Canadian Underwater Mine Countermeasures Apparatus
CVR	cerebrovascular reactivity
DAPS	Detailed Assessment of PTSD Scale
DART	Disaster Assistance Response Team
DASA	Defence Analytical Services and Advice
DCS	decompression sickness
DMFS	Directorate of Military Family Services
DRDC	Defence Research & Development Canada
DSM	*Diagnostic and Statistical Manual of Mental Disorders*
DTI	diffusion tensor imaging
DVA	Department of Veterans Affairs
$E = MC^3$	Ensemble pour Mieux Comprendre (Together to Better Understand)
EI	emotional intelligence
EMDR	eye movement desensitization and reprocessing
EMG	electromyography
EMR	electronic medical record
ENPC	Emergency Nursing Pediatric Courses
ET	exposure therapy
FABQ	Fear Avoidance Belief Questionnaire
FAC	Field Advisory Committee
fMRI	functional magnetic resonance imaging
FMS	functional movement screen
FORCE	Project Fitness for Operational Requirements of CF Employment
GNO	generalist nursing officer
GWVA	Great War Veterans Association
HC	hypercapnia
HCP	computerized hypercapnic
Heliox	helium and oxygen mixture air supply
HHD	hand-held dynamometry
HO	hyperoxic condition
HOP	hyperoxic protocol
HP R&D	Human Performance Research & Development
ImPACT	Immediate Post-Concussion Assessment and Cognitive Testing
INF	infantry occupation

IOM	Institute of Medicine
IPCP	inter-professional collaborative practice
ISTSS	International Society of Traumatic Stress Studies
$IWO_2 + SD$	in water oxygen with surface decompression
JCCA	*Journal of the Canadian Chiropractic Association*
JCE	*Journal of Chiropractic Education*
JCH	*Journal of Chiropractic Humanities*
JCM	*Journal of Chiropractic Medicine*
JMPT	*Journal of Manipulative & Physiological Therapeutics*
JRRD	*Journal of Rehabilitation Research & Development*
JTF	Joint Task Force
K-M	Kisman-Masurel
LBP	low back pain
LEFS	Lower Extremity Functional Scale
MARS OFF	maritime surface and subsurface officer
MaxBG	maximum bubble grade
MCSCS	Ministry of Community Safety and Correctional Services
MEL	medical employment limitation
MHC	Military Hospitals Commission
MOOTW	military operations other than war
MRI	magnetic resonance imaging
MSK	musculoskeletal
MSW	metres sea water
MTBI	mild traumatic brain injury
MVC	maximal voluntary contraction
MVHR	Military and Veteran Health Research
NATO	North Atlantic Treaty Organization
NCHL	National Centre for Healthcare Leadership
NFA	no fixed address
NIRS	near infrared spectroscopy
NoD	no decompression
NVC	New Veterans Charter
NVG	night-vision goggles
NYCC	New York Chiropractic College
O_2	oxygen
ODI	Modified Oswestry Low Back Pain Disability Index
OFS	Occupational Fitness Standards
$OQ^{®}$-45.2	Outcome Questionnaire -45.2
OSI	operational stress injury
OTIS	Offender Tracking Information System
PAI	personality assessment
PASL	pulsed arterial spin labelling

PC	principal component
PCA	principal component analysis
PCL–M	Post Traumatic Stress Disorder Checklist – Military Version
PCP	primary care physician
PE	prolonged exposure
PET	positron emission tomography
PICU	Pediatric Intensive Care Unit
PSP	Personnel Support Program
PTE	potentially traumatizing event
PTSD	post traumatic stress disorder
qfMRI	quantitative functional magnetic resonance imaging
RAFS	regional adaptive fitness specialist
RCL	Royal Canadian Legion
RCMP	Royal Canadian Mounted Police
Repet	repetitive
RMQ	Roland Morris Questionnaire
RMS	root mean square
SAS	Statistical Analysis Software
SCAT2	Sport Concussion Assessment Tool version 2
SFMA	Selective Functional Movement Assessment
SI	surface interval
SM	spinal manipulation
SME	subject matter expert
SPECT	single-photon emission computerized tomography
SUD	substance use disorders
TAU	treatment as usual
TE	therapeutic enactment
TSK	Tampa Scale for Kinesiophobia
TRIAGE	technique for research of information by animation of a group of experts
VA	Veterans Affairs
VAC	Veterans Affairs Canada
VFC	Valcartier Family Centre
VGE	venous gas emboli
VHA	Veterans Health Administration
VTP	Veterans Transition Program
VISN	Veterans Integrated Service Network
VistA	Veterans Health Information Systems and Technology Architecture
WHO	World Health Organization

Contributors

ALICE AIKEN, CD, PhD, is the director of the Canadian Institute for Military and Veteran Health Research. She is also an associate professor in the School of Rehabilitation Therapy, Faculty of Health Sciences, Queen's University, Kingston, ON. She does health services / health policy research in innovative models of care and disability policy as well as novel methods of knowledge translation. She has a unique focus on military and veterans in much of her research. She lectures in clinical orthopedics and military and veteran health. She received her PhD and MA from Queen's University in Kingston, her physical therapy degree at Dalhousie University in Halifax, NS, and a BSc in kinesiology at the University of Ottawa. She also proudly served in the Canadian Forces for fourteen years, first as a ship's navigator in the Navy, then as a physiotherapist.

WAYNE J. ALBERT, PhD, is a professor and dean of the Faculty of Kinesiology at the University of New Brunswick. Dr Albert's major research focus is occupational biomechanics (ergonomics) and the prevention of musculoskeletal injuries in the workplace as well as general low-back health, with research projects including (1) assessing the neuromuscular demands placed on military helicopter pilots when using night-vision equipment mounted to their helmets; (2) injury concerns in offshore industries workers who must deal with moving environments; (3) cumulative loading concerns associated with automative assembly to musculoskeletal factors; (4) biomechanical stresses of city transit workers; (5) lifting biomechanics programs in the long-term care facility workers; and 6) effects of fatigue lifting technique.

STÉPHANIE A. H. BÉLANGER, PhD, is associate scientific director of the Canadian Institute for Military and Veteran Health Research, co-editor of *A New Coalition for a Challenging Battlefield: Military and Veteran Health Research* (CDA, 2012); of *Shaping the Future: Military and Veteran Health Research* (CDA, 2011), as well as of *Transforming Traditions: The Leadership of Women in the Canadian Navy* (CDA, 2010). She is associate professor at the French Department of the Royal Military

College of Canada, where her research focuses on war testimony and soldier iden-tity. She also specializes in just war theories, topic of her monograph *Guerre, sac-rifices et persécutions* (L'Harmattan, 2010). She has served in the Royal Canadian Navy (Reserve) since 2004.

Lieutenant-Colonel MARKUS BESEMANN, BSc, MD, FRCPC, has been at the helm of the Canadian Forces Physical Rehabilitation Program since its inception in 2008. He was a general duty medical officer in the Canadian Forces prior to engag-ing in postgraduate training as a civilian in physical medicine and rehabilitation. For twelve years he was the chief of physical medicine and rehabilitation at the Regional Trauma Centre and the Regional Rehabilitation Centre in Gatineau, QC.

TIMOTHY BLACK, PhD, is an associate professor of counselling psychology at the University of Victoria. He is a co-founder of the Veterans Transition Program and is the national clinical director for the Veterans Transition Network. His research program is focused on successful veteran transition from military to civilian life.

KAIGHLEY BRETT, SLt, MD, is a family medicine resident with the Queen's Uni-versity Department of Family Medicine. She joined the Canadian Forces in 2007 as a member of the Royal Canadian Navy. She has a BSc in biomedical sciences from the University of Guelph, and a doctorate in medicine from the University of Ottawa. She is an avid scuba diver, and in addition to family medicine she hopes to pursue a career in undersea and hyperbaric medicine.

ALLIE CAREW, BSc (candidate), Loran Scholar, is an undergraduate studying bi-ology at Queen's University. Allie has worked at the Canadian Institute for Mil-itary and Veteran Health Research, where she assisted in researching veterans' health. Her research interests include veterans' health in Canada, military families, and transition from military to civilian life.

ERIC CHAN, PhD, received his PhD from the University of Calgary and completed his post-doctoral training in measurement, evaluation, and research methodology under the supervision of Dr Bruno Zumbo at the University of British Colum-bia. Dr Chan's professional interests include meta-analysis, measurement valid-ity, and test development. He is co-editing a book on measurement validity with Dr Zumbo (*When Validity Theory Meets Validation Practices*), to be published by Springer.

VICTORIA L. CHESTER, PhD, is an associate professor in the Faculty of Kinesiology at the University of New Brunswick. Dr Chester's main research focuses on the kinematics and kinetics of multi-segment foot models and upper extremity bio-mechanics. Her research program is funded by NSERC, CFI, and NBIF.

ISABELLE CÔTÉ, MD, CM, FRCPC, completed a degree in medicine from McGill University in 1985 and specialist qualifications in psychiatry from the University of Toronto in 1990. She holds the rank of lecturer in the Department of Psychiatry at the University of Toronto. She has a private practice in Hamilton, ON. She is a contractor psychiatrist at the Niagara Detention Centre, the Hamilton-Wentworth Detention Centre, and the Brantford Jail. She is also a contractor psychiatrist for thirty-two CF Health Services Centres. She has been retained as an expert witness for numerous criminal and civil cases. She has written articles related to forensic psychiatry.

DANIEL W. COX, PhD, is an assistant professor in counselling psychology at the University of British Columbia. His research focuses on the process and outcome of group and individual counselling, trauma, suicide, gender, and mental health epidemiology – with an emphasis on veteran and military populations. He received his PhD at the University of Kansas in counselling psychology. Prior to coming to the University of British Columbia, Dan was a research psychologist at the Uniformed Services University of the Health Sciences, working on several mental health studies with U.S. military members.

JAMES C. CROLL, EdD, is a professor emeritus (education) and honorary research associate (kinesiology) at the University of New Brunswick. His principal research publications have related to statistics, learning theory, and research methodology.

KARLA EMENO, MA, is completing her PhD in forensic psychology at Carleton University, Ottawa, ON. Her dissertation examines the space-time clustering of Canadian crime in order to generate prospective risk surfaces. Her other research interests include the evaluation of psychologically based investigative techniques, particularly geographic profiling. She has been conducting research for both the academic and public service sectors.

ALLAN ENGLISH, PhD, served for twenty-five years in the Royal Canadian Air Force and the Canadian Forces. He has taught undergraduate and graduate courses at the Royal Military College of Canada and at Queen's University, as well as courses in senior officer professional military education for officers in the ranks of major to brigadier-general at the Canadian Forces College, Toronto. He is an associate professor in the History Department at Queen's University, where he teaches Canadian military history. He served on committees that advised Veterans Affairs Canada, the Department of National Defence, and the RCMP on operational stress injuries.

BRENDA GAMBLE, PhD, received her PhD in medical sciences from the University of Toronto in 2006. She is an assistant professor in the Faculty of Health Sciences at the University of Ontario Institute of Technology. Prior to coming to University of Ontario Institute of Technology, Brenda was assistant professor, supervisor of studies for the Health Studies program at the University of Toronto. Research areas include health/human resources, accountability in health care, inter-professional practice/education, and the medical laboratory sector.

Captain PAULINE GODSELL, BSc (PT), has been appointed the rehabilitation phys-iotherapy coordinator for the Canadian Forces Physical Rehabilitation Program since August 2010. She joined the Canadian Forces in 2003 and received her BSc (PT) from the University of Ottawa in 2007. Upon graduation, she was the recip-ient of the Physiotherapy Foundation of Canada Entry-Level Student Research Award. Her drive and compassion were a key component to the inaugural partici-pation and success of the Joint Task Force Nijmegen 2012: Soldier On team.

KAREN E. HAINES, RN, BSCN, is a Master of Science in Nursing student at the Arthur and Sonia Labatt School of Nursing, Western University, London, ON. Karen is completing her MScN thesis, "Transitioning to Motherhood after Trauma: Experiences in the Health Care System."

MICHAEL F. HARRISON, MD, PhD, completed his PhD at the University of Regina in the area of night vision goggle–induced neck strain and injury in helicopter aircrew in the Canadian Forces. Dr Harrison completed his MD at Saba Univer-sity School of Medicine before completing a post-doctoral research fellowship at the Mayo Clinic's Preventive, Occupational, and Aerospace Medicine department, with a focus on altitude medicine. He is a resident in Henry Ford Hospital's Inter-nal Medicine / Emergency Medicine / Critical Care Medicine program in Detroit, MI, and remains a research associate at the Mayo Clinic in Rochester, MN.

Major NICHOLAS HAZLEDINE, MSc (candidate), Grad Dip PT, MCSP, MCPA, is the Canadian Forces physiotherapy practice leader for the Ontario region and the clinic team leader for the Physiotherapy Department at the Canadian Forces Health Services Centre (Ottawa). He graduated from the Joint Services School of Physiotherapy in the United Kingdom and, after serving with the Royal Army Medical Corp, immigrated to Canada. He has served in Bosnia and Afghanistan since joining the Canadian Forces.

Lieutenant-Colonel ALEXANDRA HEBER, MD, FRCPC, was a mental health nurse for nine years before entering medical school. Throughout her career, she has worked in psychological trauma. In 2006, Dr Heber enrolled in the Canadian Forces. In 2009, she deployed to Afghanistan as the officer commanding of the Canadian Forces Mental Health Clinic in Kandahar Air Field. She is clinical di-rector of Mental Health Services for the Canadian Forces Health Services Centre

(Ottawa), and head psychiatrist in their Operational Trauma and Stress Support Centre.

OLENA KAPRAL has an MA in public administration from the University of Ottawa. She obtained a bachelor of health sciences (2010) from the University of Ontario Institute of Technology and will pursue further studies in a doctoral public policy program upon completion of her master's. Ms Kapral's research interest includes inter-professional collaboration, the regulation of health-care professions, health policy, and health administration education.

KRISTEN KLASSEN, MSc, is a PhD candidate in the Applied Health Sciences program at the University of Manitoba. Her dissertation focuses on the connection between income and mental health in the military community, using secondary data analysis. She also works as the research coordinator at the Operational Stress Injury Clinic in Winnipeg, MB, a specialized outpatient mental health clinic for veterans, current Canadian Forces members, and RCMP.

NADIA KOHLER, RSW, completed her studies in social work and started her career in France. She's been working as a social worker at the Valcartier Military Family Resource Centre for six years. She has developed an expertise in the realities of military life. She counsels military families in their specific life experiences through a family systems approach. She is the author of two guides: *Children and Grief* and *Signs of Operational Stress Injury (OSI) and the Family.* She is a developer of the E = MC^3 program and is working on adapting its contents to a program suitable for children ages three to six.

JENNIFER C. LAFORCE, PhD, CPsych, is a psychologist and clinical director at the Winnipeg Operational Stress Injury (OSI) Clinic and assistant professor in the Department of Clinical Health Psychology at the University of Manitoba. She has provided clinical services and been involved in research and program development and evaluation at the Winnipeg OSI Clinic since it was formed in 2004. Dr Laforce received her doctorate in clinical psychology from Queen's University, Kingston, ON, and completed her psychology internship at SUNY Upstate Medical University in Syracuse, New York.

ANTHONY J. LISI, DC, is the director of Chiropractic Services for the Veterans Health Administration. In this role he oversees all national programmatic issues for chiropractic services in the largest integrated health-care system in the United States. In 2004 he became the first chiropractor appointed to the medical staff of the VA Connecticut Healthcare System, where he developed processes for integrating hospital-based clinical services and inter-professional clinical education. He is the chief of chiropractic service at the VA Connecticut facility, and associate professor of clinical sciences at the University of Bridgeport College of Chiropractic. He has authored or co-authored over twenty-five peer-reviewed publications and presented over twenty-five abstracts at scientific conferences throughout the United States and Canada.

MARIE S. S. LONGO, RN, BScN, is a Master of Nursing and Nurse Practitioner student at the Arthur and Sonia Labatt School of Nursing, Western University, London, ON. Marie is completing her nurse practitioner program.

CLARISSE ILDIKO MARK, PhD, Eng, is a biomedical engineer in advanced brain imaging at Queen's University Centre for Neuroscience Studies and the recipient of the Tim R. Noël Fellowship in Amyotrophic Lateral Sclerosis research offered conjointly by the ALS Society of Canada and the Canadian Institute of Health Research. After completing her bachelor in electrical engineering at McGill University, she worked two years in a start-up research company developing optical devices for medical and telecommunication applications. She then carried through a medical physics master's project on ultrasound imaging for improved radiation oncology treatment at McGill. She recently graduated with a doctoral degree from the McConnell Brain Imaging Centre of the Montreal Neurological Institute, and her post-doctoral research focuses on novel functional magnetic resonance imaging techniques that allow precise, fast, and non-invasive quantification of brain activity, of high diagnostic value to the military.

PAIGE MATTIE, MKH, obtained a bachelor of science in psychology from McGill University and master of human kinetics in sport and exercise psychology from the University of Windsor. Her research background is in mental toughness and psychological skills training for elite sport performance. Paige is research assistant in human performance within the Director General Personnel & Family Support Services of the Canadian Forces. Her research activity involves the development of occupational fitness standards and the use of incentives in increasing exercise behaviour. In addition, Paige is a certified member of the Canadian Sport Psychology Association and consults with athletes competing at the provincial and national level.

MARY ANN MCCOLL, PhD, is associate director at the Centre for Health Services and Policy Research, Queen's University. She is also a professor in the School of Rehabilitation Therapy and in the Department of Community Health & Epidemiology. Dr McColl's research interests include access to health services for people with disabilities, disability policy, spirituality and health, and community integration / social support. Before coming to Queen's in 1992, she was associate professor at the University of Toronto, Department of Occupational Therapy, and director of research at Lyndhurst Spinal Cord Centre in Toronto. She is academic lead for the Canadian Disability Policy Alliance, an association of academic, community, and policy partners committed to understanding and enhancing disability policy in Canada.

SYDNEY DALE-McGRATH, MA, is a graduate of Dalhousie University, where she obtained her BA in history. She completed her MA in history at Queen's University in 2012. Her studies have focused on Canadian military history and gender relations in colonial North America.

ALEXANDRA McINTYRE-SMITH, PhD, CPsych, is a psychologist at the Parkwood Hospital Operational Stress Injury Clinic. She provides assessment and treatment to Canadian Forces members and veterans in the Toronto area as well as consultation and education to referral sources. She completed her undergraduate training at McGill University and her graduate training at the University of Western Ontario. She is an adjunct assistant professor at the University of Waterloo. Research interests focus on the health and well-being of veterans and still-serving members; recent research projects include the impact of operational stress injuries on sexual function and predictors of suicide in treatment-seeking veterans and still-serving members.

MICHELLE MOORE, MA, completed her master's in war studies at the Royal Military College of Canada. Her research focuses on the human behaviour–related aspects of war; observing and exploring the way people act and react in the ways they do; and identifying the patterns, impacting factors, and subtle details and changes caused by the different environments throughout the Canadian Forces. She has been an intelligence officer in the Royal Canadian Navy (Reserve) since 2005.

J. PATRICK NEARY, PhD, is a professor in the Faculty of Kinesiology & Health Studies at the University of Regina. His research explores the mechanism(s) associated with cerebral, skeletal, and cardiac muscle fatigue during exercise, and factors related to muscle strain and dysfunction in aviation aircrew. His research also explores the pathophysiology of mild traumatic brain injury, with his research programs funded by NSERC, CIHR, and the Department of National Defence.

STEVEN PASSMORE, DC, PhD, earned his honours bachelor of kinesiology from McMaster University (2001), and his master of science in kinesiology with a focus on motor behaviour from the University of Nevada, Las Vegas (2003). He completed a doctor of chiropractic degree from New York Chiropractic College (NYCC) (2006) and is a PhD candidate in kinesiology at McMaster University, with a focus on perceptual learning. As a licensed clinician he practised and supervised student interns for two years in a hospital supported by an NYCC fellowship as a without compensation (WOC) chiropractor in the United States Veterans Health Administration, at the Veterans Affairs Medical Center in Buffalo, New York. He is assistant professor, holding the Canadian Chiropractic Research Foundation Professor in Spine Biomechanics and Neurophysiology in the Faculty of Medicine, School of Medical Rehabilitation, at the University of Manitoba. He is also an adjunct assistant professor in the research department at NYCC. In addition to his work on the integration of chiropractic services to publicly funded health-care systems, his primary research interests include the application of motor behaviour and perceptual motor learning paradigms as potential quantifiable clinical outcome measures and teaching tools.

GILBERT BRUCE PIKE, PhD, is the Killam Professor of Neurology & Neurosurgery and James McGill Professor of Biomedical Engineering at McGill University. He is also director of the McConnell Brain Imaging Centre at the Montreal Neurological Institute and is a national researcher of Quebec. Following an undergraduate degree in electrical engineering in his native Newfoundland, Bruce obtained his MSc and PhD at McGill University, with his research focused on stereotactic radiosurgery and magnetic resonance angiography, respectively. He then conducted post-doctoral studies at Stanford University. Dr Pike investigates magnetic resonance imaging (MRI) methods and applications for basic and clinical neuroscience research. As a primary focus, he detects and measures the physiological modulations that are associated with neuronal activation and inhibition using novel functional MRI techniques. He has used his methods to study the relationship between blood flow and oxygen metabolism in the cortex over a broad range of activation and inhibition conditions in healthy subjects and epilepsy patients. He has also developed an in vivo quantitative MR technique termed "magnetization transfer imaging" that probes the magnetic interaction between macromolecules and water and used the technique to study white matter pathology in multiple sclerosis and normal brain development.

SUSAN L. RAY, RN, PhD, CNS/APN, is an associate professor at the Arthur and Sonia Labatt School of Nursing, Western University, London, ON. She teaches in the undergraduate and graduate programs. Her research program focuses on the impact of psychological trauma on military personnel, veterans and their families, homeless veterans, military personnel transitioning to civilian life, and testing the efficacy of interventions for post traumatic stress disorder and other related co-morbidity.

STEVE ROSE, PhD (candidate), is a student in the Department of Sociology at Queen's University. His doctoral research looks at the problem of veterans' integration into civilian life and is overseen by Dr Alice Aiken and Dr Annette Burfoot. Steve also works with the Canadian Institute for Military and Veteran Health Research and the Centre for Health Services and Policy Research, where he conducts research on veterans' health and primary care needs.

MAYA ROTH, PhD, CPsych, is a clinical psychologist at the Parkwood Hospital OSIC and is involved in developing and implementing clinical outreach services within the Greater Toronto Area. Dr Roth is an adjunct member of the Yeates School of Graduate Studies at Ryerson University, and an allied scientist of the Lawson Health Research Institute in London, ON. She completed her undergraduate training at York University, and her graduate training at Queen's University and York University. Dr Roth is certified as a prolonged exposure therapist and supervisor through the Centre for the Treatment and Study of Anxiety at the University of Pennsylvania, and is CACBT-ACTCC certified in cognitive behaviour therapy. Dr Roth is involved in research examining treatment outcome in post traumatic stress disorder and mood disorders among military and veteran personnel, treatment outcome in chronic pain, as well as the examination of pain and psychological distress at end of life. Clinically, Dr Roth's practice involves the assessment and treatment of post traumatic stress disorder and other sequelae of military service, including depression, other anxiety disorders, and chronic pain.

KATE ST CYR, MSCPPH, is a full-time research associate and program evaluation officer at the Parkwood Hospital OSI Clinic in London, ON. She is also an allied scientist of the Lawson Health Research Institute in London. Ms St Cyr completed her undergraduate training in anthropology at McMaster University in Hamilton, ON, and her graduate studies in population and public health at Simon Fraser University, Burnaby, BC. Her research interests include psychiatric epidemiology and determinants of health amongst military personnel and veterans, with a focus on post traumatic stress disorder and its associated co-morbid conditions, including suicidality. Ms St Cyr is also interested in treatment outcomes–based research.

ALLA SKOMOROVSKY, PhD, obtained her doctoral degree in experimental social psychology from Carleton University, Ottawa, ON. Since 2005, she has been working as a defence scientist for the Department of National Defence, Canada. She is a team leader for the Personnel and Family Support Concepts team. Her research interests include personality, stress and well-being, wellness of military families, health risk factors, and resilience. In addition, she has been teaching psychology courses at Royal Military College and Carleton University.

Captain STEPHANIE SMITH, RN, MA, is a critical care nursing officer posted to the Canadian Forces Health Services Training Centre in Borden, ON. She instructs nursing officers and medical technicians and is actively involved with the Canadian Forces simulation training program. She recently completed a MA in disaster and emergency management at Royal Roads University, which stimulated her interest in research. She has deployed to Afghanistan on two missions and established a nursing mentorship program with the Afghan National Army in 2009. She has been involved with humanitarian work in Haiti and continues to promote clinical pediatric preparedness amongst all Canadian Forces clinicians.

MIKE SPIVOCK, PhD, obtained his doctoral degree in health promotion from the School of Public Health at Université de Montréal. His research has centred on the promotion of physical activity in a variety of able-bodied and injured populations, with particular emphasis on psychological behaviour-change models and their interaction with the built and social environment. Since 2007 he has held the position of research manager in human performance within the Canadian Forces Personnel and Family Support Services. His research portfolio includes the development of occupational fitness standards and programs, as well as several other initiatives related to monitoring and enhancing the health and fitness of CF personnel. In addition, Dr Spivock is a part-time professor in the Faculty of Health Sciences at the University of Ottawa, teaching courses in public health and research methods at both the graduate and undergraduate levels.

DANIEL THÉORET, MSc, holds a bachelor of science in human kinetics and a master of science in biomechanics from the University of Ottawa. His research interests have been focused on sports and rehabilitation biomechanics, including gait and movement analysis, functional bracing, skating, stick curvature, and snowboarding. His experience has centred on task and physical demands analysis and workplace disability management with a major Crown corporation. Since 2009 he has held the position of project manager in human performance within the Director General Personnel and Family Support Services of the Canadian Forces. Mr Théoret is the primary investigator on the Occupational Fitness Standards Project – the multi-year project tasked by chief of military personnel to develop new essential task lists that are part of the medical standards for all occupations of the Canadian Forces.

AMANDA THOMPSON, MA, is completing her PhD in psychology at the University of Ottawa. Her research interests focus on social and health psychology. She also specializes in statistics and methodology. She was the recipient of a Social Sciences Humanities Research Council Doctoral Fellowship and Ontario Graduate Scholarship. She has several years' experience conducting research in both the academic and public domains.

KIMBERLEY WATKINS, MA, completed her MA in psychology with a specialization in health psychology at Carleton University, Ottawa, in 2009. In 2009, Ms Watkins joined the Department of National Defence as a defence scientist with Director General Military Personnel Research and Analysis. She is a member of the Psychosocial Health Dynamics team, which conducts scientific research and analysis exploring the health and well-being of Canadian Forces members. Her main areas of research include transition from military to civilian life, prevention of infectious diseases, deployment stress and mental health, physical fitness trends, sources of social support, and illicit drug use in the CF.

MARVIN WESTWOOD, PhD, is a professor in the counselling psychology program at the University of British Columbia and associate member of University of British Columbia's Faculty of Medicine. In 2011 he was named to the Royal Canadian Legion Professorship in Group Counselling and Trauma at UBC. He is responsible for the development and evaluation of UBC's Veterans Transition Program. Prior to coming to UBC, he taught at McGill University. His teaching and research areas focus on group counselling and men and trauma. Invited presentations at numerous national and international conferences include the United Kingdom, Malta, Argentina, Chile, Israel, the United States, Australia, Indonesia, and Hong Kong. He received the Queen's Golden Jubilee Medal in 2002 and the Queen's Diamond Jubilee Medal in 2012.

JOHN WHELAN, PhD, is lead psychologist at Whelan Associates in Halifax, NS. Dr Whelan served in the Canadian Forces from 1977 to 1985 and began his clinical work as an intern at the Stadacona Hospital in 1993. He served as director and as clinical supervisor of addiction services at CFB Halifax from 1998 to 2005 when he entered full-time private practice. His clinical and research interests focus on the assessment and treatment of operational trauma and concurrent disorders (e.g., addiction and PTSD), and developmental trauma among serving and retired military/RCMP. Dr Whelan has developed and implemented group-based programs to VAC clients. He provides consultation and clinical supervision to private and public organizations in addiction and psychological trauma. Dr Whelan has been asked to provide advice on military and veteran mental health to the Standing Committee on Veterans Affairs, Royal United Services Institute, Canadian Psychological Association, and the Canadian Psychiatric Association.

DEBBIE WHITNEY, PhD, CPsych, is an assistant professor in the Department of Clinical Health Psychology, Faculty of Medicine, at the University of Manitoba. She is a staff psychologist and research officer for the Operational Stress Injury Clinic, Winnipeg. She obtained a BA (honours) in clinical psychology from the University of Winnipeg and then an MA and PhD in clinical psychology from the University of Saskatchewan in Saskatoon. She has many years' experience dealing with problems of trauma and recovery. She has worked with adults, couples, families, and children. As research officer, she wants to facilitate research within the clinic. Her own research interests include investigation of local norms for psychological assessment instruments and use of tele-health to expand access to service.

REBECCA WIGFIELD, MSW, has worked with individuals, couples, and families in the military community for over ten years. Throughout her career at the Valcartier Military Family Resource Centre, she has specialized with resilient military families who must deal with the lifestyle and its side effects. Her extensive training with the integrative model approach, the Military Resilience Training Program, Road to Mental Readiness, and grief training enriches her clinical work with the families. She has also participated in several American National Defence Symposiums and worked in Cyprus for troops on decompression returning from Afghanistan.

PAUL YIELDER, PhD, completed undergraduate qualifications in teaching and education at the University of Durham and in medical diagnostic radiography within the College of Radiographers in the United Kingdom. In 1979, Dr Yielder moved to New Zealand, where he assumed a senior clinical teaching position training diagnostic imaging practitioners. In 2003 he began PhD work with colleagues from the Russian State Classical Academy in Moscow and completed this degree in 2009. In 2007 he came to University of Ontario Institute of Technology to undertake teaching, and educational and research responsibilities as an assistant professor, serving as both director of health science and associate dean. Research interest includes clinical anatomy, neuroscience, and also neuropsychiatry and psychopathology associated with advanced clinical imaging techniques.

PETER ZEINDLER, Maj, MD, CCFP, joined the Canadian Forces after practising family medicine for seventeen years in a variety of locations. While in the military he has worked as a general duty physician, was in charge of the recruiting medical office, and more recently is in charge of the School of Operational Medicine and practises as a diving medicine physician. He has an MSc in occupational health, an MPH, and has completed a fellowship in undersea and hyperbaric medicine. He is deployed to Afghanistan as an advisor to the military graduate medical education program.

Index